Pain and Its Transformations

Pain and Its Transformations

The Interface of Biology and Culture

Edited by
Sarah Coakley
Kay Kaufman Shelemay

Harvard University Press
Cambridge, Massachusetts
London, England / 2007

Printed in the United States of America

Library of Congress Cataloging-in-Publication Data

Pain and its transformations : the interface of biology and culture /
edited by Sarah Coakley, Kay Kaufman Shelemay.
p. ; cm.
Includes bibliographical references and index.
ISBN-13: 978-0-674-02456-4 (alk. paper)
ISBN-10: 0-674-02456-7 (alk. paper)
1. Pain—Psychological aspects. 2. Pain—Religious aspects.
3. Pain—Cross-cultural studies. I. Coakley, Sarah, 1951–
II. Shelemay, Kay Kaufman.
[DNLM: 1. Pain—psychology. 2. Adaptation, Psychological.
3. Cultural Characteristics. 4. Spirituality. WL 704 P144355 2007]
RB127.P332142 2007
616'.0472—dc22 2007012985

For Arthur and Joan Kleinman,
with affection, admiration, and gratitude

Contents

Acknowledgments

This book is based on materials that were first presented at the Harvard conference "Pain and Its Transformations: The Interface of Biology and Culture," chaired by Arthur Kleinman and Sarah Coakley. The conference came as a climax to a two-year seminar series on the same topic led by Kleinman and Coakley and involving many of the Harvard faculty also included in this volume. After the conference Kay Kaufman Shelemay took on the co-editing with Coakley, an arduous but creative task that has involved "catching" the best moments of interdisciplinary exchange taped at the conference itself and weaving them into the unfolding narrative provided by the original conference papers (now suitably revised). The decision to proceed in this way came from the unanimous sense at the conference that new ground had been broken even as we met and exchanged ideas and perspectives. The result, we believe and hope, is a book in which the reader may actually be led afresh through the moments of insight that emerged in our interdisciplinary exchange. We make some suggestions in the Introduction and Afterword about what these insights might mean for future pain research.

Both the seminar series and the conference were sponsored by the Harvard "Mind/Brain/Behavior Initiative," an interfaculty venture at Harvard University that in recent years has piloted new strategies in interdisciplinary dialogue, research, and teaching. Without the particular generosity of James R. Houghton the conference could not have taken place. We are grateful to staff at MBB for their cheerful professional assistance, particularly to Catherine Whalen, Karen Barkow, and Cortney Langevin. We are also indebted to Zara Housmand, for editing the conference transcripts, and to Lesley Bannatyne of the Harvard Department of Music, for her considerable part in preparing the manuscript for publication. Timothy Dalrymple undertook, with meticulous scholarly care, the heroic task of bringing the style and bibliographic references in the book into conformity with the requirements of Harvard University Press. We are no less indebted to Elizabeth Knoll, Kirsten Giebutowski, Bethany Withers, and Alissa Anderson of Harvard University Press itself. Without their assistance, interest, and patience this book could not have been brought to publication. Last but not least, we thank the John Templeton Foundation for supporting our work with a subvention. We are enormously grateful to Jack Templeton himself and to Reuben Bell and Mary Ann Meyers at the John Templeton Foundation for their generosity and assistance.

Pain and Its Transformations

Introduction

1

Sarah Coakley

This book is about pain and its capacity for transformation. It is about those mysterious and variable dimensions of the human experience of pain that continue to baffle the clinicians even as molecular and systems neuroscientists get close to a definitive explanation of the somatic and neural mechanisms of it; and it is about the *meanings* of pain that different cultures, ethnicities, and religions ascribe to pain, thereby mediating—often through meditative, musical, and ritual enactment—a narrative that transcends the individual sufferer and so gives public expression to private agony. Yet if death is the great "leveler," then pain is seemingly still the great "divider"; for the variety of ways, and intensities, with which pain is individually felt and suffered continues to constitute a considerable clinical conundrum. This volume sets out to probe this mystery afresh. It does so by means of an unusual interdisciplinary conversation.

It has long been acknowledged that pain (like the brain itself) occupies a strange liminal position between biology and culture (Kleinman 1988; Morris 1991; DelVecchio Good et al. 1992; Kleinman, Das, and Lock 1997). We know, for instance, that the expressions of personal response to pain (even when measurable "objectively" under test conditions) are bewilderingly varied, not only between individuals but also between cultures. It seems that our particular sensitivity to pain, and the anxiety that attends it, is not simply a matter of genetics, physiology, and circumstance, vitally important as these are, but also one of learned "hermeneutics": the way we *interpret* our pain is all important for the mode of our suffering of it. While this facet of pain experience has long been anecdotally obvious to the medical profession (and perhaps even more so to the nursing staff than to the doctors),[1] it is only now that we are approaching a point at which it can be explained physiologically. However, it seems that even this "explanation" can only occur through a paradoxical conjoining of efforts from pain researchers who work from very different perspectives and (ostensibly) incompatible presumptions: the "bottom-up" neurobiologists studying sensation and the "top-down" neuroscientists studying modulatory systems. The former (represented in this book by Clifford J. Woolf, Chapter 3) can now explicate right down to the molecular level how a pain event occurs; they claim to be coming close to understanding the neurobiology of pain with completeness and to being able to explicate it in a physiologically reductive way that has no necessary connection with the philosophical intricacies of the "mind-brain" problem. The latter perspective (represented in this volume by neuroscientist Howard L. Fields, Chapter 4), in contrast, also makes new claims, in this case to throw crucial light on the neural mechanisms that mediate our *interpreting* of pain even as we simultaneously respond neurally to the somatic source of trauma or sickness. Such a top-down explication of the neural complexity of pain necessarily bridges the discussion into contested topics in both philosophy of mind and hermeneutics: the mind-brain problem cannot here be averted.[2]

One of the prime purposes of this book, then, is to bring these two scientific approaches to pain into conversation and even to suggest some sort of ultimate convergence. But that goal—as will be proved in the unfolding of the book's argument—cannot be achieved either quickly or simply. Indeed, it cannot be reached at all, we shall claim, without the help of other interdisciplinary assistants and interlocutors. Herein lies the specific *novum* of this volume: the claim that because the mystery of pain cannot be effectively probed merely reductively, it demands a wider interdisciplinary investigation. Ultimately, the solution to the problem requires creative forays into the arenas of philosophy, psychiatry, theological and religious studies, anthropology, literature, musicology, art, and ritual theory if all the dimensions of pain are to be tested and understood. Each of these disciplines—as we shall show—has something vital to say about the meanings of pain and the capacity of the human spirit (whether or not in purported interaction with transcendent forces) to transform it. Each, likewise, has something to say about the circumstances in which pain can be integrated into some interpersonal realm of shared significance. Although this book can only go as far as indicating the observed *correlations* between pain and these various forms of transformation, it can sketch a new and comprehensive vision of the subject and thereby provide the initial groundwork for future medical research of a precise, scientific, and explanatory nature. Indeed, the book's opening sections provide the telling neuroscientific points of entry for precisely such an extension of current clinical research. If this volume even provokes the medical imagination to such further research, it will have more than served its purpose.

Before we go further, however, we must face the first obvious, but difficult, semantic question: What *is* "pain," exactly? What is its relation to "suffering"? How many sorts of pain are there? And can physical pain finally be separated from what is colloquially called "mental" or "spiritual" pain? Or are the latter categories theoretical mistakes? Further, is pain essentially private and incommunicable, reducing us to inarticulacy, to loss of speech (Scarry 1985)? Or does it provide the axis for a potent means of communication—a bridge to empathy and a deeper recognition of the "other" in the face of suffering (Lévinas 1998; Kleinman 2006)?

It has to be admitted that there are no easy answers to these fundamental questions, and recent research and writing on pain swing wildly between the alternatives. At one reductive level of discourse, it is perhaps obvious enough what pain is: as Woolf puts it in Chapter 3, it is a "neurobiological sensory function of the brain and spinal cord," a function that Woolf and others at the helm of recent neurobiological investigation of pain claim to be coming close to explaining definitively. Yet Woolf himself admits that such an approach involves an a priori "strip[ping] away [of] the cognitive and emotional components of pain"; and as such, it might seem to involve the reductivist's presumption that thinking about pain as a "subjective" sensation already commits an implicit philosophical error—that of dualism. As Valerie Hardcastle—another ardent physicalist (and one more concerned than Woolf to make her philosophical commitments explicit)—has put it of late: "I argue that all pains are physical and localizable and that *all are created equal*" (Hardcastle 1999, 7, my emphasis). The enemy, for Hardcastle, is thus anyone who presumes that pain is a "subjective state of mind" in the first place, indeed anyone who imagines that "psychopathological pain" exists at all.

Whom, however, should we dub the real—and dubious—"ideologist" in this realm of pain? Is it perhaps the reductive physicalist such as Hardcastle herself? Or is it, in contrast, the patient investigator of the varied historic "meanings" that the so-called subjective state of pain has classically produced, meanings inextricably entangled with those "psychopathological" dimensions of pain that Hardcastle decries (see, most recently, Morris 1991; Perkins 1995; Glucklich 2001)? It is precisely this unresolved question that is raised afresh by the interdisciplinary conversation engendered in this book—but now with some real prospect of biological, neuroscientific, and philosophical solution. In order not merely to beg the ideological question, we let the debate unroll before the readers' eyes, just as it did in the original conference from which this volume is constructed. The most fascinating point of consensus that begins to emerge relates to the neurophysiological data assembled by Fields (Chapter 4), precisely in response to the molecular focus of Woolf (Chapter 3).

Woolf starts here with an exacting biological account of how ordinary physiological pain occurs at the level of "nociceptors"—pain fibers normally activated only by harmful stimuli to give an "early warning system" of danger. The same explanatory model can be extended to show how "inflammatory" pain occurs in cases where tissue has already been damaged and so becomes unusually sensitive. So-called neuropathic or pathological pain (in which some deep trauma to the whole nervous system results in regular, agonizing, and chronic pain), however, still presents the molecular pain researchers, Woolf admits, with continuing difficulties of explanation: here meanings have often seemed to fail, both scientifically and personally, although Woolf remains confident that complete molecular explanation is not far off (and he himself has played a vital role in this investigation). Fields responds, in contrast, with an account of pain that starts from a completely different angle, that of what he calls the sufferer's "projection" or "representation" of pain; and this is a dimension of the pain event, he claims, that can now be tracked neurally by fMRI imaging. Pointing to the essentially "symbolic" and patterning operations of the brain, Fields indicates how a narrowly reductive account of pain necessarily misses the crucial interaction with environmental and cultural factors that any pain event involves. A full and satisfactory account of pain (and thus also of its capacity for transformation), he argues, must chart the variable forms of involvement of the limbic system in the pain event and explain the importance of emotion, suggestibility, and trust to the production and felt effects of pain, especially in the more serious cases of inflammatory or neuropathic pain.

Both Woolf and Fields indicate areas of remaining mystery, even scientific nescience, in their differing renditions of a pain event. Does this leave any room for a potential explanatory convergence, or are we still to conclude that the two accounts ("bottom-up" and "top-down") are simply incompatible? Not necessarily, surely, if—as Fields outlines—meaning ascription in pain is itself a physiological event with identifiable neural correlates distinct from those of the somatic injury itself; for then the tired standoff between dualism and physicalism has at least a possibility here for new negotiation. Interestingly, for both Woolf and Fields the *theoretical* distinction between the base molecular components in a pain state and interpretative, "metaphorical" categories remains crucial; yet even for the physicalist Woolf (who sternly resists a "blurring" of these dimensions), there is an acknowledgment of the strange power of the latter categories, especially where the problematic—and often devastating—neuropathic pain is concerned. Perhaps on the basis of this point of potential convergence, we can begin to speak with neurological precision of pain as *intrinsically* "interpreted" (or "represented," as Fields puts it); perhaps we can agree that so-called subjective experiences of pain are not simply random (or philosophically misleading) *addita* to an "objective" physiological event (as Hardcastle would have it) but a necessary part of the pain event itself. Neurologically, in other words, we are "wired" to "interpret" pain.

If this proposal is favored, then, oddly the nondualist's desire to reduce "mind" to brain is at least partially catered for by Fields's careful explication of the neural correlates of pain in the sphere of "hermeneutics." I say "partially" because of course this move does not in itself settle the age-old debate between physicalism and dualism (a matter that this book perforce leaves open to further, and more intricate, philosophical discussion). But at least "physical" and "mental" pain are no longer set in opposition from the outset, despite their necessary theoretical distinction: there simply *is* no (conscious) physical pain that is not also neurally "interpreted."[3]

It would seem to follow, mutatis mutandis (and this is a challenging development for the harassed or puzzled general medical practitioner) that no pain can be *merely* "imaginary": a "pain interpretation" *is* a pain (so Fields). Any patient presenting with "pain," in other words, deserves to be treated with real respect and understanding even if no obvious "physical" source can be determined. But if this is so, a new clinical problem of hermeneutical *discernment* becomes the more pressing; for not all meanings ascribed to pain, clearly, are equally rational, defensible, or scientifically convincing. Some may arise wholly from false anxiety, depression, or negative expectations; others may be superstitious, gullible, or downright deluded.

At this point, physicians not only do well to reconsider the enormous power they wield personally as purveyors of reassurance or dismissive disregard (here is the effect of "meaning making" in one sense); they may also wish to join hands with chronic pain researchers in investigating religious and philosophical traditions of well-honed antiquity and efficacy in relation to pain's alleviation (reflection on meaning making in another sense). Here one may detect arenas for careful clinical scrutiny: which of these systems of meaning for pain, and attendant transformative practices, have already stood the pragmatic test of time? And which have had the particular capacity to link the individual sufferer's distress to a wider realm of shared empathy, even of "atonement"? Which, in other words, have had what Arthur Kleinman (Chapter 2) describes as "moral" force? This is the place where the theologians, religionists, ritual theorists, and musicologists insert their expertise into this book's speculative investigations of the meanings of pain. Here we seek to give at least a preliminary account of how meanings in pain experience may be mediated through religious meditative, musical, and ritual practices; and thus here we open up possibilities of careful future research on the specific neurophysiological impact of such undertakings. Again, however, we seek to avoid and avert the kind of gullibilism, both scientific and theological, that has already attended some earlier quasi-popular adventures into this realm of research.[4] To investigate the impact of religious beliefs or practices on pain, we insist, is not thereby to embrace a range of uncritical hypotheses that secular physicalists tend to associate—often dismissively—with religious commitment, *tout court.* Great care needs to be taken in developing research in this area, since theological naïveté is as likely to have a negative impact as is scientific credulity.

This fundamental stock of issues on pain and potential pain research is traced through the volume in the following way. After setting the biological and neurophysiological stage in current pain research through the expositions of Woolf and Fields, respectively, we turn in Chapter 4 to a brief retrospective assessment of the "gate theory" of pain in the work of Wall and Melzack (Melzack and Wall 1965)—a theory that had originally intrigued the Harvard seminar on pain, given its obvious openness to interdisciplinary and hermeneutical engagement. The conclusion reached here, however, with the aid of significant comments from Woolf (a former student of Wall's) and also a lengthy excursus in Fields's essay, is that the gate theory was wrong in its details but is still illuminating and worthwhile in its broad conceptual hypotheses. The mediation of pain via a mesh—of *meanings*—is indeed an integral part of a pain event. And given that this is so, then those disciplines that characteristically deal with meanings are now in business where the further exploration of pain is concerned.

This conclusion, in turn, leads to a consideration of the relation of pain investigation to "placebo" research, an area in which a number of our group have already done distinguished work, and with particular attention to the opioid effects of positive expectation of pain relief (see Harrington 1997). The intriguing results of recent research in this area make it clear that the placebo response cannot be reduced merely to the investigation of the effects of dummy pills or inert substances in the treatment of pain. On the contrary, we are up against an extremely complex range of issues that also involve at least the following factors, each of them worthy of further exacting neurophysiological research: (1) trust (or lack thereof) in one's physician; (2) trust in the immediate effect of delivered pain medications (even if spuriously concocted); (3) induced, and prophecy-fulfilling, expectations of intensified or reduced pain in controlled pain experiments; (4) reliance on religious meditative practices as pain reducers or alleviators; and (5) belief in the possibility of the impact on pain of transcendent or divine forces.[5] Each of these areas of research presents its own particular challenges of discernment (the last of course being especially problematic for secular researchers), even granted that all of them shelter under the umbrella of an investigation of pain "meanings." Again, however, the danger in these areas of investigation is one of undiscriminating "overbelief"; and the challenge, as we insist throughout our volume, is one of careful and patient discerning of the possibilities of further properly scientific testing of these purported results.

Of particular importance in this last realm is the discussion in Part II of the book of the impact of religious "meditation" practices on the experience of pain. The great pragmatic success of Herbert Benson's work at Harvard, over several decades, of pain reduction through the "relaxation response" (induced by a simple practice of repetitive, mantric dissociation) is here brought into critical conversation with Christian, Buddhist, and Jewish ascetic traditions of some complexity and depth.[6] It is argued that research on the relaxation response, important as it has proved, represents only the tip of a religious iceberg, since it restricts itself to the activities of relative "beginners" in the practices of meditation (and that of a secularized or religiously decontextualized form). Once we see that the meanings ascribed to meditation (or "contemplation" in the Christian tradition) can by no means be homogenized into a single religiously reductive category ("religion" emphatically does not *equal* "relaxation"), and that we must therefore also add the diachronic variable of different levels of religious understanding and years of meditative experience to the differences of meaning already implicit in different religious traditions, we begin to see that investigation of the effect of ascetic practices on pain experience needs to be enormously complexified in order to account for both religious and neurophysiological variations. Already, preliminary research (some of it emanating from recent investigations of Buddhist meditation by Benson's own team) has shown that *different styles* of religious meditation may alleviate pain in entirely different ways and in primary connection with different parts of the brain. That is, meditation may, on the one hand, *distract* the sufferer from the intensity of pain through a practice of a form of dissociation (Lou et al. 1999); or it may, on the other hand (and seemingly paradoxically), also alleviate pain by a quite different sort of process of intensified mental *focus*—a moving *into* the pain that at the same time reorders the way one thinks of it (Lazar et al. 2000). An equally important variable is the depth or longevity of a practitioner's religious practice: we should not expect a beginner in Buddhist meditation immediately to evidence the neural changes that may be discernible in a monk of thirty years' ascetical commitment. These kinds of differential deserve further, and more detailed, clinical investigation; they also deserve further—and concomitant—religious-theoretical explication, as the chapters on Christian and Buddhist practices in this volume attempt to unfold. The presumption, for instance, in some strands of contemplative Christianity that intimate "union" with Christ may bring intensified, rather than alleviated, pain (albeit in a changed form: so the 16th-century Carmelites), or that Christ's own passion was felt *more* painfully rather than less on account of his being the Son of God (so Thomas Aquinas), is not merely an optional "subjective" accompaniment to the pain of a committed Christian but may form the hermeneutical lifeline in an otherwise unendurable physiological state of affairs.[7]

The latter parts of this volume (Parts III–VI) move away from pain considered merely as an individual experience to set pain (particularly when accompanied by sorrow, depression, grief, or the traumatic effects of political upheaval) in various transindividual contexts. Part III is devoted to the specific affective (and concomitantly neural) transformations that music may provide in contexts of public ritualized lament or trance. Circumstantial evidence presented here from particular religious traditions (Scandinavian, Indian, African) is set into an intriguing speculative discussion with music neurology—a regrettably underfunded area of investigation in pain management. In Chapter 8 Kay Kaufman Shelemay comments incisively, by way of conclusion, that no *one*, simplistic, neurological lesson can be drawn about the effects of music on pain and its neural correlates. We need to distinguish between pain ritually expressed, shared, and transformed by music; pain that is self-inflicted in ritual religious contexts for purposes of ascetic transformation but rendered (ostensibly) painless by musically induced "trance"; and music that itself *induces* pain or neural disturbance (as in "music epilepsy"). Suffice it to say that these different interactions of music and pain are still surprisingly underresearched under clinical conditions, but it is hoped that this volume may act as a spur to more complex future experiments.

Perhaps part of the problem here, however, is the great difficulty presented for the medical pain researcher by the very idea of pain as transindividual or shared. Since one cannot, perforce, introduce whole ritual groups or theaters into an MRI machine, it is going to require ingenious research protocols to test the corporate effects of ritually transformed pain. Nonetheless, the cumulative anthropological, religious, and psychiatric evidence is formidable, as the latter sections of this book explore. On the one hand, we have existing non-Western systems of medical theory, such as the Chinese Confucian, based on a theory of *qi* that links the individual sufferer or practitioner through varying levels of community and social interaction right to the level of the cosmos (see Tu Weiming, Chapter 9). Perplexing as such metaphysical conceptions may be to existing Western biomedicine, they do at least deserve close clinical attention, given the long-established efficacy of some Chinese remedies and pain treatments. On the other hand, we have examples of effective social and psychic transformation, after traumatic political upheavals, through intentional ritual activity in which painful memory is summoned and its "affect" narratively redirected (see Jennifer Cole, Chapter 10). Such a capacity of painful memory to be shifted and purged by ritual presents, as Stanley Tambiah comments in Chapter 10, an interesting social parallel to individual psychotherapy; and in each case, as Kleinman points out, bodily "narrativization" is linked with specifically moral meanings—what he terms the "somatomoral" dimension of pain.

In Part V, this dimension is further probed by examining the conditions of the very possibility of the aesthetic "representation" of pain. In Chapter 11 Elaine Scarry asks, Does *intense* pain render such artistic or literary representation impossible? Or are there ways of "doubling," or transferring, pain such as to make it representable—and so communicable? When does pain obliterate communication or speech, and when does it render empathy and compassion the more developed in the sufferer? While no definitive neurological answer is arrived at in response to this question in this section of the book, a hypothesis is at least suggested by Richard K. Wolf in his analysis, in Chapter 12, of Shi'ite drumming and self-flagellation in the annual ritual memorialization of the death of Husain. Here there is a whole series of doublings or displacements of pain: from internal to external, from past to present, from imaginary (or remembered) to real and self-inflicted, and from body to ritual instrument (the drum). These shifts and displacements, argues Wolf, augur a transformed capacity for expression and externalization; they render pain in some sense newly manageable or controlled precisely by shared expression of emotion. In this sense pain is manipulated to fuel new solidarity, moral fervor, and compassion.

The last section of the volume, from here, moves to confront head-on the pressing philosophical question of pain's possible moral *worth*. Since Woolf had raised at the start of our conference the expectation of a possible world without pain (given the speed and success of his own and others' current biological researches), we were bound to ask in closing whether such a possibility would be a welcome one. *Should* pain always be avoided or obliterated? asks Nicholas Wolterstorff in Chapter 14. And if not, when and why is pain a "moral good"? Is the complete aversion to pain a peculiarly modern American aberration (as Kleinman suggests in Chapter 2)—a sign of moral weakness or spiritual wimpishness? Do we *need* pain in some circumstances, not only to signal that something is awry physically but just as much to effect moral or spiritual transformation in ourselves? While Wolterstorff examines this question through the lens of a classic philosophical treatment in the work of Augustine, Laurence J. Kirmayer treats it psychiatrically in Chapter 13, arguing finally that "pain is *good* to think with" because "[we] cannot [even] think and act morally without an intimate understanding of others' pain." In short, while surely everyone welcomes the prospect of effective palliative relief for cases of agonizing temporary, chronic, or terminal pain, this volume raises significant questions, both religious and philosophical, about the possible intrinsic value of certain sorts of *unsought* pain, a question that is to be distinguished from that of the power and control that may be mobilized by self-imposed religious "discipline" or flagellation (see Asad 1993; Glucklich 2001). The book ends, therefore, with a reminder that any future research on pain that is to be informed by the interdisciplinary questions we have raised in this volume should be as alert to the questions of the moral ambiguity of pain as it is to the crucial roles of the sufferer's interpretation, expectation, and sense of narrative meaning.

A chronic pain sufferer (with intense and continuous pain caused by a sports injury suffered as a young student) recently remarked to me that amid all the pain regimens and treatments and strategies and medications offered to him over the many years since his original accident, no doctor or therapist had ever asked him what his pain *meant* to him—existentially, communally, let alone religiously. Since he is a deeply religious person, a Christian of strong commitment, the theological issue of providence—and the Christological issue of the meanings of "passion"—has all along exercised him greatly in his suffering; but so far it has been completely repressed in discussion with his physicians. If this book achieves nothing more, we trust it will alert both pain sufferers and pain researchers to the multileveled significance of such meanings (religious or otherwise) in the experience and transformation of pain; to the remarkable circumstantial evidence of musicologists, religionists, and ritual theorists about the alleviation and transformation of pain through religious and aesthetic undertakings; and therefore to the great potential for further exacting clinical research in the areas suggested by our interdisciplinary interchange. As Fields remarks in Chapter 4, the explanatory study of the biological components of pain is "advanced," whereas the "[interdisciplinary] study of the context-determined components" of pain is "in its infancy." This volume aims to nourish that promising "infant" and so engender further creative medical research on pain and its transformations.

Notes

1. An interesting but emblematic divergence may be found here between an accepting view (provided in a nursing journal by a nurse) of a dying patient's refusal of pain medication as a result of religious meaning-attribution (Kumasaka and Miles 1996) and two physicians' account of the "problem" of religious belief as "a barrier to the pharmacologic control of cancer pain" (Bosch and Baños 2002).

2. For recent introductory accounts of the mind-brain problem, see, inter alia, Warner and Szubka 1994; Heil 2004; Kim 2006.
3. It could be argued that the material presented in this book, as a whole, as it unfolds suggests a subtle gradation, or spectrum, of *levels* (let us call them L1–L6) of approach to pain. Although the technical philosophical argument cannot be made in this book, such an approach could be used to support an "emergentist" solution to the philosophy of mind issues encoded here and to seek to overcome in this way a stark physicalism/dualism divide. On such a view, we have a cumulative, perspectival set of accounts of pain that only together can do justice to pain in all its dimensions and jointly span the "emergence" of "mind" from "body": the biological investigation of pain (L1); the study of the central nervous system (CNS) in pain (L2); the explanation of the mental "representation" of pain (understood initially prehermeneutically, in purely neurological terms) (L3); the explication of the neural correlates of pain in the actual sphere of "hermeneutics" (L4); the study by psychologists and anthropologists of the experience of pain as felt and expressed by the subject (and worried about by the family) (L5); and the explication of theological or metaphysical beliefs encoded in religious practices that claim to deal with pain (L6). Reflection on the different levels of approach to pain can thus aim to avoid a stark *disjunction* between "physical" and "mental" accounts. However, the problem remains as to how to explicate the precise relation of these levels and how to clarify the point at which "mind" ostensibly "supervenes" on (or "emerges" from) "body." For a succinct account of the variety of different theories of supervenience in current philosophy of mind, including an older-style "emergentism," see Kim 1994. For more recent accounts specifically of the emergentist option in the philosophy of mind, its advantages, and remaining problems, see Johnson 2001; Clayton 2004; and for more general accounts of the problem of emergence and science, see Morowitz 2002; Gregersen 2003.
4. A particularly unfortunate (but well-publicized) version of such tendencies is Neuberg, d'Aquili, and Rause 2001, a volume that makes such statements as " 'God' will not go away—He is caught by . . . neurological events" (53). The argument thereby manages to be simultaneously theologically and scientifically reductive: "God" is reduced to certain events in the brain ("a deeper, more spiritual part of ourselves"), and these particular "God" events are seemingly neurally *locatable.*
5. These different factors are touched upon seriatim throughout this volume. For representative introductory discussions of the various issues distinguished here, see: (1) on patient/physician "trust," Moerman 2002; (2) on the impact of dummy pain medications, Harrington 1997; (3) on spurious pain impositions resulting in actual (even intense) "pain" under experimental conditions, Bayer et al. 1991; (4) on religious meditative practice as

effective for pain relief, Lou et al. 1999 and Lazar et al. 2000; (5) for a recent survey of the existing psychological research on the effects of "spirituality" and "prayer" on illness in general, and pain in particular, Miller and Thoresen 2003. The latter article, introducing a whole issue of the *American Psychologist* devoted to health and religious beliefs, reveals many of the reductive problems and questionable methodological procedures (both scientific and theological) that have so far attended attempts to investigate "transcendent interactions" in relation to pain and recovery. That is not to say that such problems could not *in principle* be overcome by the development of much more exacting and subtle experiments and theoretical frameworks.

6. For Benson's meditative technique and its accompanying theory of the "relaxation response," see Benson 1975, 1984, 1996. This current book wishes to give all credit to Benson for his pioneering work in the area of "meditation" and pain relief but to query and *complicate* his theories both about meditation and about belief.
7. For a discussion of "union" with Christ in relation to pain states, see Sarah Coakley's chapter "Palliative or Intensification?" in this volume. For the idea that Christ felt human pain more intensely, not less, qua Son of God, second "person" of the Trinity, see Aquinas 1948, 2264–2265 (*ST* III, Q. 46, art. 6): "Christ's sense of touch, the sensitiveness of which is the reason for our feeling pain, was most acute. His soul likewise, from its interior powers, apprehended most vehemently all the causes of sadness."

References

Aquinas, T. 1948. *St. Thomas Aquinas: Summa theologica. Complete English Edition in Five Volumes,* vol. 4. New York: Benziger Brothers.

Asad, T. 1993. "Pain and Truth in Medieval Christian Ritual." In *Genealogies of Religion.* Baltimore: John Hopkins University Press, 83–124.

Bayer, T. L., P. E. Baer, and C. Early. 1991. "Situational and Psychophysiological Factors in Psychologically Induced Pain." *Pain* 44: 45–50.

Benson, H. 1975. *The Relaxation Response.* New York: Morrow.

———. 1984. *Beyond the Relaxation Response: How to Harness the Healing Power of Your Personal Beliefs.* New York: Times Books.

———. 1996. *Timeless Healing: The Power and Biology of Belief.* New York: Scribner.

Bosch, F., and J. E. Baños. 2002. "Religious Beliefs of Patients and Caregivers as a Barrier to the Pharmacologic Control of Cancer Pain." *Clinical Pharmacology and Therapeutics* 72: 107–111.

Clayton, P. 2004. *Mind and Emergence: From Quantum to Consciousness.* Oxford: Oxford University Press.

DelVecchio Good, M.-J., P. E. Brodwin, B. J. Good, and A. Kleinman, eds. 1992. *Pain as Human Experience: An Anthropological Perspective.* Berkeley: University of California Press.

Glucklich, A. 2001. *Sacred Pain: Hurting the Body for the Sake of the Soul.* New York: Oxford University Press.

Gregersen, N. H., ed. 2003. *From Complexity to Life: On the Emergence of Life and Meaning.* Oxford: Oxford University Press.

Hardcastle, V. G. 1999. *The Myth of Pain.* Cambridge, Mass.: MIT Press.

Harrington, A., ed. 1997. *The Placebo Effect: An Interdisciplinary Exploration.* Cambridge, Mass.: Harvard University Press.

Heil, J. 2004. *Philosophy of Mind: A Contemporary Introduction,* 2nd ed. New York: Routledge.

Johnson, S. 2001. *Emergence: The Connected Lives of Ants, Brains, Cities and Software.* New York: Scribner.

Kim, J. 1994. "Supervenience." In S. Guttenplan, ed., *A Companion to the Philosophy of Mind.* Oxford: Blackwell, 575–583.

———. 2006. *Philosophy of Mind,* 2nd ed. Boulder, Colo.: Westview.

Kleinman, A. 1988. *The Illness Narratives: Suffering, Healing and the Human Condition.* New York: Basic Books.

———. 2006. *What Really Matters: Living a Moral Life amidst Uncertainty and Danger.* New York: Oxford University Press.

Kleinman, A., V. Das, and M. Lock, eds. 1997. *Social Suffering.* Berkeley: University of California Press.

Kumasaka, L., and A. Miles. 1996. "My Pain Is God's Will." *American Journal of Nursing* 96: 45–47.

Lazar, S. W., G. Bush, R. L. Gollub, G. L. Fricchione, G. Khalsa, and H. Benson. 2000. "Functional Brain Mapping of the Relaxation Response and Meditation." *Neuroreport* 11: 1581–1585.

Lévinas, E. 1998. *Entre Nous: On Thinking-of-the-Other.* New York: Columbia University Press.

Lou, H. C., T. W. Kjaer, L. Friberg, G. Wildschiodtz, S. Holm, and M. Nowak. 1999. "A 150-H20 PET Study of Meditation and the Resting State of Normal Consciousness." *Human Brain Mapping* 7: 98–105.

Melzack, R., and P. D. Wall. 1965. "Pain Mechanisms: A New Theory." *Science* 150: 971–979.

Miller, W. R., and C. E. Thoresen. 2003. "Spirituality, Religion and Health: An Emerging Research Field." *American Psychologist* 58: 24–35.

Moerman, D. 2002. "Explanatory Mechanisms for Placebo Effects: Cultural Influences and the Meaning of Response." In H. Guess, A. Kleinman, J. W. Kusek, and L. W. Engel, eds., *The Science of the Placebo.* London: B. M. J. Books, 77–107.

Morowitz, H. J., ed. 2002. *The Emergence of Everything: How the World Became Complex.* Oxford: Oxford University Press.

Morris, D. B. 1991. *The Culture of Pain*. Berkeley: University of California Press.

Neuberg, A. B., E. d'Aquili, and V. Rause. 2001. *Why God Won't Go Away: Brain Science and the Biology of Belief*. New York: Ballantine Books.

Perkins, J. 1995. *The Suffering Self: Pain and Narrative Representation in the Early Christian Era*. London: Routledge.

Scarry, E. 1985. *The Body in Pain*. New York: Oxford University Press.

Warner, R., and T. Szubka, eds. 1994. *The Mind-Body Problem: A Guide to the Current Debate*. Oxford: Blackwell.

Opening Remarks
Pain and Experience

2

Arthur Kleinman

Pain is an elemental aspect of experience. On that point, almost all are agreed. So encompassing is the idea of "experience" that the biomedical researcher's vision of pain as a universal, prelinguistic, neurological condition and the clinician and anthropologist's understanding that pain is felt, lived, and dealt with in the intimate context of a person's life and local world can be together accommodated as different sides of experience. The recognition that pain transforms condition and network also lends itself to a unified vision running from material neuronets to embodied social relations and moral meanings.

So much depends on how we understand "experience." Like many of you, I have "experienced" pain. But that sense of a personal reality that we have had happen to us is not an adequate way of formulating what I take experience—including the experience of pain—to be.

Experience for me is a flow of interpersonal actions, reactions, resistance, and change. It is the medium of everyday life where we interact with others, feel, remember, and do things. In the sense I hold of it, experience is simultaneously within me and between me and others. It is constituted out of smiles, stares, gestures, stories. Experience is the pain I communicate to you with my grimace, and it is taken up and made up out of my efforts to explain (or deny) what I feel, and out of your efforts to hear me, help me, or avoid me. In the way metaphors extend from physical body to social body, I can feel and remember you as my pain. And in the way emotion resonates across intimates, I may feel your pain in my head, my abdomen, my back.

My prayer makes the memory of your pain come alive within me, just as your sensibility of Christ's sorrow and hurt on the cross makes your body the locus of religious ritual. When I see Roman Polanski's *The Pianist,* the Holocaust's world of pain is not only an image before me but takes on life within my feelings and memories. I experience something of it, am brought into its nightmarish reality, just as that reality finds its place in me. And when I resist, avoid, or rework the lived memory of someone's pain, the same thing happens: I am caught up in resistance, avoidance, and reworking as a mode of experiencing my world.

I have come to regard this flow of experience within me and between us as moral. It is moral because there are things that are deeply at stake for me (for us), that matter greatly, which orient how I (we) perceive, interpret, and respond. What is most at stake for me (us) can be highly idiosyncratic, but it also can be shared with others in my (our) local world: family, network, neighborhood, wider community. It is because experience is moral, because affect, memory, and social value are so intimately connected, that pain can be regarded as moral experience.

Pain can express what is culturally at stake, such as the decidedly American idea that pain prevents a person from "naturally" enjoying life or the medieval Christian idea that pain can be suffering divinely ordained that prepares us for salvation. Pain can also express what is particularly at stake for a person, such as the felt notion that my pain is deserved as a punishment for a shameful act that I committed or that my pain is the badge of injustice in a cruel world of betrayal, inequality, and underserved misery. My pain can be your misfortune or my test of your commitment. Pain communicates my moral status, which does in part reflect your inattention and blame, responses that, as the Chinese put it, make me lose face.

The local world we inhabit is the site of moral transformation. Pain may make me exalted or humiliated because of how I and my pain are regarded by you and by others who matter. You may not want to hear my pain, denying me acknowledgment. That reduces my moral status—and perhaps yours as well. Alternatively, simply listening, witnessing, and acknowledging my pain may transform my (and your) moral status from passive victim and absence of presence to active engagement among moral agents. Stigma, in this perspective, might be thought of as a negative transformation of the moral experience of a member of a local world by others in that world.

A fundamental transformation of the local world may transform the moral experience of the person in pain. How did ordinary nurses and doctors under the Nazis end up killing their child patients who were suffering from, among other conditions, the pain of rheumatoid arthritis, and their chronically mentally ill patients whose psychic pain was just as obvious and compelling? Judith Perkins (1995) shows how early Christians in the second century transformed pain and their local worlds by fashioning a religious ideology of the suffering self as salvific and created with it hospitals, hospices, and a movement of political resistance to the imperial Roman state, for whose stoic ideology pain had an entirely different significance. In 1949, as the Chinese Communist Party took control of China, it unleashed a revolutionary campaign of "speaking bitterness" through which peasants were compelled to express the pain of living under the feudal regime and to direct their rage at landlords, who were then humiliated, beaten, and killed as class enemies. Pain became an instrument of political mobilization.

None of this contradicts the neuroscience vision of pain. To the contrary, the more we learn about the biology of pain, the more we may come to understand how that biology itself becomes a local biology underwriting these painful transformations of moral experience. Political and economic change shift collective and personal poles of experience under the influence of shifting cultural meanings and moral conditions. Emotional and moral transformations transform bodily experience. Pain experiences are remade as local clusters of biological reactions, moral meanings, and social relations. And something very much like this must also occur in the healing process. What Daniel Moerman (2002) calls the "meaning response," and what I have referred to as the "remoralization of pain patients," must involve such changes in the local clusters of the moral and medical aspects of pain. We might say that what we look for is "enabling languages" in the response to the problem of pain, which will allow us to talk about the interactions between society and biology in terms that are as rich for the humanistic and social sciences as they are for biology. If we can achieve a kind of interactivity across domains by building concepts and relating them to experience in this way, I think we shall have advanced substantially in this meeting.

References

Kleinman, A. 1988. *The Illness Narratives*. New York: Basic Books.

———. 1999. "Experience and Its Moral Modes." In G. B. Peterson, ed., *The Tanner Lectures on Human Values,* vol. 20. Salt Lake City: University of Utah Press, 357–420.

Moerman, D. 2002. "Explanatory Mechanisms for Placebo Effects." In H. Guess et al., eds., *The Science of the Placebo*. London: B. M. J. Books, 77–107.

Perkins, J. 1995. *The Suffering Self: Pain and Narrative Representation in the Early Christian Era*. London: Routledge.

Schwarcz, V. 1997. "The Pain of Sorrow: Public Uses of Personal Grief in Modern China." In A. Kleinman, V. Das, and M. Lock, eds., *Social Suffering*. Berkeley: University of California Press, 119–148.

Response:
Enabling Strategies—A Great Problem Is Not Enough

Anne Harrington

A great problem is necessary to gather the kind of talent that we have at this conference and to motivate us to come and spend three days together. But one of the things that I learned from my previous experience organizing a conference on the placebo effect with the Mind/Brain/Behavior Initiative (Harrington 1997) is that a great problem is not enough unless you have "enabling languages," as Arthur Kleinman has challenged us to find. I would like to add to the idea of enabling languages some other enabling *strategies* that will help us to see more than isolated points of interest. When I leave here in three days, I will have seen a mosaic of interesting ideas and points of view, but in the end, will I know how to do my work any differently than I did before, or will these ideas remain undigested provocative fragments? How can we enable something more interesting than that?

I have three approaches to thinking about what it might mean to "enable." The first was offered by Arthur when he talked about enabling language. I want first to flesh that out a little bit because he didn't actually give us any explicit examples of what enabling language might be. But as people were talking, some possibilities for enabling language were put on the table, so I wrote them down.

One of them is suffering. An example of enabling language is a word that makes sense to us in our domain but also makes sense to other people in a different domain. "Suffering" is a word that appears to overlap domains but potentially points us in different directions. It means something in Howard Fields's domain, and it actually points him toward the ways in which the brain parses and differentiates the experience of pain into different systems. Suffering in Arthur Kleinman's world points him toward questions about moral economy. You can fill in other examples from very different enterprises, and then you begin to see how each use of the word "suffering" might enable us to ask different kinds of questions of that word and its role in our own world. "Meaning" and "representation" are two other examples of potentially enabling language that were put on the table. Both of these apparently mean something in our different domains.

Another strategy, for which our task is laid out for us, is enabling models. We want a brain model that is both generous enough to encompass the kind of phenomena, in all their specificity and complexity, that we want to do justice to, and rigorous enough to benefit from the insights that a tenacious reductionist perspective can yield for us.

This group started, historically, with an interest in the fate of the gate control theory of pain, and though some of us may now criticize that theory quite radically, we would still like to build on some of the insights of the gate control theory and take it someplace else.[1] There is a need not only for a model from the brain sciences but also for an equally explicit model for articulating the processes of cultural mediation so that one can begin to see how they might interface with biology and brain processes. Laurence Kirmayer (1992) has talked about a potential mediating model that would focus on metaphor. Metaphor is something that makes sense when we think about the world of culture, but it also appears to make sense when we look at the way experience manifests itself physiologically. Maybe there is the kernel of a model that one could begin to articulate here.

The last strategy is on a different level: it's the idea of an enabling attitude. I got this idea as I was listening and noticing moments when people around the room began to talk like those in another disciplinary camp. For example, Judith Becker said she was interested in the fact that when people go into a trance, they become analgesic. Here is an ethnomusicologist suddenly talking like a neurologist. What if that was not just an accidental figure of speech, but you actually stopped at such moments and explicitly practiced a neurobiological attitudinal or analytic stance that would allow you to probe more deeply? What would it mean to think neurobiologically about culture, and conversely, what would it mean to think anthropologically or ethnomusicologically about the brain? Could we enable each other by teaching this attitude to each other?

Note

1. Early in its work the group discovered the classic nook for their reflections in the gate control theory of Melzack and Wall (Melzack and Wall 1965; also see Melzack 1993). For a further discussion of this (now widely criticized) theory, see the discussion by Howard Fields, Elaine Scarry, and the group in Chapter 4, and the editorial introduction in Chapter 1.

References

Harrington, A., ed. 1997. *The Placebo Effect: An Interdisciplinary Exploration.* Cambridge, Mass.: Harvard University Press.

Kirmayer, L. J. 1992. "The Body's Insistence on Meaning: Metaphor as Presentation and Representation in Illness Experience." *Medical Anthropology Quarterly* 6(4): 323–346.

Melzack, R. 1993. "Pain: Past, Present and Future." *Canadian Journal of Experimental Psychology* 47(4): 615–629.

Melzack, R., and P. D. Wall. 1965. "Pain Mechanisms: A New Theory." *Science* 150: 971–979.

Pain at the Interface of Biology and Culture

I

Deconstructing Pain

A Deterministic Dissection of the Molecular Basis of Pain

3

Clifford J. Woolf

Stripping Pain to Its Physiological Essentials

Pain has multiple faces. It is both a metaphor for an existential angst of the spirit and an unpleasant physical experience. In this chapter I will attempt to strip away the cognitive and emotional components of pain and ignore the transforming aspects of the experience of pain to reveal it as a neurobiological sensory function of the brain and spinal cord. In short, I shall take a consciously "reductive" approach, which will doubtless be contentious in this company but which will best expose the work on pain I do at the molecular level.

Pain, defined as the conscious awareness of a sensory experience that is unpleasant, distressing, or disturbing, remains incredibly complex but ultimately reducible to scientific scrutiny. This pain is amenable to a deterministic dismantling of the molecular components of the nervous system. We are now finding "pain" genes without having to consider the metaphysical aspects of pain. This is not to belittle suffering or spiritual unease, just to say that they are altogether different experiential categories, ones that happen to share through metaphorical allusion the word "pain." When pain is used in a literary, religious, or symbolic context, it is infused with a meaning that is fundamentally different from that of neurobiological sensory pain, and there is no *mechanistic* commonality.

Sensory Pain

What, then, is the meaning of pain as a sensory experience? Sensory neurobiology is concerned with understanding the relationship between a stimulus and a response. Consider, for instance, photons falling on the retina and visual perception, the movement of hair cells in the inner ear in response to changes in air pressure and the sensation of sound, or an excess of protons on the tongue and a sour taste. Common to all these are the encoding of the quality, intensity, duration, and location of the stimulus as well as special features such as color, pitch, or texture. Beyond a threshold level, increasing the intensity of the stimulus produces a greater response until a ceiling is reached. Sensory pain has all these features—it is a sensation. We readily appreciate that a light touch to the skin usually elicits a response that is quite different from a jab of a needle and that a stab wound is "worse" than a needle prick.

What makes pain different from all other sensory experiences, though, is that the sensation is linked inescapably and integrally with a conscious awareness of its unpleasantness. Pain is always painful! We may find certain visual or auditory experiences unpleasant, such as the paintings of Francis Bacon or techno music. But this is a different unpleasantness from that of sensory pain. Disliking Bacon is a matter of taste, convention, culture, and experience and is subject to individual disagreement. Pain is unpleasant because that is its biological imperative. It is a sensation all normal individuals experience in response to an intense or noxious stimulus. The unpleasantness of pain originated and has been elaborated and retained by evolution because it has survival value. The unpleasantness of pain is irreducible from its adaptive function because it is the key to its adaptive function.

Pain Is Good

There is an inherited neurological condition, fortunately rare, called congenital analgesia in which patients feel no pain. The condition is caused by a mutation in the gene encoding a growth factor receptor that is essential for the survival of sensory neurons that act as the first relay station in the "pain pathway." But this chance deletion of the peripheral sensory apparatus for pain is not a boon; it is a disaster. The tips of the fingers of the affected individuals are typically lost through repeated trauma, their tongues and lips are usually mutilated by chewing, and their life spans are significantly shortened. Although these individuals can go to the dentist without fear or sail through childbirth without a grimace, they cannot differentiate a potentially damaging from an innocuous stimulus. They cannot feel the difference between warmth and scalding hot, and therefore they are at constant risk of being scalded. We need pain to survive.

All living organisms from the simplest unicellular creature to primates need to detect whether their environment is hostile or damaging and, if it is, to get out of there quickly! A single-celled creature does this without any conscious awareness, and humans too retain an automatic response to noxious stimuli. Although we have, through the evolution of the brain, acquired the capacity to be self-aware, we flick our hand away from contact with a burning-hot surface without knowing—we move before we think. Such brisk withdrawal reflexes from a noxious stimulus are retained in individuals with spinal cord injury, indicating the complete independence of these reflexes from the brain and sensation. They have many features of the form of pain without the content—pain without awareness.

However, the experience of pain enacted by the cortex of the brain enables a response that goes beyond simple withdrawal from a noxious stimulus. Through its unpleasantness, it drives us to try to avoid noxious stimuli, rather than just simply reacting to them. Through our conscious appreciation of the unpleasantness of pain, we can and do anticipate pain (cringing in anticipation of a flu shot) and adopt complex behavioral strategies to avoid it. These may include behaviors as simple as recognizing situations that have previously resulted in pain and refraining from them (do not touch a red-hot surface) or using our intelligence and capacity to control the environment to protect ourselves from potentially injurious stimuli by, for example, wearing shoes when walking on stones or using tools.

To work well as a protective mechanism, the sensory awareness of the noxious stimulus must be accompanied by a very strong feeling of hurt and unpleasantness. A neutral pain sensation would not serve as an adequate driving force to prevent damage. The emotional color of the sensation has to be so strong that it overrides other mental activities. In this sense it resembles other biological drives essential to survival such as thirst, hunger, or the need to procreate. To work, pain must dominate our awareness. A good analogy is a fire alarm. If the noise of fire alarms is irritating rather than intolerable, we soon learn to ignore them, believing that they are likely to be false alarms, and we carry on with our "important" business rather than attending to yet another fire drill. To compensate for this, effective fire alarms have to be so loud that we are forced to leave the building. To be effective, pain also has to be so unpleasant that we are forced to pay attention. For this reason we do not habituate to pain; if anything, we increase our sensitivity to it. The unpleasantness of sensory pain makes it an ideal metaphor to express other forms of physical or psychic suffering. A clinical problem, though, is the reverse, when patients suffering from severe organic pain feel that they are somehow being punished for some wrongdoing rather than being the unfortunate victim of an illness of the nervous system. Pain can also be subverted and distorted into other complex psychological needs in a manner that retains no link with its protective role—the self-inflicted pain of the religious fanatic or sadomasochist comes to mind.

Pain as an early warning device is not the only kind of sensory pain. There are distinct pains that occur when tissue damage cannot be avoided, such as when the protective capacities of the early warning device system are overwhelmed, as in postoperative or posttraumatic pain, or when pains are an expression of the abnormal function of the nervous system, true pathological pains. These sensory pains are clinical pain syndromes, in contradistinction to the protective pain, which is a normal physiological function.

How Does Pain Work?

To begin to address this question, we first need to ask, "Which pain?" The mechanisms for physiological, inflammatory, and pathological pains are different. Just because we use a common word to describe the sensation we experience, this does not mean that the neurobiological operations that result in the sensation are the same.

Physiological pain has three key elements: *transduction, transfer,* and *processing.* Transduction is that process whereby an external stimulus—be it heat, a pinch, or a chemical irritant—acts on a neural element to produce an electrical signal in that nerve cell. For pain the neural elements that interact with the environment are the primary sensory neurons. These are highly specialized nerve cells that transfer electrical signals from the peripheral targets like skin, muscle, joints, or internal organs to the spinal cord (in the case of the body) or the brain stem (in the case of the face and head). These are the input component of the pain sensory apparatus. Their specialization for this job comes from the fact that they are activated only by intense, potentially damaging stimuli. Other sensory neurons have lower activation thresholds and contribute to innocuous sensations like touch, vibration, movement of hairs, position of a limb, and warmth.

The "pain fibers" technically are called "nociceptors" because they are normally activated only by noxious stimuli. We should avoid the term "pain fiber" or "pain pathway" to describe the neural apparatus that generates pain because it confuses the stimulus with the response. Not all noxious stimuli result in pain (patients may suffer from diminished sensitivity due to nerve damage but still have pain, or may fail, in times of danger, to experience pain in response to injury where this offers a survival advantage due to the recruitment of powerful neural inhibitory mechanisms); and pain may result from stimuli that normally generate innocuous sensations—a very common feature of clinical pain—as in the movement of a joint of a patient with arthritis.

Heat Pain Exposed

How do nociceptors act to detect noxious stimuli? We now have a pretty good idea, and it is a useful illustration of the power of the molecular approach to the analysis of pain. I will use as my example heat pain. If the skin is slowly heated from room temperature (typically about 20°C), then the stimulus will start off feeling neutral, then warm, then hot, then painful, and finally intolerably painful. The temperature at which there is a transition between hot and painful sensations is between 42° and 44°C, and that is true—provided the same skin area is tested by the same probe—in men or women, "stoic" Swedes, or "hysterical" Italians. This transition, measured in such psychophysical experiments, constitutes the heat pain threshold. Recordings from individual sensory fibers in laboratory animals or in human volunteers show several quite distinct populations of fibers: one, for example, that is activated maximally at about 30–40°C, and one that begins to respond at about 42°C, with maximal firing at 50–55°C. The former are warm fibers and the latter, heat pain fibers.

How do they differ? The heat pain but not the warm fibers produce a protein that is inserted into the outer membrane of the peripheral terminals of nociceptors innervating specific target organs like the skin. This protein is a transducer protein. When it is subjected to a heat stimulus of 42°C or above, its shape changes, opening a channel; and this channel enables sodium ions to enter the terminal through the membrane. This passage of charged sodium ions constitutes a current, a flow of electricity, and is the key step in the translation of a hot stimulus into electrical activity in the nervous system. If enough current flows, it initiates an explosive in-rush of sodium ions through other ion channel proteins, and a pulse of electricity, the action potential, travels from the periphery to the central nervous system, carrying the information that a hot stimulus has been detected in a certain location at a certain time. The number of action potentials encodes the intensity of the stimulus.

The molecular identity of at least one of the heat pain transducer proteins has been identified; it is a channel called VR1 (Caterina et al. 1997), cloned by David Julius and colleagues at the University of California in San Francisco. If the messenger RNA for VR1 is injected into a frog egg cell (a favorite living tool for molecular biologists), then the human protein is made and inserted into the frog egg membrane. Heating the frog egg now produces a sodium current with a threshold of 42°C, which is identical to your or my heat pain threshold—the mindless/brainless frog egg acts to detect heat just like us. This is true molecular determinism! The VR1 channel is activated not only by heat but also by the pungent ingredient in chili peppers, a chemical called capsaicin. The reason peppers feel hot when we eat them is that they act on the same receptors that react to heat! The nervous system is "fooled" into "thinking" it has been activated by a heat stimulus. Similar analyses have been made for many irritant chemicals, and progress is well advanced in understanding how mechanical stimuli are converted to electrical signals.

Pain Hypersensitivity: Reduced Threshold and Increased Responsiveness

The VR1 receptor clearly has a key role in the "tripwire" "early warning detection," or physiological role of pain. But it also contributes to inflammatory pain. A feature of damage to tissue and the inflammatory reaction is the liberation of a number of compounds by the inflamed tissue—the inflammatory mediators—that act on the peripheral terminal of the nociceptor to sensitize it. This literally means to make it more sensitive. A good example of this is acute sunburn. UV light induces an inflammatory response in the skin, making it red (on account of increased blood flow). This is accompanied by increased heat sensitivity. A warm shower now feels burning hot. The reason for this is that the heat pain threshold has been reduced. The molecular mechanisms involved are now understood. There is production of inflammatory sensitizing chemicals including prostaglandin E2 and bradykinin, and these act on the nociceptor terminal to switch on a cascade of chemical changes in the terminal that makes it both hyperexcitable and that also act on the VR1 receptor to reduce the temperature at which its pore opens. The commonly used over-the-counter aspirin-like analgesics work by blocking production of PGE2, reducing the sensitization.

Apart from changes in the excitability of the peripheral ends of the nociceptor with inflammation or tissue injury, the central nervous system also shows a remarkable capacity to modify its chemical makeup and function in these circumstances. There are two general kinds of change, one that is driven by electrical activity (activity-dependent plasticity) that alters the function of neurons and one that relies on chemical signals to change gene expression in the neurons. Together they produce changes in the excitability of central neurons, a phenomenon known as "central sensitization." This is analogous to turning up the volume control in the sensory pathway so that stimuli that would not normally produce pain, like lightly touching the skin, begin to do so.

Central sensitization is also the reason we feel tenderness or soreness in a skin area outside of an area of injury where there is no peripheral sensitization. In this circumstance, pain is no longer reflecting a specific sensory response to a noxious stimulus but is an amplified or exaggerated response of the central nervous system to a normal innocuous stimulus that now feels like pain because the central nervous system is reacting to it in an abnormally hyperexcited way. This reveals that pain reflects the functional status of the nervous system at any particular moment, rather than just detecting the presence of an intense stimulus. What is normally not painful can become so. The reverse is also true: there are powerful inhibitory mechanisms that can damp down the responsiveness of the central nervous system so that normally painful stimuli are no longer so. As with peripheral sensitization, enormous progress has been achieved in the understanding of the molecular mechanisms responsible for central sensitization, most of which operate in the spinal cord. This is certainly going to lead to the development of newer, more effective analgesics.

Pathological Pain: When the System Fails

Physiological pain has an obvious protective role. Inflammatory pain hypersensitivity can be argued teleologically also to represent an adaptive and useful feature of the nervous system, in this case not protecting the integrity of the organism from danger or damage but dealing with a situation where such damage could not be avoided. In other words, if the defenses implicit in the physiological pain system have been overwhelmed, resulting in a traumatic injury, what is it in the organism's best interest to do? The answer is to allow repair and healing to occur. An important way to do this is to increase the sensitivity of the system such that instead of reacting only to noxious stimuli, the system now reacts to innocuous stimuli as if they were noxious, until the damaged tissue has healed.

Pathological pain, in contrast, is pain with no adaptive function: the pain is the expression of pathology. The pain is the disease. This pain usually results from a lesion to the peripheral or central nervous system and is called "neuropathic pain." Examples of neuropathic pain include phantom limb pain after amputation of a limb, postherpetic neuralgia, AIDS neuropathy, diabetic neuropathy, poststroke pain, and the pain of spinal cord injury. Multiple mechanisms can produce neuropathic pain, and these can involve abnormal excitability of injured sensory fibers, neurodegenerative changes, and a structural reorganization of the connections of the nervous system. In most of the patients the injury of the original insult has long disappeared, but the pain remains, typically consisting of explosive bursts of shocklike pain and exquisite burning pain to even the lightest of touches of the skin. This is the pain that, by virtue of its persistence and severity, as well as by its resistance to most analgesics, represents such an enormous challenge to understanding and treatment.

Conclusion

Pain as a sensory experience is a complex phenomenon subject to our learned experiences and culture as well as our genetic makeup; and this in itself may predispose some, and not other, individuals to develop chronic pain. In spite of pain's complexity, we are making very good progress in unraveling the neurobiological mechanisms responsible for it, and this is revealing a new and rational basis for the treatment of pain. We will soon look back with amazement at the enormous ignorance that physicians have had about the pathophysiology of pain and the crudity and relative ineffectiveness of treatments that have tended to blur biological with psychic pain even though they *are* distinct.

References

Basbaum, A. I., and C. J. Woolf. 1999. "Pain." *Current Biology* 9: R429–R431.

Caterina, M. J., M. A. Schumacher, M. Tominaga, T. A. Rosen, J. D. Levine, and D. Julius. 1997. "The Capsaicin Receptor: A Heat-Activated Ion Channel in the Pain Pathway." *Nature* 389: 816–824.

Doubell, T. P., R. J. Mannion, and C. J. Woolf. 1999. "The Dorsal Horn: State-Dependent Sensory Processing, Plasticity and the Generation of Pain." In R. Melzack and P. D. Wall, eds., *Textbook of Pain*, 4th ed. Edinburgh: Churchill-Livingstone.

Woolf, C. J., and M. Costigan. 1999. "Transcriptional and Posttranslational Plasticity and the Generation of Inflammatory Pain." *Proceedings of the National Academy of Sciences U.S.A.* 96, no. 14: 7723–7730.

Woolf, C. J., and R. J. Mannion. 1999. "Neuropathic Pain: Aetiology, Symptoms, Mechanisms, and Management." *Lancet* 353: 1959–1964.

Woolf, C. J., and M. W. Salter. 2000. "Neuronal Plasticity: Increasing the Gain in Pain." *Science* 288: 1765–1768.

Setting the Stage for Pain

Allegorical Tales from Neuroscience

4

Howard L. Fields

The growth of knowledge and scholarship in biology, the social sciences, and humanities in the recent past has been remarkable. A by-product of this growth is the creation of a multitude of experts. The sheer expanse of knowledge challenges the capacity of individuals to maintain their expertise without losing touch with areas outside their own discipline. The increasing isolation of disciplines that have significant potential to inform each other is particularly unfortunate. Because advances in understanding often occur at the boundaries between academic areas of scholarship and research, it is essential to create a venue for interdisciplinary collaboration. The choice of pain as a focus for such collaboration is both imaginative and prescient. Pain is a powerful force in human behavior, and the biology of pain is a fairly advanced science. However, biological explanations are often not satisfying to scholars in the social sciences and humanities. The problem is in the area of meaning. The humanists do not find meaning in discussions of neural activity, and the neuroscientists usually are not looking for it.

On the other hand, the distance between the two camps is not that great. Because the impact of pain is so highly dependent on the meaning ascribed to it by the individual, a fuller understanding of pain in human beings requires an interdisciplinary approach that transcends the usual biomedical model. A major limitation in our ability to relieve the suffering of patients with chronic pain is an insufficient understanding of the role of meaning.

In this chapter, "meaning" will refer primarily to a set of associations. For example, a sound may initially have little meaning for an individual. It acquires meaning over time through the process of association. We first learn that the sound "mama" is associated with a particular person. The meaning could be general, coming to signify a general relationship of a female to a child. It could, in a different context, refer to a particular person. In the latter case, the meaning is enriched by a potentially very large set of associations related to the individual's life. Clearly, associations build over time, are context dependent, and can be culturally determined. A major challenge in neuroscience is to determine how the neural connections that underlie associations are made and maintained by the central nervous system.

To the extent that we seek to understand the human experience of pain as fully as possible we must address the issue of meaning. This requires constant interchange between neuroscience, the social sciences, and the humanities.

Meaning and Brain Activity

The brain provides the interface of biology with culture. Although the brain is a bodily organ, it has the unique property that its operation is completely symbolic. Patterns of neural activity are representational. Some patterns produce sensations; others produce language and memory. Unique patterns of neural activity represent the body, the external world, and memories. Although these activity patterns symbolize very different things, the representations themselves are all ontologically identical. They are all messages written in the same code, that is, spatiotemporal patterns of neural activity. Because they are coded in the same way, they can interact. Whether conscious or unconscious, bodily or cultural memories, current perceptions, and imagined futures are written in the same language, that is, electrochemical changes in nerve cells. The evolutionary history of the species as recorded in its nucleic acid, the accumulated icons of culture and clan, and the narrative of the individual are all written in the language of neural activity. The brain translates these different aspects of individual experience and weaves each of them into the seamless web of subjective experience and behavior.

Although few dispute that the nervous system is the organ of mental activity, the impact of this idea in the social sciences and humanities is minimal. Even natural scientists rarely delve into the broad implications of this idea. Since all human endeavors, from breathing to philosophy, depend on a set of rules governing the action and interaction of nerve cells, understanding brain function can inform a broad range of disciplines from aesthetics and history to anthropology and political science. Conversely, knowledge of neural activity and connectivity is insufficient to provide a complete understanding of the function of the human brain. Such understanding requires knowledge of concurrent contextual factors as well as the past experience and the goals of the individual. While not ignoring the power of genetics to explain individual differences, it is clear that the moment-to-moment experience of each person is interpreted with reference to his or her individual narrative and belief system. Furthermore, because of the rich tools that have evolved for human communication, our past histories include information derived in symbolic form from other people. This information is represented in the nervous system and has a profound effect on brain function. What we see is only partly shaped by what we are looking at. It is also determined by our past experience, which influences what we are looking for and which, in turn, is conditioned by what we want. Beyond our biological needs for survival, what we want depends on who we are. Who we are is constrained by our biology, but it is also shaped by cultural, interpersonal, and experiential factors.

The Natural Science of Meaning, or Why the Brain Is Not Like Other Organs

In the era of modern neuroscience, the triumph of the reductionist method is magnificent and undeniable. We have learned how nerve cells communicate with each other, how the right anatomical connections are determined during development, and how the strength of these connections is altered during learning. Insofar as brain cells are like cells in other organs, our knowledge is extensive and is growing exponentially. We are very close to having the entire human genome described. With this knowledge in hand, it becomes technically feasible to know the amino acid sequence of every protein in the body. We will then know all the building blocks that go into nerve cells. To the extent that we can stick electrodes into it and take pieces out of it, we have made enormous strides in understanding *how* the brain works. We are close to knowing how it works; the question is, *What does it do?* What is the meaning of brain activity? Analyzing the connections and electrical properties of nerve cells in isolation would not answer this question, because the meaning of neural activity lies *outside* the brain *(vide infra)*. It is this crucial insight that enables the interdisciplinary project.

Brain activity can be understood, that is, has meaning, only to the extent that it is a representation of the state of the body, of the external world, or of a potential behavior. Just as it would be pointless to analyze a book by investigating the chemical composition of paper and ink, a reductionist analysis of brain activity, that is, taking it apart and analyzing its nucleic acids, enzymes, receptors, and ion channels, fails to explain what brain activity accomplishes. The neuroscience of meaning requires experiments that study brain activity as the body moves through the world or as people describe their experience.

In an operational sense, the function of the brain has more in common with that of language than with that of other bodily organs. Because the brain operates symbolically, objects and events encoded by neural activity are not constrained by space or time. Brain activity can represent things experienced in the past or in an anticipated future. Furthermore, since representations can interact and be combined in novel ways, they are not constrained by objective reality. Neural activity can represent completely imaginary things like unicorns or a moon of blue cheese.

The Symbolic Brain: Neural Activity, Networks, and Representations

The minimal meaningful unit of nervous system function is the *network*. A network is a set of interconnected neurons whose coordinated activity produces an observable action or a subjective experience. The spatiotemporal pattern of *activity* of neurons in a network that produces an action (or perception) is a *representation*. Neuroscientists say that representations *encode* such things as stimuli or intended movements. Thus, representations relate to things and/or events external to the brain. The very concept of the representation depends on the thing that is represented. Although representations can be unrelated to the external world (e.g., those associated with introspection, imagination, expectation), even these representations are usually understood in the context of things external to the brain. Since our subjective experience of self, body, and world is an *emergent property* of dynamic networks of coordinated neural activity, the brain must contain representations of the body, the self (mind), and the external world. These representations give rise to the ongoing subjective experience of the individual.

Representations are a neural (physical) embodiment of meaning that is often understood in the context of intention. Intention assumes goals; goals imply values. A major task of the brain is to make choices between goals, and this in turn depends on values and predictions of consequences. Since biological, cultural, and personal factors play a major role in the determination of value, value is another critical area for the interdisciplinary enterprise.

In summary, the nervous system is poised at the interface of organism and environment. It is made up of bits of the body that generate a dynamically changing representation of the environment and body in relation to each other. The organism's biological program for survival and reproduction is reified in the neural analysis of this virtual body / virtual context relationship. This analysis of representations guides the physical organism through the external environment. The interacting dyad of brain and context is the canvas upon which "we" continually create ourselves. The brain is the site where culture and biology interact. It is an interface constrained by the laws of physics but liberated by imagination and hope.

The Fallacy of the Faithful Representation: Vision and Television

Old ideas fade slowly, particularly simple, elegant ideas that are consistent with our personal experience. One such idea is that the brain generates sensations by recreating an image of an object in the external world. This idea implies that a process occurs in the brain that is conceptually similar to what happens when a television camera monitors an object and converts it to (i.e., encodes as) a set of electrical signals that is then decoded by the tuner. The tuner then produces a visual image on the television screen that looks like the object in the camera. In this case the wavelength and pattern of light coming from the object completely determine the shape and color of the image on the television screen. The object is the ultimate cause of the image.

Many people, including some neuroscientists, assume that the human visual system works in a roughly analogous manner. In other words, that the object we are looking at completely determines the image we perceive. To a certain extent, this attitude is reinforced by certain arbitrary properties of the brain. Thus, for example, the visual cortex contains topographically accurate maps of visual space, and some cells in the visual cortex respond to lines of specific orientations, while others respond to specific colors. It is not a huge leap from these observations to the idea that there is a unique neural representation of the visual image that is completely determined by the wavelength and spatial pattern of light arriving at the retina from the external object. This representation would then generate the perceived image.

Although simple, this idea is hard to reconcile with the fact that people have vivid visual imagery during dreaming, when no visual stimuli impinge upon the retina. Hallucinations induced by drugs, trance, or mental illness are also difficult to reconcile with the brain as television monitor. These are only the most dramatic examples of processes that are in continual operation coloring our moment-to-moment experience. A purely bottom-up explanation of sensory experience is inconsistent with the facts.

The Perceptual Process: Selection or Reconstruction?

In fact, sensory stimuli impinge on a brain that is conditioned by genetics and learning. The process that leads from visual input to a subjectively experienced image is more akin to a computation about the likely cause of the stimulus than a photographic reproduction of the object. It is more selective and synthetic than reconstructive.

Dramatic and compelling evidence for this idea are the observations of Wilder Penfield and others who electrically stimulated the cerebral cortex in awake patients undergoing surgery for epilepsy. Depending on the location of the electrodes, stimulation could produce a variety of projected sensations (Penfield 1958; also see Gloor 1990). Of greatest interest were the effects of stimulation of the temporal lobes, which elicited complex narrative reports with strong emotional coloring. It is unlikely that the neural activity producing the experience is localized to the small area actually stimulated. What is more likely is that the stimulation activated a set of "prepackaged" representations. These representations could have a genetic component, but it is likely that they evolve over time through a combination of sensory experience and synthesis. The point is that, rather than passively reproduce images from sensory stimuli, the brain actively uses these inputs to combine and shape images that are selected from a potentially large but limited preexisting file.

Here is another potential interface for neurobiology: the social sciences and the humanities. Each individual will have a nervous system that is shaped by his or her unique experience. This is powerfully influenced by language, religion, and other cultural factors. A key point is that this influence is a two-way street: not only do bodily and environmental factors create central representations; these representations strongly influence the interpretation of ongoing experience. I will expand upon this point later.

Projection and the Illusion of the Mind-Body Dichotomy

The studies of Penfield as outlined above illustrate the process of *projection*. The process of projection is critical to understanding the experience of pain. Penfield's studies proved that electrical stimulation of the brain can elicit fully formed experience that is projected beyond the body to a "virtual" external world. Electrical stimulation of pain-transmitting neural pathways results in an experience of pain that is projected onto a specific body part (see, e.g., Craig and Dostrovsky 1999). In this case, there is nothing happening in that body part. The only thing that is "happening" is electrical activity in nerve cells activated either directly or indirectly by electrical stimulation. A neural representation has been activated and has produced the subjective experience of pain. The same thing happens when there is actual tissue injury (e.g., due to a broken bone), and the pain pathways are activated by the usual route. The experience of pain is the result of activating a neural representation in the brain and is projected in space to the site of tissue injury. The point is that the pain is generated at a site distant from the injury but is perceived to be at the injury site due to projection. The pain is generated in the brain. It is neural and mental. It is physical pain in the sense that nerve cells and their activity are physical. It is mental pain in the sense that it is subjectively experienced "in" what we generally call the mind.

Two illustrative examples of the phenomenon of projection are phantom limb and referred pain. Following amputation of an arm or leg, the amputee continues to feel the presence of the limb even though he knows it is not present. Of course, this is not surprising since the brain's representation of the limb is intact. Over time, the perceived size of the experienced phantom limb shrinks as the brain's representation changes (Flor, Elbert, and Muhlmickel 1998). In the case of referred pain, projection is also at work. The gall bladder is located just below the liver, but when it is inflamed, it often generates a pain that is felt as if it were in the right shoulder. This is because the sensory fibers from the gall bladder enter the nervous system along with the sensory fibers from the shoulder. Under normal conditions there is almost never a neural signal from the gall bladder, but when it is inflamed, it generates a signal that activates central pathways that are frequently activated by sensory input from the shoulder. The mislocalization of the source of the pain is due to the projection of the sensation to the usual source of the sensory signal.

Once one understands and accepts the concept of projection, it becomes obvious that all pain is mental. Furthermore, what most people call mental, or emotional, pain is ontologically identical to what they call organic, physical, or bodily pain. This point is counterintuitive, and failure to appreciate it has compounded the confusion about the nature of pain. Once this point is appreciated, many confusing phenomena, such as the placebo response, somatization, psychologically induced headache, and analgesia in trance, become less surprising and arcane.

Projection is a psychobiological phenomenon of great relevance to the interdisciplinary project (see my concluding remarks). It illustrates dramatically the metaphorical nature of neural activity. Furthermore, it reveals to us that everyday life requires an ongoing suspension of disbelief as our brains displace our subjective experiences from their intracranial generators (representations) out to our bodies and the external world. It seems to me that understanding these aspects of brain function provides one "humanities-friendly" ground of neuroscience.

The Neurobiology of Pain and Suffering: Pain as Sensation, Pain as Emotion

Up to this point I have focused on properties of brain function that relate to perception in general. This section will focus specifically on the neural mechanisms of pain perception. This will be a traditional bottom-up approach, covering brain areas that mediate different components of the pain experience. I will suggest how the meaning of pain associated with tissue damage can be shaped by personal and cultural factors. I will then discuss the evolution of current ideas about how activity in neuronal circuits elicited by tissue-damaging stimuli give rise to pain. This brief introduction to the neurobiology of pain transmission will be followed by a review of top-down factors that influence pain: specifically, the pain modulatory networks through which contextual factors interact with pain pathways to suppress, enhance, or even create the sensation of pain.

The rough outlines of the pain sensory system have been known since the late nineteenth century. Tissues are innervated by sensory nerve fibers that respond selectively to intense, potentially injurious events. These nerves propagate messages to the central nervous system. These messages activate numerous parallel circuits in the central nervous system that produce a variety of objective and subjective responses. For example, if you inadvertently touch a hot iron, you will automatically turn toward the iron and pull your hand away well before you experience a painful sensation. If you cannot pull away quickly enough, your blood pressure and heart rate will rise. Each of these responses depends on a separate circuit in the central nervous system; none requires the cortex.

Turning to the subjective experience: there are three distinct components (Melzack and Casey 1968; Fields 1999). First, there is the purely

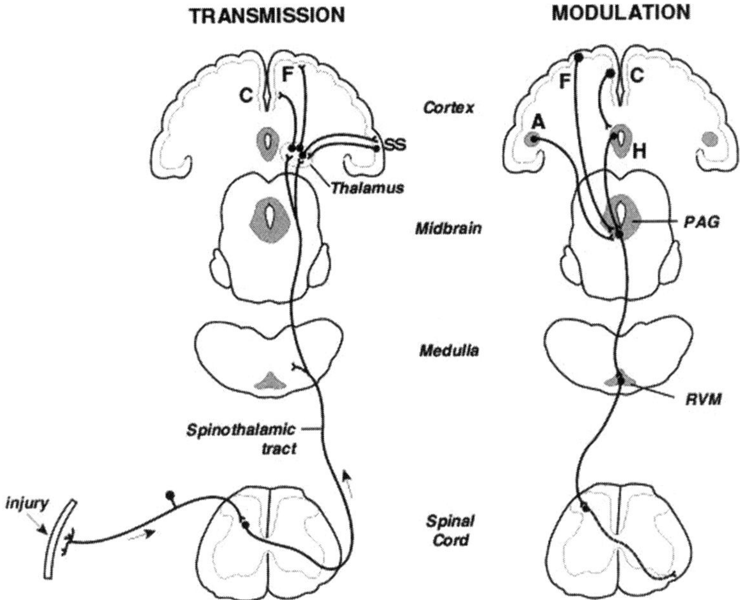

Figure 4.1. Pain Transmission and Modulation. Left: transmission pathway. Tissue injury activates primary afferent sensory fibers that relay information to the spinal cord. Initial processing takes place at the level of the dorsal horn and is then conducted in the spinothalamic tract to the thalamus. At this level, the pathway diverges into a medial projection to the front lobe (F), which includes the anterior cingulate cortex (C), the lateral pathway that projects to the somatosensory cortex (SS). Right: modulation pathway. Signals depending upon memories and contextual cues arise from the frontal cortext and amygdala (A) and project to the midbrain periaqueductal gray (PAG), which controls the spinothalamic pathway via the rostral ventromedial medulla (RVM).

discriminative part that includes recognizing the quality of the sensation as a burn and localizing it to your hand. Second, there is the motivational aspect associated with the desire to pull your hand away or to terminate the sensation. Third, there is an evaluative component—the thought of the damage that has been done to your hand and how that will affect your life in the hours and days ahead. All three subjective components of the pain experience are triggered by activity in peripheral nerves that enter the spinal cord and activate cells that project to the contralateral thalamus (see Figure 4.1, Transmission). This is the spinothalamic tract, which is required for all components of the sensation of pain in normal individuals. At the level of the thalamus, the pain signal diverges into separate pathways that underlie the different components of the experience. The discriminative component (what and where) largely involves the somatosensory cortex. In contrast, forebrain areas known as the limbic system mediate the motivational and emotional component of pain (how bad it feels). The limbic system includes the cingulate gyrus and anterior insula of the frontal cortex and the subcortical structure known as the amygdala. The neurobiology of the evaluative component is still an open question.

In addition to its role in pain perception, the limbic system mediates emotional responses to a variety of factors including personal loss, anticipation of harm, and so on. The dysphoric states such as depression and anxiety share limbic system circuits with somatic pain. It is thus no accident that the word "pain" is often used to denote emotional pain that has no somatic component. For the purposes of our multidisciplinary project, it is important to keep the distinction between somatic and emotional pain clear. Although somatic injury can produce both somatic and emotional pain, the neural representations of these two aspects of the experience are largely separate. For example, patients with frontal lobotomies selectively lose the motivational (suffering) component of pain, but the discriminative component is spared. When these patients sustain tissue injury, they report intense pain and can give a precise description of its quality and location and yet have no emotional response to it (Fields 1999).

The motivational and evaluative aspects of pain are tightly bound. Imagine the difference between a headache sustained after a bout of heavy drinking and an equally severe headache the week after learning that one's identical twin brother with a similar headache was diagnosed with a malignant brain tumor. In these two examples, although a similar peripheral signal was at work, the meaning was completely different. The point is that the response to the "pain" signal does not occur in a vacuum, and the cognitive response to it depends in large part on the context in which the pain arises. Since the context depends on interpersonal dynamics, cultural factors, and the individual's personal narrative, their analysis requires the tools and concepts of the social sciences.

The Evolution of Ideas about the Neural Mechanisms of Pain

The focus on pain as a sensation as opposed to an emotion stimulated research on specific pain pathways. The success of these studies on sensation reinforced the tendency of investigators to focus on this aspect of pain. In the early nineteenth century the pioneering work of Bell and Magendie had established the differences between sensory and motor nerves (e.g., see chapter 5 in Keele 1957). The definition of a distinct system for somatic sensation, including pain, fit in well with the law of specific nerve energies proposed by the German physiologist Muller. This law postulates that each sensory modality (vision, smell, hearing, somatic sensation) is subserved by a distinct set of neural structures in peripheral nerves and in the brain. This idea received strong confirmation through the mid-nineteenth-century experimental and clinical studies of Brown-Sequard that clearly identified the anterolateral quadrant of the spinal cord as a discrete spinal pathway for pain. More specialized anatomical techniques allowed later investigators to determine that the thalamus is the relevant target for this pathway.

Primary Afferents for Pain: The Rise and Apparent Fall of Specificity Theory

Pain sensation requires primary afferents to transform tissue pathology (e.g., injury and inflammation) into a code (nerve impulses) that can be interpreted by the brain (see Chapter 3). Primary afferents are neurons that have their cell bodies in the dorsal root ganglia near the spinal cord. They send one process (axon) out to innervate the peripheral tissues, and another axon carries the message into the spinal cord. By the late nineteenth century, anatomists had discovered a variety of different skin specializations innervated by cutaneous primary afferent nerves. These discoveries led von Frey to propose that each anatomical specialization conferred specific sensitivity to a specific type of stimulus energy (e.g., warm, cold, touch, pain, itch). Perhaps because of its elegance and simplicity, this idea held sway until the mid-twentieth century, when it was thoroughly discredited by anatomical studies showing a dissociation between any of the known skin specializations and the sensations of cold, warm, and pain. On the other hand, von Frey's idea that a class of primary afferent is specialized to encode information about intense, tissue-damaging stimuli was ultimately vindicated, but not until after a period of strong controversy.

After World War II, a new method emerged that revolutionized neuroscience. This was the ability to record the activity of single nerve cells. This method enabled investigators to determine precisely what stimuli a given nerve fiber responds to optimally. The first rush of data stimulated specific theories. As is often the case, the first interpretations were based on incomplete information. The earliest studies found few primary afferent nerve fibers specialized to respond to intense tissue-damaging stimuli. Furthermore, the first pain-responsive neurons studied in central pain pathways responded across a broad range of stimuli, including innocuous mechanical stimulation. These findings appeared at odds with the dominant idea of a labeled line that consisted of specialized primary afferent receptors and central pathways for pain sensation. In addition, there were behavioral studies in animals, clinical observations, and human psychophysical data that were at odds with the idea of a simple one-to-one relationship between stimulus intensity and perceived pain intensity. First, there were the experimental studies of Russian physiologist Ivan Pavlov. When he trained dogs by consistently preceding food administration with tissue-damaging stimulation, over time, they began to salivate instead of whining and cowering when the noxious stimuli were applied. Somehow the pairing of the intense stimulus with food changed its meaning. These findings were complemented by the observations in people that psychological factors such as fear and expectation could powerfully alter pain perception. The most famous of these were the reports by Beecher (1959; see also 1946) of American soldiers in World War II who denied feeling pain despite grievous injuries. Not only do these observations illustrate the importance of learning and context; they clearly imply that the brain has mechanisms that allow it to suppress typical responses to intense, tissue-damaging stimuli, including the perception of pain. Finally, peripheral nerve lesions or selective blockade of large myelinated axons in peripheral nerve were shown to produce exaggerated responses to stimuli that were normally innocuous or only mildly painful. This suggested that the large myelinated fibers inhibited central pain pathways.

This evidence of interaction of stimuli from different sensory channels smacked of pattern theory, that is, the idea that sensation has as much to do with the interactions and *patterns* of neural activity as with their specific sensitivity. As it turns out, both ideas were eventually incorporated into our current concepts of the neural coding relevant to pain perception.

The Gate Control Hypothesis in Perspective

In 1965, Melzack and Wall suggested a specific neural model, the gate control hypothesis, to account for these and other findings at odds with specificity theory. This model was revolutionary in that it was the first serious attempt to incorporate the puzzling clinical features of pain and the newly emerging data from studies of single neurons. Their theory was consistent with what was known at the time, and it was simple, highly specific, and testable. At that time it was generally accepted that the smaller-diameter, most slowly conducting primary afferents had the highest threshold for activation, and the larger-diameter fibers responded maximally to light-innocuous stimuli. The core of Melzack and Wall's idea was as follows: (1) the different primary afferents responding to either innocuous (large-diameter primary afferents) and noxious stimuli (small-diameter primary afferents) converge onto, and directly excite, pain transmission neurons (T cells) that produce responses to pain-including sensation; (2) there is also an interneuron (SG cell) in the spinal cord dorsal horn that inhibits both types of primary afferent by preventing neurotransmitter release from their terminals onto the T cells; (3) the SG cell is inhibited by the small-diameter primary afferent and excited by the large-diameter afferent. Excitation of SG interneurons by large-diameter fibers suppresses pain responses. Furthermore, the model predicts that strong inhibition of the SG cells by the small-diameter primary afferents would block the inhibitory effect of the large-diameter fibers so that they would *produce pain* rather than inhibiting it.

This last prediction presented the greatest challenge for specificity (labeled line) theory, since the large-diameter myelinated fibers do not respond differentially to intense stimuli. In fact, subsequent research has shown conclusively that selective stimulation of large-diameter fibers in awake human beings under normal conditions produces a nonpainful vibratory or tingling feeling but never pain. However, following selective activation of small-diameter fibers, selective stimulation of the same large-diameter fibers produces a burning pain. The activation of the small-diameter fibers has produced a change in the pain pathways so that the large myelinated fibers now have access to it. There has thus been a modality shift such that the same fibers that produce an innocuous feeling of touch under one condition can produce pain when tissue damage has occurred. There is no way that this robust finding can be accounted for by a labeled central line for pain. Modality shifting is the ultimate vindication of a core concept of the pattern theory idea because it clearly demonstrates that the perceptual impact of activity in a primary afferent can be robustly changed by activity in other primary afferents.

It is difficult to overestimate the impact that the Melzack/Wall hypothesis had. By proposing a specific and testable neural hypothesis for pain perception, it stimulated an explosion of experiments and invigorated the field of pain research. By providing a neural explanation for the paradoxical dissociation of stimulus and perception, it not only shook the foundations of specificity theory, but it brought the most clinically relevant aspects of pain out of the realm of pure psychology and into the realm of neuroscience. A corollary of this was to provide enhanced respectability for pain patients, for the physicians who cared for them, and for the scientists working in the field. Instead of asking, "What's wrong with this person?" the question became, "What's wrong with his/her nervous system?" The latter question is clearly more susceptible to investigation with the tools of modern biological science. The gate control hypothesis was a heuristic success.

Despite the huge impact of the gate control hypothesis, critical observations upon which it was based were either incomplete or misleading, and most of its specific assertions have crumbled under the weight of investigation. Later discoveries provided better explanations for most of the phenomena that the model addressed. First, it turns out that there are, in fact, many primary afferents that respond selectively to intense, tissue-damaging stimuli. More problematic for the hypothesis is the discovery of dorsal horn neurons that respond selectively to noxious and to thermal stimuli. The prolonged excitatory changes in pain transmission neurons are now known to result from changes intrinsic to the primary afferents and the central transmission neurons as opposed to inhibition of inhibitory SG interneurons. Thus, many primary afferents show increased sensitivity and spontaneous activity following intense tissue damage or when they themselves are damaged. Furthermore, most substantia gelatinosa neurons are excitatory, not inhibitory, and the weight of evidence indicates that the shift in modality of large myelinated fibers from touch to pain is due to long-term excitation of the pain transmission (T) cells themselves, not disinhibition (Doubell, Mannion, and Woolf 1999). While there are some inhibitory SG neurons, there is no evidence that they are inhibited by small-diameter primary afferents, which is a key component of the gate control model. Finally, and most relevant to our multidisciplinary project, there is no compelling evidence to support a role for the dorsal columns in the "central control trigger."

In summary, our understanding of the primary afferent nociceptor and the spinal transmission neurons they excite has evolved dramatically. A subset of primary afferents responds selectively to tissue-damaging stimuli and shows lowered thresholds and spontaneous activity when exposed to prolonged or repeated intense stimuli or when damaged. The spinal neurons (T cells) activated by nociceptive primary afferents also become sensitized following prolonged or repeated intense stimuli. When (and only when) the second-order (T) cells are sensitized, they can be activated by light (normally innocuous) mechanical stimuli that only activate the large myelinated fibers. It is this sensitization that accounts for the modality shift from touch to pain in large-diameter primary afferents, which was a major impetus for the gate control hypothesis. Nearly four decades after the theory was proposed, we have better explanations for most of the observations that it attempted to explain. Yet its impact is undeniable. The advances in our understanding since mid-1965, while dramatic in their cumulative effect, have been incremental, and none have had anything like the revolutionary impact as the gate control hypothesis. Specificity theory is now generally understood to be inadequate. The importance of convergence and plasticity in the connections to spinal cord pain transmission neurons remains unchallenged, as is the idea that forebrain control is exerted via descending connections to a spinal "gate."

Top-Down Influences on Pain: Modulatory Systems

A major impetus for the gate control hypothesis was the recognition that learning, attention, expectation, and mood can exert powerful control over pain. At the time of the original proposal, much less was known about these top-down factors than about primary afferent nociceptors and spinal cord pain processing. Melzack and Wall clearly realized that unless these factors could be accounted for, any theories of pain would be woefully inadequate. Pain research was able to progress precisely because scientists doing psychophysical studies could control these modulating factors and isolate the mechanisms specific to the bottom-up sensory process. To a certain extent, the emphasis on the ascending sensory pathways remains the dominant theme in pain research. However, there is a growing interest in studying the neural systems that underlie the top-down modulatory factors.

While descending pathways were known to impinge on and control spinal cord pain transmission neurons, their origin and function were unknown (Fields, Basbaum, and Heinricher 2006). The gate control hypothesis incorporated these descending pathways by proposing a vague "central control trigger." The central control was activated by a bodily stimulus that, via large-diameter afferents in the dorsal column, triggered an evaluative forebrain process that generated a signal sent back down to the spinal cord "gate" to close it before the slowly conducting input from the small fibers arrived. This idea has not been supported by experiment. No bodily stimulus is required for activation of evaluative processes known to precede and modify pain. Furthermore, there is no compelling evidence that the dorsal column pathway contributes significantly to pain modulation.

The study of pain modulation began in earnest about five years after Melzack and Wall published their hypothesis, and our knowledge in this area has since grown explosively. Briefly, brain regions comprising the limbic system (the cingulate and prefrontal cortex, the medial temporal lobe and amygdala, and the hypothalamus) connect via neurons in certain brainstem structures that descend to and control the dorsal horn neurons that receive inputs from the primary afferents that specifically respond to noxious stimuli (Fields and Price 1997; Fields, Basbaum, and Heinricher 2006; see again Figure 4.1, Modulation). The structures in this pain-modulating circuit are linked by endogenous opioid peptides (endorphins), and the evidence is compelling that the circuit mediates the pain-relieving effect of powerful narcotic analgesics such as morphine. In addition to suppression of pain, neurons in the circuit can *facilitate* pain. In other words, pain modulation is bidirectional. The impact of our improved understanding of pain-modulating systems has been extraordinary and rivals that of the gate control hypothesis and subsequent research in pain transmission. Research on pain modulatory systems has been crucial for increasing understanding of how centrally acting analgesic drugs relieve pain, how drug tolerance develops, and how cognitive factors modify pain.

The Brain as a Hypothesis Machine: The Biological Function of Reward and Punishment

After this brief introduction to the basic neurobiology of pain, let us return to more general issues. It is essential to put the neurobiology of pain into a broader functional perspective in order to move toward a rigorous dialogue with the humanities. This requires identifying points where the neurobiology of pain informs such key interdisciplinary bridging concepts as meaning and expectancy. Up to this point, we have focused on the subjective experience of pain. After all, pain is defined in those terms, and most scientific work on pain to date has focused on mechanistic explanations of the perceptual experience. However, a deeper and broader understanding requires that we put the subjective experience into a biological perspective. To ask, "What is the biological purpose of the neural systems that mediate and modulate the experience of pain?" is clearly quite a different matter than to ask, "What are the neural mechanisms underlying pain sensation?" The former question requires us to address the general issue, "How does the brain use sensory information?"

Earlier in this chapter we discussed representation and projection and put the relationship of stimulus to perception in perspective. As mentioned earlier, representations are best understood in the context of goals, which in turn imply a set of values. Biological values are determined by the survival and reproductive success of the individual. Nervous systems are designed to enable an organism to respond to potentially tissue-damaging or life-sustaining objects or processes in the internal or external environment. As the repertoire of potential responses expands, more complex neural computations are required to choose the response most likely to be beneficial. Whether to run, fight, or pay someone else to fight, the more options there are, the more possibilities to "succeed." The brain gathers all the information and makes a computation about which course of action is most likely to achieve the desired end. In other words, the computation leads to a prediction of consequences in the form of a hypothesis: If I carry out action A, the consequence will be B. If I carry out C, the consequence will be D. B is more desirable than D; therefore I will carry out A. The role of pain (and pleasure) is to inform the organism of the cost (and benefit) of the chosen action. This information allows the brain to reevaluate the accuracy of its predictions. The point is that the sensory system is not a passive conduit for transmitting information about stimuli. The sensory system is active in the context of goal-directed behaviors and provides data the brain uses to evaluate the consequences of specific actions. The brain is not passive; it is actively probing and exploring. At any given time, what the brain "perceives" depends as much on what questions it is asking and what happened in the past as it does on what stimuli are presented to it. The modifications that take place can be thought of as transformations of the meaning of the neural activity produced by tissue-damaging stimuli.

Pain Transforms Meaning, Meaning Transforms Pain

Although our interdisciplinary project is still in a nascent stage, it is not too soon to ask whether we can conceptualize a neurobiological model for the transformative process. How could pain transform meaning, and how could meaning transform pain? There is no doubt that these transformations occur, but we have yet to develop a common language. First we have to agree on what the phenomenon is that we want to explain. Consider this section a preliminary attempt to get the conversation going.

One aspect of this conversation is straightforward. By the process of association, pain can transform the meaning of contextual cues, intentions, and behaviors. It is no accident that the Latin root of the word "pain" is punishment. Punishment is a core interpersonal transaction that leads to social control and the reinforcement of cultural norms. For example, take the dictum Honor thy parents. Parents may inflict pain on their children if they lie, deliberately break things, or simply act in a defiant manner. Through the agency of punishment, the (actual or intended) performance of the punished act acquires new meaning. One could argue that obedience becomes a good because of its association with the avoidance of pain. The threat of pain can become incorporated into cultural myths that serve the same purpose as punishment. For example, in some ideas of hell, physical pain plays a prominent role. Conversely, pain can transform behaviors in the opposite direction. You might say that defiance is transformed from disrespect to courage when it is done in the anticipation of physical punishment. What the parent views as evil, the child's peers might view as a good. In this case, the concept of courage (or defiance) requires cultural insights and is usefully informed by anthropology and/or sociology. Courage is generally thought to be good, but again, good and bad are not scientific constructs. Here one must call on scholars in philosophy and religion. Through the analysis of such specific behaviors, the interdisciplinary project of the Mind/Brain/Behavior Initiative can be advanced.

How can we inject neurobiology into this conversation? In this specific case it would be difficult. At some point it might be possible to develop a neurobiology of courage; however, the neurobiology of culturally defined personal qualities is virtually nonexistent. What is possible, now, is to find a model for a *behavioral* transformation produced by pain.

An Animal Model to Study the Neurobiology of Pain-Induced Transformation: Conditioned Fear and Pain-Modulating Pathways

An excellent animal model of transformation is *conditioned fear* in rodents. One rodent response to threat is to freeze and become analgesic.

Presumably, the biological significance is that the rodent is less likely to be seen by a predator if it is absolutely still. In the conditioned fear paradigm, rodents are exposed for a few seconds to a painful stimulus in a small box from which they cannot escape. After a couple of brief exposures to such stimuli, when the rodents are returned to the box in which they had previously been shocked, they freeze and become completely analgesic. What has happened is that the sensory features that are unique to the shock-box have been transformed. Where once the box was considered safe, it is now threatening. In other words, through associative conditioning the contextual stimuli (color, texture, odor of the box) have acquired new meaning. One can do the same thing by cueing the shock with an innocuous tone or light.

From the neurobiological standpoint, the mechanism of conditioned fear is well understood. The underlying circuit includes the endogenous opioid-mediated pain-modulating pathway described earlier (e.g., see Helmstetter and Tershner 1994). Furthermore, the sites of plasticity that underlie the "transformation" in meaning of the cues that have been paired with the shock have been localized in specific limbic system structures. The synaptic changes underlying the learning are partially understood. The point is that we have a model for discussing meaning at a biological level. The nervous system objectively embodies meaning and renders it accessible to scientific study. By virtue of the physical interaction of representations, new representations emerge that change behavior and perception. When referring to this process, substitute the word "learning" for "transformation," and neuroscientists become comfortable.

How Meaning Modifies Pain

Because it is such a powerful motivating force, and can signal the threat of irreversible harm, it is not surprising that pain has transformative power for individuals. What is surprising, however, is the power of symbolic manipulation to change the experience of pain. The placebo analgesic response is an excellent example of the power of expectation to alter the pain experience (Fields and Price 1997).

There is compelling evidence that placebo analgesia requires the same opioid-mediated pain-modulating circuitry that underlies the analgesic effect of conditioned fear in rodents. In human subjects with experimental pain, placebo analgesic responses are associated with activity in brain areas that largely overlap those activated when opioids are administered (Petrovic et al. 2002). This circuitry is homologous to that activated by opioids and conditioned fear in rodents. In view of the fact that placebo analgesia in humans is blocked by the opioid antagonist drug naloxone, this observation demonstrates the importance of specific pain-modulating circuitry in mediating the suppressing effects of meaning and expectancy on pain. It seems to me that the placebo analgesic effect, with its powerful cultural and personal determinants, and a partially described neural mechanism, is an ideal place to focus an interdisciplinary discussion.

Another dramatic example of the power of verbal instruction to alter pain perception is a study by Dworkin and colleagues at the University of Washington. They used the method of tooth pulp stimulation to deliver a standard noxious stimulus in normal human volunteers (Dworkin et al. 1983). Subjects were stimulated at an intensity adjusted to produce the same reported subjective pain intensity. Following this, all subjects were given nitrous oxide. The independent variable was what the subjects were told. One group was simply told they were receiving nitrous oxide; the other group was told that nitrous oxide actually enhanced awareness. Those told simply that they were receiving nitrous oxide reported significant pain relief, whereas those told that nitrous oxide enhanced awareness experienced a significant increase in their pain levels. In this case, the physical manipulations resulted in different outcomes based on different verbal instructions.

Even more dramatic is the study by Bayer and colleagues (Bayer, Baer, and Early 1991). They examined normal volunteers who had electrodes placed on their temples. The subjects were told that they would receive electrical stimulation at increasing intensity and were to report the level of pain they experienced. The stimulus intensity was signaled by an intensity gauge that the subject could view and by a tone whose pitch increased in increments that were parallel with the

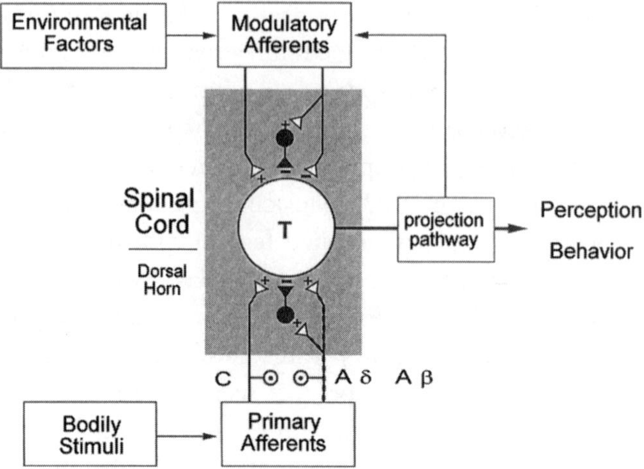

Figure 4.2. Top-down Factors in Pain. Pain depends on both potentially injurious bodily stimuli and the context in which those stimuli are given. The pain transmission system integrates both somatic stimuli (shown coming up from below to contact the T, or transmission neuron). Of equal or greater importance are top-down inputs from modulatory systems that are determined by behavioral state (both internal motivations and external contextual cues). Cultural factors can be powerful determinants of the state of the T neuron. Aδ and C fibers include nociceptors, while Aβ fibers are activated by light, normally innocuous stimuli. Bottom-up and top-down systems can be either inhibitory (acting via the small, dark inhibitory neurons) or excitatory.

gauge readings. One hundred subjects were included in the study. They were divided into five groups and given different instructions. Although no stimulus was actually delivered (the electrodes were not connected to a power source), up to 50 percent of subjects reported pain at the electrode site, and up to 25 percent requested pain medication. This study is very important because severe pain was elicited in the absence of any stimulation. It illustrates the power of meaning to influence the pain experience. There is evidence that the pain modulatory systems described here may be involved in these cognitively generated pain responses. The pain modulatory system is known to exert bidirectional control; that is, it can generate as well as suppress pain. Furthermore, recent functional imaging studies are consistent with the notion that brain regions identified as part of this system are activated during the time when a painful stimulus is expected (Hsieh, Stone-Elander, and

Ingvar 1999; Sawamoto et al. 2000; Tracey et al. 2002; Keltner et al. 2006).

Although a complete understanding of contextual influences on pain is many years in the future, a general model is emerging. The basic idea is that through the process of association environmental stimuli gain the ability to exert powerful influences on perceived pain intensity. The process of association changes the neural representations (meaning) of the relevant contextual stimuli. Consequently, the contextual stimuli gain the power to change the neural representations elicited by actual or anticipated tissue-damaging stimuli. These changes are exerted via a specific pain-modulatory system with links in limbic forebrain, amygdala, and brain stem. This circuit projects to, and selectively controls, pain-transmitting spinothalamic tract neurons. Thus the old view that the experience of pain is a bottom-up process determined largely by the stimulus must be revised. In the current view, activity in the pain pathways is determined not only by tissue injury but by expectation (see Figure 4.2). This, in turn, is conditioned by the individual's past history and by current contextual stimuli. In this view, pain normally has both stimulus-bound and context-determined components. The study of the stimulus-bound components is advanced and is largely the province of neurobiology. The study of the context-determined components is an inherently interdisciplinary endeavor and is in its infancy.

References

Bayer, T. L., P. E. Baer, and C. Early. 1991. "Situational and Psychophysiological Factors in Psychologically Induced Pain." *Pain* 44: 45–50.

Beecher, H. K. 1946. "Pain in Men Wounded in Battle." *Ann. Surg.* 123: 96–105.

———. 1959. *Measurement of Subjective Responses: Quantitative Effects of Drugs.* New York: Oxford University Press.

Craig, A. D., and J. O. Dostrovsky. 1999. "Medulla to Thalamus." In P. D. Wall and R. Melzack, eds., *Textbook of Pain,* 4th ed. Edinburgh: Churchill-Livingstone, 183–214.

Doubell, T. P., R. J. Mannion, and C. J. Woolf. 1999. "The Dorsal Horn: State-Dependent Sensory Processing, Plasticity and the Generation of

Pain." In P. D. Wall and R. Melzack, eds., *Textbook of Pain,* 4th ed. Edinburgh: Churchill-Livingstone, 165–182.

Dworkin, S. F., A. C. C. Chen, L. LeResche, and D. W. Clark. 1983. "Cognitive Reversal of Expected Nitrous Oxide Analgesia for Acute Pain." *Anesth. Analg.* 62: 1073–1077.

Fields, H. L. 1999. "Pain: An Unpleasant Topic." *Pain* supplement 6: S61–S69.

Fields, H. L., A. I. Basbaum, and M. M. Heinricher. 2006. "Central Nervous System Mechanisms of Pain Modulation." In S. B. McMahon and M. Koltzenburg, eds., *Wall and Melzack's Textbook of Pain,* 5th ed. Edinburgh: Elsevier Churchill Livingstone, 125–142.

Fields, H. L., and D. D. Price. 1997. "Toward a Neurobiology of Placebo Analgesia." In A. Harrington, ed., *The Placebo Effect: An Interdisciplinary Exploration.* Cambridge, Mass.: Harvard University Press.

Flor, H., T. Elbert, and W. Muhlmickel. 1998. "Cortical Reorganization and Phantom Phenomena in Congenital and Traumatic Upper-Extremity Amputees." *Exp. Brain Res.* 119: 205–212.

Gloor, P. 1990. "Experiential Phenomena of Temporal Lobe Epilepsy: Facts and Hypotheses." *Brain* 113: 1673–1694.

Helmstetter, F. J., and S. A. Tershner. 1994. "Lesions of the Periaqueductal Gray and Rostral Ventromedial Medulla Disrupt Antinociceptive But Not Cardiovascular Aversive Conditional Responses." *J. Neurosci.* 14: 7099–7108.

Hsieh, J. C., S. Stone-Elander, and M. Ingvar. 1999. "Anticipatory Coping of Pain Expressed in the Human Anterior Cingulate Cortex: A Positron Emission Tomography Study." *Neurosci. Lett.* 26 (262): 61–64.

Keele, K. D. 1957. *Anatomies of Pain.* Oxford: Blackwell Press.

Keltner, J. R., A. Furst, C. Fan, R. Redfern, B. Inglis, and H. L. Fields. 2006. "Isolating the Modulatory Effect of Expectancy upon Pain Transmission: An fMRI Study." *J. Neurosci.* 26: 4437–4443.

Melzack, R., and K. L. Casey. 1968. "Sensory, Motivational, and Central Control Determinants of Pain." In D. Kenshalo, ed., *The Skin Senses.* Springfield, Ill.: C. C. Thomas, 423–439.

Melzack, R., and P. D. Wall. 1962. "On the Nature of Cutaneous Sensory Mechanisms." *Brain* 85: 331–356.

———. 1965. "Pain Mechanisms: A New Theory." *Science* 150: 971–979.

Penfield, W. 1958. *The Excitable Cortex in Conscious Man.* Springfield, Ill.: C. C. Thomas.

Petrovic, P., E. Kalso, K. M. Petersson, and M. Ingvar. 2002. "Placebo and Opioid Analgesia: Imaging a Shared Neuronal Network." *Science* 295: 1737–1740.

Sawamoto, N., M. Honda, T. Okada, T. Hanakawa, M. Kanda, H. Fukuyama, J. Konishi, and H. Shibasaki. 2000. "Expectation of Pain

Enhances Responses to Nonpainful Somatosensory Stimulation in the Anterior Cingulate Cortex and Parietal Operculum / Posterior Insula: An Event-Related Functional Magnetic Resonance Imaging Study." *J. Neurosci.* 20: 7438–7445.

Tracey, I., A. Ploghaus, J. S. Gati, S. Clare, S. Smith, R. S. Menon, and P. M. Matthews. 2002. "Imaging Attentional Modulation of Pain in the Periaqueductal Gray in Humans." *J. Neurosci.* 22: 2748–2752.

Wall, P. D., and R. Melzack, eds. 1999. *Textbook of Pain,* 4th ed. Edinburgh: Churchill-Livingstone.

Response:
Is Pain Differentially Embodied?

Anne Harrington

I want to respond to Howard Fields's suggestion that we don't need the "body" to have pain. I understand that in one sense the "body" exists virtually inside the brain. But I want to argue that at the very least the external body might be an important analytic reference point. It might turn out to be very important to differentiate pain, at least phenomenologically, by how it manifests itself within the body *differentially.*

Last summer when I was in China, I was privileged to be invited to witness an operation in Shanghai on a woman who was having a tumor removed from her thyroid without any anesthesia or medication at all. The only intervention she received was a form of so-called *chi gong* therapy (see Cohen 1997) by a traditional Chinese medicine practitioner. It was evident that she was not in pain, but she was not completely without any sensation. At one point the sheet on her shoulder became uncomfortable or annoying for her, and they had to adjust it. But when blood spurted across the room onto the white coat of one of the surgeons, that didn't seem to have any effect. It was quite amazing.

At a debriefing session with the surgeons after the surgery, we talked about what kind of operations they use this *chi gong* therapy for. They said they don't use it for anything that deals with abdominal organs; then they bring in the heavy artillery, pharmacological anesthesia. There was no particular explanation why pain can be managed with traditional methods—mind and culture—when removing a tumor from the thyroid but not when dealing with tissue in the abdominal cavity. There is certainly a story here about the way in which all pain in the body is not the same, and the body therefore must matter if we're going to understand how biology and culture interface in the varied experiences of pain that are our lot. In short, different *parts* of the body may have different meanings and significance in different cultures and religious systems.

Reference

Cohen, K. S. 1997. *The Way of Qi Gong: The Art and Science of Chinese Energy Healing*. New York: Ballantine Books.

Response:
Pain and the Embodiment of Culture

Elaine Scarry

I will also address the topic of cultural perspectives, but with a slightly different emphasis. Like most of you, I see pain as underscoring the connection between "body" and world. But I also want to insist on a slightly more restricted sense of pain, limited to the physical. Many of you talk about suffering, grief, or depression as pain, and I recognize the accuracy of that and salute it. But I think that on some levels physical pain is distinguishable from these other things, and by separating it you emphasize the interesting interactions between body and world that pain calls attention to.

Virginia Woolf talked about the fact that we have no language for physical pain: "The merest schoolgirl, when she falls in love, has Shakespeare or Keats to speak her mind for her; but let a sufferer try to describe a pain in his head to a doctor and language at once runs dry" (1948 [1930], 11). We have many centuries of literature that has profound expressiveness for romantic heartache, for horrible forms of depression, for different kinds of psychotic pain, and so forth, but the number of works expressing the brute fact of cancer pain, burn pain, extreme headache, et cetera, would probably fit in an ordinary binder. Compare that to Thomas Mann's statement that he couldn't write an encyclopedia volume on the literature of suffering because every piece of literature in the world is about suffering. But the books about physical pain would really fit right here.

Once you acknowledge the fact that pain is so resistant to language, it seems odd that at the same time it is so revelatory of memory and interaction between the body and the world. Since it resists language, even destroys language, reducing us to cries and moans and the kinds of expression we make anterior to learned language, we would expect it to be resistant to culture, something happening prior to culture.

But yet we know that isn't true. We know it can be culturally shaped. Just by looking around the table, it's clear that I shouldn't even address this since all of you have such intricate specific knowledge about pain in different cultures. We also know that pain confirms the deep presence of culture in the body. When immigrants come to the United States from different countries and progressively lose all of their cultural habits, the last to be lost is the cultural disposition to express or not express physical pain in a certain way. It's not obvious that that would be the case; you might think it would be the first thing to go. But it is consistent with its resistance to language; if you don't have a lot of poems and artworks describing physical pain, then whatever your learned responses are, they won't be continually renegotiated.

That's the end point that culture doesn't reshape, but there's also a starting point. The gate control theory is not the only model for pain, and as we have heard, it needs major modifications, but I think that it will eventually be the model for a lot of perceptual events that we don't understand; in fact, it has started being applied to things like visual experience. But here again, culture comes in at a very early point. Melzack's argument in the gate control theory of pain is that even before you begin to feel the pain, or to amplify or diminish it, your brain has already localized it and brought to bear certain cultural predispositions.

The idea of the brain as a membrane between the body and the world often appears in art as the notion that the body interiorizes all of our great cultural artifacts. When Richard Selzer describes doing an operation on the abdomen, pushing back the layers of the body, he will say something like, "You go in through this layer, and then you pull back the fat in this layer, and then finally you get to where it's so ancient . . ." The image you expect is something ghastly and organic, like a primeval worm, but actually, he says, "so ancient that you expect to find a cave painting on the wall" (see Selzer 1996).

There is an insistent belief that the body contains not physical matter but all the world out there. We see this happening again and again in Renaissance texts of poetry, medicine, and philosophy, where the great cultural artifacts are pictured inside the body. Many of you know John Donne's poem about the lovers being turned into a pair of compasses, "A Valediction Forbidding Mourning" (Donne 1896), where he has embedded one of the most potent instruments of the age inside the body of two lovers. In "The Damp," where Donne is addressing his mistress, he says,

> When I am dead, and doctors know not why,
> And my friends' curiosity
> Will have me cut up to survey each part,
> When they shall find your picture in my heart....

Other poems place a beehive, or a newly invented window glass, in the body. A lot of medical case histories from that period do the same thing, as does the philosopher Nicholas Cusanus. Leonardo's drawings are similar. Inside the drawing of a leg he puts text and a drawing of compasses. There are equivalents in much more modern texts as well. This just reinforces what many people here have said, that the boundary at the edge of the body is very porous, and pain heightens our awareness of that.

References

Donne, J. 1896. *Poems of John Donne,* vol. 1. Ed. E. K. Chambers. London: Lawrence & Bullen.

Selzer, R. 1996. *Mortal Lessons: Notes on the Art of Surgery.* New York: Harcourt.

Woolf, V. 1948 [1930]. "On Being Ill." In *The Moment, and Other Essays.* New York: Harcourt, Brace, 9–23.

Discussion:
Is There Life Left in the Gate Control Theory?

CLIFFORD WOOLF: The antecedents of the spinal gate control theory lay in a debate about how the sensory system works, which emerged out of nineteenth-century German studies of sensation. The big debate was between the specificity theory and the pattern theory of sensation. In other words, do we experience touch, pain, or any other sensation as the result of the activation of a fixed, determined line that produces that sensation, or is there a pattern that itself is responsible for the generation of a sensation? The spinal gate control theory was the most articulate expression of the pattern theory. Unfortunately, it was wrong from a neurobiological point of view.

At the time the theory was put forward, no one had identified sensory nerve cells that responded to particular pain stimuli such as heat or noxious stimuli. Patrick Wall's contribution to the theory, to a large extent, was an attempt to describe how activity in different kinds of fibers could interact through a gating mechanism to produce the sensation. In fact it turned out—and this is one of the reasons why the theory fails—that there are very specialized sensory fibers that respond to very specific aspects of the environment. They filter out the environment right at the periphery in ways that are independent of the spinal gate.

The strength of the theory was that it indicated that there aren't labeled lines. The brain does not work like a telephone switching system. At that time in the sixties, the technological framework of information processing was based on hardwired systems, which now looks like an old-fashioned analog perspective. This was before the software revolution that shaped the way we now think of information processing.

What Wall and Melzack showed us, which was an enormous conceptual breakthrough, is that active processing occurs very early and involves information from multiple sources. I think this is fundamental and important. What was wrong were the specific predictions about which cells were responsible and how the process happened. The details are wrong, but the conceptual framework remains correct that there is processing, modulation, and interaction at all different levels.

SARAH COAKLEY: And cultural meanings can also be a part of that processing?

WOOLF: Absolutely. But the specific diagrams of the interactions they mapped don't exist. Those were wonderful mind experiments, but they weren't based on data.

LAURENCE KIRMAYER: As an undergraduate student of Melzack's, I should say that the way he taught the gate control theory was not about the specifics at all. That was a hypothesis he tendered that fell by the wayside. The key insight was the notion of central control of peripheral processes: that afferent control occurs at many different levels. That provided a natural conceptual framework to begin to integrate cognitive, psychological, and ultimately social and cultural processes. He continued to use that framework to make models of various kinds of different processors.

COAKLEY: That's interesting. Maybe the question now is whether the gate theory in that *wider* sense has still got life in it.

KIRMAYER: We could turn that into a more specific question: Is there control from central processes at the spinal level? In other words, are there afferents at the spinal level that can modulate incoming signals in a significant way, so that even though a pathway is very specifically coded as intense heat, for example, which could not be interpreted differently at higher levels, it could be dampened or modulated peripherally in some way?

WOOLF: Without doubt.

KIRMAYER: To me that's a very important fact.

HOWARD FIELDS: That is basically the research that Alan Basbaum did, to which I contributed (see Fields and Basbaum 1999). It was an elaboration of what was then the gate control hypothesis.

Reference

Fields, H. L., and A. Basbaum. 1999. "Central Nervous System Mechanisms of Pain Modulation." In P. D. Wall and R. Melzack, eds., *Textbook of Pain,* 4th ed. Edinburgh: Churchill-Livingstone, 309–329.

Discussion:

The Success of Reductionism in Pain Treatment

CLIFFORD WOOLF: As our token reductionist, what can I say to convince you of the value of breaking the system down to its smallest elements? Is this a meaningless exercise, or can it tell us something profound about the pain experience? Can this have any influence on our understanding of pain mechanisms and on our treatment of patients? I think the answer is, without a doubt, yes, although it does not in any way exclude the fact that we need to see pain in a broader context as well.

One measure of the success of this approach is conventional pain treatment. Pain treatment at the moment is almost entirely driven by empirical discoveries, and many of these actually had antecedents in folk medicine. The use of opiates as both sedative and analgesic has been known for as long as recorded history is available, so there are many millennia of experience in narcotics.

The other mainstay of treatment is the nonsteroidal anti-inflammatory drugs like aspirin. Again, if one looks into history, the bark of the white willow was used in folk medicine as an analgesic antipyretic, reducing fever and inflammation for many hundreds of years. That willow bark is filled with salicylate, which is the basic ingredient of aspirin, acetylsalicylic acid.

The third major treatment for pain is local anesthetics. One of Freud's great contributions was not his insights into our id or ego but his discovery that extracts of the coca leaf when applied to the cornea cause the absence of sensation by blocking neural activity. Cocaine was recognized as one of the first local anesthetics.

The discoveries that opium is analgesic, that local anesthetics block sensory input, and that extracts of the willow bark have an anti-inflammatory action all came without any understanding of pain or the mechanisms of action of any of these drugs. What has molecular biological analysis taught us? Do we understand now, at the beginning of this new millennium, how these treatments work? Yes, we do.

The opiates work by binding with a very specific receptor protein called the mu opiate receptor. Although there are endogenous compounds in the brain that interact with this receptor, the endorphins, their activity is rather subtle compared to the powerful and universal action of opium. Opium derivatives, such as morphine, remain the gold standard of treatment for pain management. One major reason for that is, in addition to reducing pain, they make many people feel euphoric. An interesting issue that we need to pursue is the biological nature of happiness as well as the unpleasant and dysphoric nature of pain—and the fact that we can switch both moods on pharmacologically.

How this opiate receptor developed over the course of evolution in vertebrates is an interesting question, as if it knew that there was an extract of the poppy seed out there waiting to interact with it. Charles Darwin didn't discuss that in his book. Maybe someone has some bright ideas?

Once it was recognized that drugs work by interacting with receptors and that almost certainly morphine would interact with a specific receptor, this became one of the big challenges of biological science in the seventies. Almost every big laboratory working in this area, both in Europe and in America, set out to search for the opiate receptor.

What about the nonsteroidal anti-inflammatory drugs—the aspirin-type drugs, including Tylenol, Naprosyn, and Advil, which constitute a multibillion-dollar market? Again, we now know exactly how they work, by inhibiting an enzyme called cyclo-oxygenase. In fact, the major breakthrough that has occurred in pain therapy in the last ten years has been the recognition that there are two forms of this enzyme and that one of them is responsible for the gastric disturbances and bleeding side effects of aspirin and the other one for its analgesic and anti-inflammatory actions. This led in the late 1990s to the introduction of Cox-2 selective inhibitors. These block the production of prostaglandin, an inflammatory mediator that sensitizes the periphery of primary sensory neurons so that they respond more readily during inflammation. Cox-2 inhibitors initially represented an enormous market. In terms of the number of prescriptions and the amount of money spent in a year, Celebrex, the first of the Cox-2 inhibitors, was the most successful introduction of any new drug ever in the history of the world, outselling even Viagra by an enormous amount. Unfortunately, as many millions of patients were exposed to this class of drugs, an increased risk of cardiovascular side effects was noticed, leading to the withdrawal of Vioxx. Drugs actively marketed as being side-effect free rarely are, and all medicines involve a cost-benefit analysis.

What about the local anesthetics? In the last ten years we've discovered how they work. They act to block a very complicated series of proteins called sodium ion channels. The problem with the currently available local anesthetics is that they block all sodium ion channels. They have therefore tremendous side effects because there are ion channels in the heart and throughout the nervous system and vascular systems.

One exciting area of molecular biology has been looking at different families of sodium ion channels. We have found a family of sodium channels that is present only on those fibers that encode noxious or pain stimuli. This offers the possibility of selectively blocking ion channels in pain fibers so that an epidural or local anesthetic could block the sensation of pain without causing a loss of motor function. Imagine a childbirth where you could still move and feel but would not have the pain experience. That is not inconceivable; on the contrary, it is very likely in the not-too-distant future.

A reductionist approach to the molecular mechanisms involved in the generation of pain will almost certainly lead to the development of new targets. Current pain therapy has been largely empirically driven, but we're now in a transition from that phase to one where the treatment will be targeted to very specific mechanisms. That will lead to a totally different way of approaching the patient. Instead of trying treatments on an empirical basis to see what the patient will respond to, we'll be able to identify what mechanisms are present and then treat the patient accordingly. So enormous effort is being made to study how pain is generated. The mechanisms turn out to be immensely complicated. Unfortunately, the same mechanism may manifest as different kinds of pain, and the same pain may be produced by different mechanisms. This is not an easy issue, and there are no shortcuts.

A hundred years ago, shortly after Sigmund Freud indicated that cocaine was a local anesthetic, you could buy cocaine as a treatment for toothache for fifteen cents. The German company Bayer also made two major discoveries a hundred years ago. One was the chemical synthesis of aspirin, of which they are very proud; the other was the synthesis of heroin. We need to be cautious about cures, because today's cure may turn out to be tomorrow's problem.

In short, there are deep ethical and societal issues entangled with the investigation of pain, and we shall have to come back to these later.[1]

Note

1. See especially Chapters 13 and 14.

Beyond "Coping"

Religious Practices of Transformation

Palliative or Intensification?

Pain and Christian Contemplation in the Spirituality of the Sixteenth-Century Carmelites

5

Sarah Coakley

In the important scientific contributions of Clifford J. Woolf and Howard L. Fields to this volume, we have already heard two strikingly different accounts of the relation of biological and neural events to "subjective" responses in the experience of pain. Woolf's account might be called a "bottom-up" one: it focuses on the molecular levels of the explanation of pain and attempts—at least initially—to bracket out questions of personal interpretation and evaluation. From this perspective, "physical" pain so understood could, at least in principle, be *obliterated* altogether if we could finally understand all its micromechanisms; and that goal, Woolf has hypothesized, may not now be so far off. Fields's approach is, in contrast, a "top-down" one; it attempts to explain—albeit still speculatively—what Fields has dubbed in conversation the "mysterious gap" between the actual physical trauma (and its particular neural accompaniments) and the full subjective "experience" of pain. It does this by highlighting the crucial part played by *interpretation* in the experience of pain and the distinctness of the neural pathways that convey this "hermeneutic" response. On this view, even if pain from a physical site of injury could be blocked altogether, the interpretative dimensions of pain might still be excruciating; from this perspective, "physical" and "psychic" pain can, for the sufferer, only notionally be rent asunder. It follows, seemingly, that the more the biographical and contextual dimensions of such interpretation of pain are explicated—the more one understands the *particular* repertoire of learned skills, practices, and narratives the pain sufferer has to apply her agony to—the more we may be able to account for the notable differences in "felt" responses to pain. And this, not unnaturally, is where reflection on religious responses to pain and suffering may have an especially important and revealing role to play in future medical investigations.

My task, then, is to attempt to complexify our understanding of that relation of psychic or spiritual pain to "physical" pain yet further by considering some features of the writings of two of the greatest exponents of the Christian "mystical" tradition,[1] the sixteenth-century Carmelites Teresa of Ávila (1515–1582) and John of the Cross (1542–1591). The interest of these authors for our purposes lies partly, first, with the detailed way in which they both chart the progress of Christian prayer from scriptural "meditation" via "contemplation" to achieved "union": their systematic accounts are more complex and nuanced than earlier exponents' narratives, and their insistence that union with Christ can be a sustained and irrevocable condition, novel. As such, their expositions of the ascent of the human soul to God have achieved a certain normative status in the history of Western "mystical theology," and their concomitant accounts of various forms of pain can be seen as placed in an interpretative narrative of progressive spiritual deepening.

Second, however, Teresa and John command our particular attention in the medical context because of their interesting historical location on the cusp of "modernity" in that last, saturatedly religious generation before modern science takes the intellectual stage with full hegemony. They write as early modern authors in the heated inquisitional atmosphere of the Spanish Counter Reformation but as ones who, as Michel de Certeau has been wont to hypothesize, represent the *subversive* "mystic" voice of those being pressed to the margins of society:[2] Teresa, because she was a dominant and strident woman in an ecclesiastical culture increasingly skeptical about female "mystical" graces and was of suspicious Jewish (conversos) ancestry to boot;[3] John, also probably of part-Jewish ancestry and from an impoverished and dispossessed background, because of his irritatingly fearless commitment to the monastic reform begun by Teresa, a reform that necessarily discomforted both the ecclesiastical establishment and his own religious order.[4]

But third, and perhaps most significantly for this book's purposes, these authors are worthy of our scrutiny because they give us such interesting clues about the relation of physical pain and suffering to spiritual pain and suffering and thus about that mysterious, aforementioned gap between physical manifestations and subjective response; herein lies the particular, practical rub for our interdisciplinary and medical interests in this volume. For the clues the Carmelite authors provide about this relation, as I hope to show, vastly *complicate* the currently held perceptions of the mind-body nexus held by those in the medical profession who have embarked in the last generation on exploring this spiritual dimension of pain and its transformations. (I am thinking here especially of the work of Herbert Benson and his highly acclaimed "relaxation response," involving the use of a simple form of mantric meditation that has had remarkable palliative effect on many pain sufferers.)[5] To put my central thesis boldly in anticipation: what our sixteenth-century authors show us—if we give them credence—is that a lifetime's commitment to prayer, and especially to the higher stages of "infused" contemplation, is more likely to *intensify* spiritual "pain" than to alleviate it (after a perhaps rosy first stage of meditative delight), but that this purgative pain may eventually give way—in most cases after long years of struggle—to the qualitatively higher state of transformed "union." Even such union, however, does not promise the cessation of pain and suffering altogether; rather, what has occurred is a form of appropriation of Christ's life and sufferings, such that the physical and psychic symptoms that might previously have signaled the disease of distance from God now, in changed affect, signal the union of the self with Christ's self so that the self is knit into the very life of the Trinity. Thus the transformation, by implication, does not have merely individual but communal significance: that one is thus transformed reorders the narrative of those about her and realigns the community toward a universal and Christological truth about the transformative capacity of suffering. Individual, community, and political transformation hang together.

It is also worth stressing here that Teresa and John were people not unfamiliar personally with states of intense physical pain and sickness; but it would seem unthinkable for them to reflect on such without it being imparted implicit spiritual meaning. In Teresa's case, especially, we know from her autobiographical first work, *The Book of Her Life,* that in her earlier years in religion she suffered fainting and dizziness spells, heart pains, and at one point an almost total paralysis and generalized pain for some long time;[6] other symptoms (that she herself describes as religious "raptures" or "touches" of union) may perhaps suggest an epileptic condition.[7] (I shall leave open for the moment here whether these symptoms can be reductively explained as neurotic or psychosomatic or whether an alternative diagnosis of true epilepsy would thereby evacuate her narrative of theological significance; my own view is that it would not.)[8] John, somewhat differently, underwent severe malnourishment from intense poverty in his early youth as an orphan (one of his two brothers died at the same time); and later he was imprisoned by some of his Carmelite confreres who opposed his and Teresa's reforms and kept him in a state of sensory deprivation and extreme physical discomfort in a dark lavatory for nine months before he managed to escape. It was during that time that he nonetheless composed much of his extraordinary mystical love poem, *The Spiritual Canticle.* Finally, John died at the relatively young age of forty-nine after a fever and the outbreak of excruciating spreading gangrenous sores, one reaching from his thigh to his instep.[9] In short, we are dealing here with two people who are fully cognizant of physical ailments and their challenges but whose narratives deliberately smudge the line between physical and spiritual pain. Indeed, as we shall shortly chart, their language for "pain" and "suffering" is extraordinarily rich, fluctuating, and varied; the metaphors they employ to express it range from those of punishment and assault through those of curative medical intervention, to that of sexual union. Unlike some of their earlier Christian predecessors in the narration of martyrdom,[10] however, their discussion of pain or suffering rarely sees pain as a *good in and of itself*[11] or as a self-imposed penance designed to be consciously instrumental in spiritual advance. Rather, it is viewed, usually retrospectively, either as a curative part of the divine purpose for the soul's good; or—contrariwise—as a sign of the soul's straying from the path set rightly before it but disobediently evaded; or—finally—as a serendipitous event that can nonetheless be woven purgatively into God's plan. In short, there is a subtle and multivalent attitude to pain in these authors, but not one (if I read them aright) in which it is a morbid or masochistic point of fascination.

So much by way of brief introduction. The countercultural import of those who can write about pain positively and purgatively, not least for the modern medical profession rightly bent on the alleviation if not on the "conquering" of pain, need hardly be stressed. What, one wonders, would Teresa or John think of the possibility of the *obliteration* of physical pain such as speculatively raised by Woolf? Let us just raise that enticing question now but return to it at the end of this chapter, for it bears careful consideration. But let me now turn to some of the salient and more detailed points about "pain"—in the ramified sense we have indicated—in the two writers individually.

I shall address John of the Cross first, even though he is the slightly later writer, for a particular reason. John writes in the established third-person style of earlier patristic and medieval mystical theologians; he does not impose his experiences on us autobiographically but rather charts a complete and objective vision of the progress of the soul (any soul) to God, a progress he represents diagrammatically as an ascent up the slopes of Mount Carmel.[12] He is able to write in this way, to be sure, on account of his status as an educated male; but one of the outcomes is relatively little attention to what Arthur Kleinman would term the *individual* "somatization" of his transformation.[13]

Teresa, in contrast, is in much more danger (as an unschooled woman) of inquisitional attack if she attempts a foray into mystical theology in the elite, educated sense of an account of engagement with God that goes beyond normal intellectual apprehension. Consequently, although she does lay out stages in such an engagement, she feigns ignorance (in what Alison Weber calls her artful "rhetoric of femininity") of the whole mystique of negative theology and especially of the scholastic divisions of the parts of the soul.[14] Instead, she provides in her *Life* what we may call the first "modern" account of mystical *states*—the first anticipation of James's psychologizing approach to what he would generalize as "mysticism"—by focusing on the particular bodily and psychological effects of her own experience as a charter of development in the life of prayer.[15] As a result of this novel trait, she has been derided by some modern spiritual directors and theologians as presenting an inferior, naive, or intrinsically "female" form of John of the Cross's superior and "objective" theory of ascent.[16] Such assessments remain willfully uncomprehending of the factors of ecclesiastical and gender politics under which she was operating, as well as fail to appreciate the *theological* importance of the fascinating details she vouchsafes us about the somatic accompaniments of her claimed transformation into the life of God.

But let us now look briefly, and comparatively, at the two authors' accounts of pain and its transformations. Although they have much in common theologically, they also present distinctive differences of emphasis and expression.

John of the Cross on the Nights of Sense and Spirit

John uses many words for "pain" and associated experiences. As well as "pain" itself, such synonyms (or "family resemblance" terms) as "suffering," "affliction," "torment," "desolation," "infirmity," "misery," "abandonment," "annihilation," "assault," "woundedness," and "melancholia" are common occurrences in his text.[17] But it would be a mistake to see his recurrent usage of such terms as indicating a fixation on pain; indeed, it is "desire" more than "pain" that constitutes the orienting category of his theory of prayer and transformation into God. As is explained in his diagrammatic account of the ascent of Mount Carmel, it is the purgation and *redirection* of desire toward God that animates his entire spiritual program; various sorts of pain and discomfort necessarily attend such a redirection but do not (as I read John) constitute an end in themselves.[18]

John's theory of ascent involves a journeying though two "dark nights": the "night of sense" and then the (much rarer) "night of spirit." The progress is charted in two complementary ways: in *The Dark Night of the Soul* (which describes what God is doing to the soul throughout), on the one hand, and in *The Ascent of Mount Carmel* (which describes what we are to do in response), on the other; and each account is built around John's entrancing poem *The Dark Night,* which forms the irreducible fundament of both commentaries. Both "nights" involve distinct forms of spiritual pain, though of different sorts. In the first, the "night of sense," the pray-er moves, after a period of satisfying enjoyment of scriptural meditation (a form of praying by thinking imaginatively about a biblical text), into a disorienting transition into "infused contemplation," characterized by intense "aridity" and a lack of sensual satisfaction. Prayer will now seem, says John, like "wasting time," so dry and imperceptible are the effects of God on the prayer (*Dark Night* I, 10.4: Kavanaugh and Rodriguez 1991, 382); but in fact what is happening is that God is taking away pleasure in the things of God precisely in order to purge the senses of an inappropriate attachment to anything other than God in Godself. At this time, John tells us, the greatest suffering arises from imagining that one has lost one's way: "Spiritual persons," he says, "suffer considerable affliction in this night, owing not so much to the aridities they undergo as to their fear of having gone astray. Since they do not find any support or satisfaction in good things, they believe there will be no more spiritual blessings for them and that God has abandoned them" (*Dark Night* I, 10.1: Kavanaugh and Rodriguez 1991, 381). Although the empty contentless prayer that John describes at this stage is not hugely different in practical terms, it might seem, from the techniques of Herbert Benson's "relaxation response," the effects could hardly be more different.[19] Far from bringing obvious palliative relief from physical or psychic discomfort, or providing a means of "coping" or warding off pain, this stage is marked for John by characteristic feelings of painful aridity and "emptiness . . . in the senses" (*Dark Night* I, 9.6: Kavanaugh and Rodriguez 1991, 379) even though John assures his readers that all that they need do is to "liberate themselves from the . . . fatigue of ideas" in a "loving and peaceful attentiveness to God" (*Dark Night* I, 10.4: Kavanaugh and Rodriguez 1991, 382). Everything seems to be going wrong; but in fact one is being led by a way of unknowing that cancels one's previous reliance on positive feeling states: the senses are, as John puts it, being brought into conformity with the spirit.

The much rarer second night (described in *The Dark Night*, Book II) is the deeper stage of purgation of the spirit itself. This involves a truly fearful level of spiritual pain as the self comes to confront the darkness in itself and its distance from the God it seeks. But this is (paradoxically) all the result of the brightness and light of contemplation impinging profoundly on the innermost self. As John puts it, "Since this divine infused contemplation has many extremely good properties, and the still unpurged soul that receives it has many extreme miseries, and because two contraries cannot coexist in one subject, the soul must necessarily undergo affliction and suffering. . . . When this pure light strikes in order to expel all impurity, a person feels so unclean and wretched that it seems God is against him and that he is against God."[20] In a memorable extended metaphor, John describes the process the soul is now going through as the burning of a log and its gradual expulsion of dross so that it can be fully transformed into the fire. Needless to say, this is hardly a comfortable process: the soul feels that "all blessings are past," that it is "full of evil," and that it is "alone, empty and weak" (*Dark Night* II, 10.8, 11.7: Kavanaugh and Rodriguez 1991, 418, 421). Fear and self-loathing are characteristic effects of this latter process of transformation; yet, again paradoxically, what is being heightened throughout is the deep and passionate love of God, which can only be completed and brought to fruition in the receptacle of human "weakness" (*Dark Night* II, 16.11: Kavanaugh and Rodriguez 1991, 434). As John puts it with a final medical metaphor: "the soul as it were is undergoing a cure to regain its health, which is God Himself" (*Dark Night* II, 16.10: Kavanaugh and Rodriguez 1991, 433). So the "wound" that it feels is actually the wound of love, destined, when finally cauterized, to be filled with God.

Thus is it that the intense "pain" of cautery can be identified, paradoxically, with the "delicate touch" of divine erotic consummation in "union." As John writes in his great poem on union, *The Living Flame of Love:* "O living flame of love that tenderly fills my soul in its deepest center! Since now you are not oppressive, now consummate! If it be your will: tear through the veil of this sweet encounter!" (*Living Flame*: *Stanzas the Soul Recites,* in Kavanaugh and Rodriguez 1991, 639). The second stanza of this poem is particularly revealing for our purposes; in it John describes the "sweet cautery" of "union" that is also the "delicate touch that tastes of eternal life." He goes on to explain that "there is a difference between this loving cautery and the one generated by material fire. The wound left by material fire is only curable by other medicines, whereas the wound effected by the cautery of love is incurable through medicine; for the very cautery that causes it, cures it, and by curing it, causes it. . . . The more wounded the lover, the healthier he is, and the cure love causes is to wound and inflict wound upon wound, to such an extent that the entire soul is dissolved into a wound of love."[21]

The coincidence of renewed "wounding" and renewed "loving" must thus be contrasted with the earlier "pain and detriment" of the soul's undergoing of moral and spiritual purgation—and yet again, with mere physical, "material" wounding. "Pain" at this level of "union" must thus be read as only *metaphorically* related to "normal" physical pain by a series of spiritual rarefications, and yet nonetheless the metaphor remains indispensable: it is the meaning-structure of union with Christ's life and suffering that supports the whole narrative.[22] It is thus in his commentaries on *The Spiritual Canticle* and *The Living Flame* that John asserts that the transformed soul has, in "union," been brought into a "deified" state such that it may "love through the Holy Spirit, even as the Father and the Son love one another."[23] That is, it has achieved an objective state of incorporation into the life of the Trinity itself. "Pain," although never completely removed in this bodily life, has been transformed—interpretatively overlaid—by "delight" in God.

Teresa of Ávila on Spiritual and Physical Pain

Now when we compare all this with Teresa's accounts of the process toward union, there are both intriguing similarities (unsurprising since there was considerable mutual influence between the two reformers) and notable differences. Like John, Teresa employs a rich vocabulary of "pain" in her writings, although the range of terms is not exactly coterminous with John's: "infirmities," "afflictions," "torments," "sufferings," and "distress" are frequently used words, but John's developed theory of the "nights" is absent and particularly his starker language of divine "assault" or "annihilation" in the second book of *The Dark Night*.[24] But the most important stylistic difference from John in *The Book of Her Life* (Teresa's earliest work written under the close—and nervous—supervision of her then-spiritual adviser)[25] is that already mentioned above: Teresa does not give us, like John, a measured third-person—and two-tiered—account of progress (thereby charting the difference between what the soul thinks is going wrong and John's assurance that all is actually going right); rather, she provides a chronological and autobiographical description of her own experiences of both pain and transformation, of both difficulty and progress.

The result is a much messier and more confusing story than John's, but one in which Teresa's physical as well as spiritual pains are closely attended to. Not that they are separated: we first hear of years of physical discomforts, trials, and mistakes that to Teresa, looking back, signal her spiritual dis-ease and separation from God.[26] Once she gets on track with prayer again, however, after some years of poor direction and lapsing,[27] the narrative is again full of physical effects. There is frustrating aridity now, to be sure, as she struggles to maintain scriptural meditation long after it dries up on her; but there are also direct touches of union, which at this point result in the suspension of her faculties into unconsciousness or immobility. Hence, in the account of her spiritual development in *The Life,* Teresa actually charts her progress according to how much effect on her mind and body is produced. In the famous "four waters" of chapters 11–18 of *The Book of Her Life,* for instance, in which she develops the metaphor of a garden being watered with increasing ease (and finally with a downpour of rain) in the growth in prayer, she likens biblical meditation (the "first water") to lugging buckets of water arduously round the garden (*Life* 11: Kavanaugh and Rodriguez 1987, 110–119), but states of physical rapture (the "fourth water") as the "union of all the faculties" and "no power [remaining] in the body" (*Life* 18.1: Kavanaugh and Rodriguez 1987, 157). She says, "[T]he soul . . . feels with the most marvelous and gentlest delight that everything is almost fading away through a kind of swoon in which breathing and all the bodily energies gradually fail . . . in such a way that one cannot even stir the hands without a lot of effort" (*Life* 18.10: Kavanaugh and Rodriguez 1987, 161).

At the time of writing *The Book of Her Life,* Teresa evidently thought that this "rapture" represented the final physical implication of "union"—and very inconvenient at that![28] But by the time she wrote *The Interior Castle* (and had come strongly under the influence of John of the Cross), she had completely changed her mind.[29] The adjustment is noteworthy for our interests. Changing her fundamental metaphor for struggle and ascent, Teresa now no longer speaks of the laborious task of tending an arid Spanish garden until the rain comes; instead, it is a matter of moving through the various rooms (or "mansions") of a castle in which the self is attempting to find the innermost place of encounter with Christ (and thus with the true "self"), notwithstanding the distracting presence of various reptilian forces that constantly threaten to throw it off course. Now the final stage of achieved (and maintained) union, described in the seventh "mansion" of *The Interior Castle,* is a state no longer involving physical immobility or incapacity, as in *The Book of Her Life,* but rather a consummated "marriage" between Christ and the soul-body that nonetheless enables it to go on with its ordinary duties.[30] A fundamental and irreversible change has occurred in the self, metaphysically and personally; but life goes on, and the busy round of duties, burdens, and irritations in community life—and beyond—continue unabated.

There are communalities here—but also contrasts—with John's distinctive account of ascent, pain and, union; and these are worthy of comment. As with John, first, so here in Teresa, pain and suffering are undeniably a purgative *precondition* of the final transformation: "When our Lord is pleased to have pity on this soul that He has already taken spiritually as His Spouse because of what it suffers and has suffered through its desires, He brings it . . . into His dwelling place which is this seventh."[31]

And again, as with John, such union involves a new understanding of the internal life of the Trinity—and not just an understanding but an internalization in the self of the active life of Trinity: "Each day this soul becomes more amazed, for these Persons never seem to leave it any more, but it clearly beholds . . . that they are within it," actually incorporated into "some place very deep within" (*Interior Castle* 7, 1.7: Kavanaugh and Rodriguez 1980, 430). However, a distinct contrast with John's account comes in the relatively matter-of-fact narrative of consummated union in the climax of *The Interior Castle.* This union is characterized now, in the seventh "mansion," not by any swooning ecstasy or delight, nor even by that ostensibly oxymoronic combination of intense pain and joy that we have seen is so distinctive in John's *The Living Flame,* but rather by a more matter-of-fact acknowledgment that an irreversible change has taken place in the soul's status of desire; for now the marriage with Christ has been "consummated." Even this, however, does not guarantee immunity from continuing discomforts, difficulties, institutional frictions, and even the risk of minor forms of sin.[32] The soul, says Teresa, has been so specially "favoured" in union *only* in order to strengthen it in its further imitation of Christ and his suffering; and so the final test of this change can only be the "fruits" of "good works," humdrum as they may be.[33] This rather stringent conclusion has led some to comment that Teresa's greater length of life, and longer experience of union, can perhaps therefore be seen to exhibit a stronger "incarnational" maturity even than John's.[34] Certainly in her descriptions of union in *The Interior Castle* she exhibits deep concern to keep her fellow sisters' feet on the ground, both literally and metaphorically, and to stress that even in these heights of spiritual attainment the surest test of authenticity is an almost *ordinary* perseverance in the business of "love."

These conclusions on Teresa, union, and pain may seem surprising, however, and even misplaced, to those strongly affected by Bernini's famous statue of Teresa in ecstasy—an image that now seems to dominate the popular modern understanding of mysticism and its ostensibly erotic states.[35] A word of further explanation on this matter is therefore called for, for it may indicate another subtle point of difference between Teresa and John on the matter of pain and transformation. The statue illustrates a particular passage in *The Book of Her Life,* chapter 29 (Kavanaugh and Rodriguez 1987, 246–253) that Teresa herself treats—even at this earlier stage of her writing career—with some diffidence. She recounts her vision of an angel's spear piercing into her innermost being alongside other "visions" that she is attempting to categorize as either authentic or potentially misleading. That is why it appears in this section of *The Book of Her Life,* which is particularly concerned with the pressing questions of discernment between different sorts of visionary event and of the distinct possibility of delusion.[36] But seemingly this particular vision of an angel is not intended by Teresa as an *apex* of union or indeed as even an especially significant moment in growth—it was simply one of the many side effects of Teresa's intense spiritual development at this turbulent time. However, the importance for our purposes of this passage is its stress—anticipatory of John's in *The Living Flame*—on the coincidence of pain and bliss as the angel plunges his spear into Teresa's heart several times: "The pain was so great," writes Teresa, "that it made me moan, and the sweetness this greatest pain caused me was so superabundant that there is no desire capable of taking it away; nor is the soul content with less than God. The pain is not bodily but spiritual, although the body doesn't fail to share in some of it, and even a great deal" (*Life* 29.13: Kavanaugh and Rodriguez 1987, 252).

Teresa then gives no further emphasis to the experience in later work, preferring, as we have seen, to insist on practical outworkings rather than experiential climaxes.[37] But what is fascinating is that John later alludes to the same event in *The Living Flame* 2.9–10 (though without specifying Teresa as its source) and adjudicates its place as something short of complete or lasting union—more like an "intellectual" vision that gives an intense moment of anticipation of his "cautery" of union (Kavanaugh and Rodriguez 1991, 660–661). We may well hypothesize that Teresa had sought John's advice on the matter, and perhaps been more chastened herself by his dampening approach to prideful dangers of visions in general than *he* was in his assessment of its relatively "high" significance as a momentary anticipation of union. Be that as it may, the effects of overconcentration on this passage in *The Life,* and on Bernini's visual interpretation of it, have inevitably tended toward a crude reductive "sexualization" of Teresa, suggesting even a sadomasochistic reading of the passage rather than its appropriate placing in the context of Teresa's own maturation of thought about pain and union.[38] Ironically, then, as we have tried to show, it is John's account of the coincidence of pain and union in divine "cautery" that fills out the hints given here in *The Life,* chapter 29; while the mature Teresa herself—precisely heeding John's teaching on the dangers of visions and ecstasies[39]—sees continuing, *ordinary* "sufferings" in the state of union as much less dramatic or noteworthy. One must perhaps surmise that Teresa's body has, by this time, become more accommodated to divine closeness: the "pain" of union is less now an ecstasy than a simple *given* of intimacy with Christ.

To sum up: in the course of this chapter we have already seen how difficult it is, in our current postmodern culture of "commodified desire," *either* to comprehend the ascetical complexity of a life devoted over the long haul to prayer and transformable "pain" *or* to relate that wisdom to a medical context in which, even in a proposed "mind-body" treatment, almost instantaneous results are expected. In the former case, the ascetic life can be salaciously reduced to a twisted form of sadomasochistic sexuality; in the latter, the demand for short-term, identifiable outcomes can distract altogether from the possibility of significant longer-term effects. Let us take these problems as a charter of the difficulty the contemporary exponent of mystical theology may have in credibly exegeting the final significance of "pain and its transformations" in these Carmelite writings, where—as we have seen—a purged and transformed eroticism in the tradition of the *Song of Songs* provides the finally indispensable metaphor for union with God. The interpretative problems for today's culture are formidable. But *nil desperandum*, nonetheless; and hence I close with three comments that I hope may generate further reflection and discussion among pain specialists in the light of this material.

Conclusions and Questions

I trust it will have become clear, even in the brief course of this chapter, that no *one* theory of "pain" can be attributed to Christianity *tout court*, and even between the two sixteenth-century Carmelite authors we have investigated we have found subtle but important differences of opinion on the relation of pain to spiritual transformation and union. Moreover, "pain" is itself a confusingly multivalent term and, once blended into the more encompassing category of "suffering," extremely hard to pinpoint precisely: in the case of the Carmelites we have seen how it can be applied to many things, from a recurrent physical malady or inconvenience to an extremity of spiritual agony or joy. But what is distinctive to their narratives is the presumption that no such "pain" is without spiritual *meaning;* pain is not only a necessary part of embodied life, but particularly it is part of the life of those bent on Christian sanctity. This is not to say that it should be actively sought: life supplies it in abundance without any active courting, and—as we have noted—both John and Teresa urge some caution against those who seek to apply it to themselves artificially or manipulatively.

Yet the *valorization* of pain as a means of spiritual transformation is an undeniable strand in Christian history, and is something that has been rightly questioned in modernity from many directions and with greatest point recently by twentieth-century feminist critiques of Christian traditional atonement theology.[40] In order to meet this critique, the most obvious theological ploy is to draw careful distinctions between physical pain that is personally or societally avoidable (especially abuse meted out on powerless people), and pain that is unavoidable and capable of producing transforming spiritual qualities. So far, so good. But that of course assumes that physical and spiritual pain can be neatly divided—and therein lies the rub, as the case of the Carmelites has surely shown. For them, and especially for Teresa (as we know from the nature of her "somatized" narrative in *The Book of Her Life*), physical and spiritual pain are inexorably welded together. As Howard L. Fields has well put it, the role of "meaning" in the explanation of pain is what is most crucial and satisfying, and the Carmelites certainly give us that: whatever is happening to them neurologically or physiologically, their "subjective experience"—to use Fields's phrase—is of a progressive transformation into God, even if only retrospectively understood. So our first closing question in this chapter for the medical fraternity is this: Are the Carmelite accounts "satisfying" explanations of pain, to use again Fields's language, or are they merely cloaks of delusion or neurosis? Can pain investigation and research accommodate itself *positively* to the variables of different religious meaning systems? Can it perhaps apply Teresa's spiritually pragmatic criterion of "fruits," or "good works," to an analysis of different pain strategies that might take religious narratives, rituals, and meanings into account? And can we, in the future, devise further medical investigations of the neural events that accompany the religious practices of *long-term* adherents and their distinctive approaches to pain?[41]

A second point follows on immediately from here and reengages with the important mind-body work of Herbert Benson. My question is whether the notion of "relaxation response," complemented by what Benson calls the "faith factor," will do sufficient justice to the ramified accounts of long-term "meditation" (or "contemplation," as it is termed in the Christian context) such as we have discussed in this chapter. Benson is of the opinion that the faith factor enhances the effects of the relaxation response (see Benson 1996, 155) but that different faith factors pretty much amount to the same thing. This I do question, given that—as I have shown—narratives of spiritual development such as the Carmelites' effectively "remake the world," placing pain in doctrinal, communal, and even—one might say—cosmic significance for the sufferer; and it is not at all obvious—as Luis O. Gómez demonstrates in Chapter 6—that different Buddhist remakings of the world do the same thing as Christian ones (or indeed even that intra-Christian variations on the theological significance of pain are strictly compatible with one another).

What I am again interested in here is whether the *long-term* nature of a suffering person's meditative or contemplative or sacramental practice can palpably affect the felt quality of her physical pain; for this is a qualitatively different matter from the use of simple meditative "techniques" to alleviate tension and anxiety, important and effective though these may be. Dying Christians often, for instance, ask to hold a crucifix. Are we to dismiss this as merely talismanic? Or are they, in the mode of the Carmelites, repositioning themselves imaginatively, symbolically, and transformatively into Christ's pain? If this is a real possibility of which contemporary medicine should be taking account, then we need to be asking how its effects could be measured scientifically.

Finally, we have been struck in this volume by Clifford Woolf's ready admission that a world without pain would not only be dangerous but morally evacuated. With that the Carmelites would of course most readily agree! As John of the Cross writes in one of his spiritual maxims, "The purest suffering produces the purest understanding."[42] But need the pains and sufferings of the Carmelites have been so extreme? And if we were ever in the position to obliterate most physical pain, would it be wise to do so? What would then be the spiritual and moral cost? For we are also left with a conundrum raised by Elaine Scarry in Chapter 4: if it is true, as Virginia Woolf tells us, that physical pain is the one thing in the modern world that is hard to thematize verbally,[43] then perhaps the secular impoverishment of our current medical meaning systems for pain would need attention before we could hope to answer that bigger moral question that Woolf speculatively raised for us.[44] To say this is not in any way to condone the continuation of curable pain or to invite medical neglect; rather, it is a plea to *enrich* medical reflection on pain and pain management with a deep consideration of the ethical and spiritual questions that narratives such as the Carmelites' lay before us.

Notes

1. In what follows I prefer to use the technical term "mystical theology" (as utilized by the Carmelites themselves) over the modern term "mysticism," with its primary emphasis on passing psychological phenomena and high-point "experiences" (James 1960 [1902]). For a succinct historical account of the difference in these two terms (and a somewhat barbed critique of the latter), see Louth 1983.
2. De Certeau (1986, 1992) has argued that the "mystic voice" in the particular period of the sixteenth and seventeenth centuries tends to come from the margins of society (in a time of great political and economic transformation) and to represent a particular kind of "turn to the subject" *in God,* an interim phase between the dramatic splits in Christendom at the Reformation and the onset of a truly secular "modernity" at the Enlightenment.
3. For illuminating accounts of these dimensions of the life of Teresa, see Weber 1990 (ch. 1) and Williams 1991 (ch. 1).
4. The classic biography of John, for such details as this of his life, is still Crisógono 1958; shorter treatments are to be found in Peers 1943 and Kavanaugh 1999.
5. Benson 1975 represents Benson's first and most famous account of this technique. Some attempts to relate the technique more closely to particular religious traditions are to be found in Benson 1984 and Benson 1996.
6. See Kavanaugh and Rodriguez 1987, 63, 66, 70–80.
7. Teresa's views about such "raptures" (discussed in connection with what she calls "union" in *The Book of Her Life:* see Kavanaugh and Rodriguez 1987, 157–184) change in subsequent writing, as we shall shortly discuss. If Teresa was an epileptic, there is little to suggest the condition bothering her in later life.
8. See Payne 1990, Part II, for a careful analytic defense against psychologically reductive understandings of John of the Cross's mystical theology. Teresa's case is more complicated since, from a modern medical perspective, her earlier life would certainly seem to involve at least neurotic and probably also neurophysiological problems.
9. For further details of these life events, see again: Peers 1943; Crisógono 1958; Kavanaugh 1999. The paradoxicality of John's writing of the delights of spiritual "betrothal" and "union" in the oppressive and physically distressing conditions of imprisonment is especially noteworthy; and the mode of John's last illness, and his bearing of it, is also particularly poignant for our theme of transformed "pain."
10. Compare Judith Perkins's account of the motivational dimensions of early Christian martyrdom (Perkins 1995); and see Arthur Kleinman's brief discussion of this point in Chapter 2 of this volume.

11. It is true that the use of the "discipline" is passingly discussed by John in his correspondence (see *Letter 14,* Kavanaugh and Rodriguez 1991, 749); but it is not part of his own formal program of spiritual advance, and his emphasis is always more closely on *spiritual* mortification in the form of "detachment." For further cautions from him on the inappropriate or forceful use of physical penance, see *Ascent* I, 8.4; *Dark Night* I, 6.1–2 (Kavanaugh and Rodriguez 1991, 136; 371). Teresa appears on the whole to have been even more skeptical than John of the positive value of such self-inflicted penances, fearing the intensification of what we would now call "neurotic" tendencies in her nuns.
12. The Carmelites historically associate themselves with Elijah's sojourn on Mt. Carmel (see 1 Kings 18.42 ff.). For John of the Cross's pictorial diagram of the spiritual "ascent" up Mt. Carmel, see Kavanaugh and Rodriguez 1991, 110–111; and see also 150–151, for his commentary.
13. For this theme of "somatization," see Arthur Kleinman's contributions to this volume and also Kleinman 1988. Despite John of the Cross's (relative) lack of expatiation on bodily effects, it is important not to fall prey to a crude gender stereotyping of him as a "male intellectual mystic" inherently despising of body (such as is suggested by Grace Jantzen's feminist account of the Christian "Dionysian" tradition: Jantzen 1995). Alain Cugno's more sensitive reading of John of the Cross (Cugno 1982), written from the perspective of contemporary continental philosophy, rightly stresses that bodiliness is consistently *implied* by John's pervasive discussion of "desire," even though not experientially spelled out in autobiographical terms.
14. See Weber 1990, esp. ch. 2, for an acute feminist analysis of Teresa's rhetoric of feigned "feminine" ignorance at the time of the writing of *The Book of Her Life;* yet note that Teresa was in fact not lacking in knowledge of what classical Christian mystical theology entailed: influence from the pseudo-Denys almost certainly came to her through her reading of the Spanish mystical writers Laredo and Osuna, as well as through interaction with her confessors. For Teresa's discussions of mystical theology at this stage in her career, see *The Book of Her Life,* chs. 10.1, 11.5, 12.5, 18.2, and cf. 18.14 (Kavanaugh and Rodriguez 1987, 105, 112, 121, 158, and cf. 163).
15. See Louth 1983 (negatively) and Williams 1991 (more positively) for this line of assessment of Teresa.
16. Abbot John Chapman's account (see Chapman 1917) is a particularly grievous, and now classic, example of this stigmatization of Teresa as an inferior "female mystic"; but he has clearly influenced others in the English-speaking world such as Dicken (1963), and even Louth (1983), who tend also to interpret Teresa as an inadequate "female" version of the "superior" John of the Cross. The capacity to read Teresa as sui generis, and in some respects

arguably more mature and "incarnational" on "union" than John, is a more recent development in Anglophone interpretation of the Carmelites: see Williams 1991, ch. 5.

17. In checking the use of these English terms in the Kavanaugh and Rodriguez (1991) translation of John of the Cross against the Spanish original (see Rodriguez 1980), one confronts a complex of Spanish terms not always exactly related to the use of "pain" or "suffering" in the English: these include a rich mixture of the verbs *padecer, penar, afliger, atormentar, aniquilar, ebestir,* and *herir;* and related nouns such as *dolor, pena, afliccíon, enfermedades, miseria, aniquilada, llegas,* and *melancolía.* It is important to stress that in some cases where the English translation inserts the word "suffering," John's Spanish text leaves the actual word unsaid, although he implies it: for example, at *Ascent*, Prologue; *Spiritual Canticle* 13.1; or *Living Flame* 4.12 (Kavanaugh and Rodriguez 1991, 115, 520, 712). I am grateful to Brenna Moore, Harvard doctoral student in theology, for assistance in tracing these correlations in the Spanish.
18. The *nada, nada* ("neither, nor") of John's diagram of the ascent of Mt. Carmel, warning of false "attachments" (see again note 12), is often misunderstood as *repressive* of all joy or pleasure; in fact, the proper purgation of "desire" may ultimately lead to the full joy of union. For a critical account of such repressive misreadings of John, see the second chapter of Coakley 2002.
19. A comparison between Herbert Benson on "meditation" as "relaxation response" (Benson 1975) and Thomas Keating on "contemplation" (Keating 1995 attempts to popularize and psychologize contemplative prayer of John of the Cross's sort for contemporary applications) is instructive here. Keating stresses that contemplative prayer, if undertaken daily over a significant period of weeks and months, is as likely to induce anxiety as to relieve it: such is its intrinsic "purgative" logic.
20. *Dark Night* II, 5.5: Kavanaugh and Rodriguez 1991, 402. John goes on in chapters 6–8 to detail other pains and afflictions that characterize the "second night."
21. *Living Flame* 2.7: Kavanaugh and Rodriguez 1991, 660. Also see *Living Flame* 4.12: Kavanaugh and Rodriguez 1991, 712–713, where John explains that the reason the soul does not "faint" in union is twofold: first, the lower part of the soul is by now "highly purged" and thus no longer feels the same "pains" of imperfection; and second, the touch of God is thus now experienced, truly, as "gentle." (Similarly, in *The Spiritual Canticle,* John will talk of the flame of God as "painless" in this state [*Spiritual Canticle* 39.14, in Kavanaugh and Rodriguez 1991, 627–628], although he admits here that in this life not *all* "pain" can be removed, given that the full "beatific transformation" has not yet occurred and that the "strength

and height of so much love" remains overwhelming to our "natural weakness.")

22. Toward the end of *The Spiritual Canticle* John finally makes explicit the intrinsic logical connection between the "hypostatic union of the human nature with the divine Word" in Christ and the "corresponding union of human beings with God": it is the former that makes possible the latter (*Spiritual Canticle* 37.3: Kavanaugh and Rodriguez 1991, 615).
23. *Living Flame* 3.79–82: Kavanaugh and Rodriguez 1991, 706–707; see also *Living Flame* 4.17: Kavanaugh and Rodriguez 1991, 715. The same theme of incorporation into the Trinity is memorably, and daringly, treated in *Spiritual Canticle* 39.3–14: Kavanaugh and Rodriguez 1991, 622–628.
24. The Spanish terms include *enfermidades, afflicíon, tormento, pena, dolores,* and *inquietas,* and the verbs *padecer, pasarse, sufrire,* and *afligire.* On occasion Teresa will herself distinguish between different sorts of "pains": those that are fleeting or passing and those that constitute a form of "death" en route to "union" (see, e.g., *Interior Castle* 5, 3.4–5: Kavanaugh and Rodriguez 1980, 349–350).
25. The chief spiritual adviser in the production of *The Book of Her Life* (1562–1565) was the Dominican García de Toledo. For a brief account of Teresa's early confessors, and of the process of her writing of the *Life,* see Kavanaugh and Rodriguez 1987, 33–37.
26. *Life,* chs. 4–7: Kavanaugh and Rodriguez 1987, 64–94.
27. Her return to prayer was at this point initiated by reflection on the suffering Christ: see *Life* 9.1: Kavanaugh and Rodriguez 1987, 100–101.
28. Teresa does at one point make a distinction between physical "rapture" and "union," rather strangely describing rapture as "of a higher degree" since it effects both interior and exterior features, while union takes place only in the "interior of the soul" (*Life* 20.1: Kavanaugh and Rodriguez 1987, 172). The physical raptures experienced by Teresa at this stage of her life caused her not only deathly pain but at times considerable embarrassment: she would ask her sisters to hold her down physically, for instance, lest she levitate during Mass and cause disturbance (*Life* 20.3, 20.5: Kavanaugh and Rodriguez 1987, 173, 174).
29. *The Interior Castle* was written in 1577 at a time when the *Life* was being adjudicated by the Inquisition. (Since the production of the *Life,* Teresa had also composed *The Way of Perfection* and *The Meditations on the Song of Songs.*) For the background to the writing of *The Interior Castle,* see Kavanaugh and Rodriguez 1980, 263–279. Although one can probably detect an influence from John of the Cross in Teresa's new account of the relatively passing significance of bodily rapture, Teresa's new account of achieved union also has significant differences from that of John, as we now chart.

30. See *Interior Castle* 7, 3.12 (Kavanaugh and Rodriguez 1980, 442), which reports that "raptures" are now almost never a problem, and so on; the whole of book 7 is given over to a discussion of union in this new sense, allowing continuation of normal duties and trials even as the state of spiritual "marriage" is maintained.
31. *Interior Castle* 7, 1.3 (Kavanaugh and Rodriguez 1980, 428). Note that "desire" is again the key category here. In the preceding last sections of book 6 of the *Interior Castle* (6, 11.2–4: Kavanaugh and Rodriguez 1980, 422–423), Teresa has just described the most intense pain of "affliction" that the soul suffers just before union in which it thinks it is actually dying.
32. See *Interior Castle* 7, 2.9–11, 4.1–3 (Kavanaugh and Rodriguez 1980, 436–438, 444–445), where Teresa mentions continuing "pain," "trials," "fatigue," "tumult," and even "disturbance" and temptation to "venial sins"; but she has already insisted (*Interior Castle* 7, 1.8: Kavanaugh and Rodriguez 1980, 430) that in union the soul is not idle but "much more occupied than ever before with everything pertaining to the service of God." Note that John of the Cross, in contrast, explicitly mentions the "fittingness" of "withdrawal" from "business" in states of "union": *Living Flame* 4.15 (Kavanaugh and Rodriguez 1991, 714).
33. See *Interior Castle* 7, 4.6 (Kavanaugh and Rodriguez 1980, 446). Also see *Interior Castle* 5, 3.11 (Kavanaugh and Rodriguez 1980, 352), where Teresa has already insisted that one of the best tests of good prayer is "compassion"—the capacity to feel the "pain" of another.
34. This assessment is hinted at by Williams 1991, ch. 5 (see again note 16).
35. William James's view of "mysticism" (James 1960 [1902]) has greatly contributed to this concentration on high-point "states"; and Jacques Lacan's sexualization of Teresa has become even more notorious ("you only have to go and look at Bernini's statue in Rome to understand immediately that she's coming, there's no doubt about it": see Mitchell and Rose 1985, 147). These presumptions tend to be taken on, unfortunately, by otherwise insightful commentators on "pain" (see, e.g., Morris 1991) who appeal to the example of Teresa and use Bernini's statue as their icon (Morris uses it on his front cover).
36. See the whole relevant section in *Life*, chs. 22–29 (Kavanaugh and Rodriguez 1987, 191–253), which is concerned with the problem of discerning the significance and source (whether divine or demonic) of unusual bodily effects in prayer—"locutions" as well as various sorts of "visions."
37. However, as we have already noted (note 31), in *The Interior Castle* 6, 11.2–4 (that is, in the "mansion" just before "union"), Teresa describes an experience of very great pain—a "deep wound," a "blow," which seems—in retrospect—to be a preparatory for "union" proper: see Kavanaugh and Rodriguez 1980, 422–423.

38. On this point, see Amy Hollywood's recent feminist account (Hollywood 2002) of the "sexualization" of "mysticism" in twentieth-century psychoanalytic thought in France and its implications for the reading of Teresa.
39. *Ascent* II, 10–12 (Kavanaugh and Rodriguez 1991, 178–189). I am grateful to Michael Buckley, S.J., for a fruitful discussion on this point about John's apparent assessment of Teresa's vision of the angel in *Life* 29.
40. See, among other relevant feminist literature, Grey 1989; Thistlethwaite 1989; Imbens and Jonker 1992.
41. Recent neurological studies of different kinds of meditation (using fMRI and other means of brain imaging) suggest that different kinds of meditational techniques (or, in Christian terms, "meditation" *or* "contemplation") can result in different sorts of ameliorative responses to pain. On the one hand, there are religious practices that are, roughly speaking, *dissociative,* reducing concentration, anxiety, and thereby pain, by throwing reflection away from "self" and conscious attention (i.e., by distracting the subject); these practices tend to show a reduction in activity in the frontal cortices (Lou et al. 1999) and an increased blood flow in the posterior artery (Litscher et al. 2001). On the other hand, there are meditational practices that *intensify* attention, thought, and concentration by activating frontal structures; and they—ironically—can also ameliorate pain (see Lazar et al. 2000), seemingly by an intentional moving into it, facing it, and—putatively—giving it new meaning. See the Introduction to this volume for suggestions on further research that might be attempted in this crucial area of recent discovery.
42. Kavanaugh and Rodriguez 1979, 678, "Spiritual Maxim" no. 48. (I have been unable to find this same saying in their 1991 revised edition, in which some of John's ephemeral material has been reordered and renamed.)
43. See Scarry's remarks in Chapter 4; but note that Virginia Woolf's views on the incommunicability of pain run into the philosophical conundrums discussed by Ludwig Wittgenstein under the rubric of "the private language" problem: see Wittgenstein 1968 [1953], paras. 269 ff., 289 ff., 302 ff., 665 ff.
44. Nicholas Wolterstorff's contribution to this volume, Chapter 14, attempts a philosophical reflection on the moral value of pain. As such, it supplies a first answer to Clifford Woolf's question on whether it would be *good* to obliterate pain altogether.

References

Alvarez, T. de la Cruz. 1971. *Obras completas: Santa Teresa.* Burgos: El Monte Carmelo.

Benson, H. 1975. *The Relaxation Response.* New York: Morrow.

———. 1984. *Beyond the Relaxation Response: How to Harness the Healing Power of Your Personal Beliefs.* New York: Times Books.

———. 1996. *Timeless Healing: The Power and Biology of Belief.* New York: Scribner.

Chapman, J., O.S.B. 1917. "Mysticism (Christian, Roman Catholic)." In J. Hastings, ed., *Encyclopaedia of Religion and Ethics,* vol. 9. Edinburgh: T. and T. Clark, 90–101.

Coakley, S. 2002. *Powers and Submissions: Spirituality, Philosophy and Gender.* Oxford: Blackwell.

Crisógono de Jesús, S., O.C.D. 1958. *The Life of St. John of the Cross.* London: Longman, Green and Co.

Cugno, A. 1982. *St. John of the Cross: The Life and Thought of a Christian Mystic.* London: Burns and Oates.

de Certeau, M. 1986. "Mystic Speech." In *Heterologies: Discourse on the Other.* Minneapolis: University of Minnesota Press, 80–100.

———. 1992. *The Mystic Fable,* vol. 1: *The Sixteenth and Seventeenth Centuries.* Chicago: University of Chicago Press.

Dicken, E. W. T. 1963. *The Crucible of Love: A Study of the Mysticism of St. Teresa of Jesus and St. John of the Cross.* London: Darton, Longman and Todd.

Grey, M. 1989. *Redeeming the Dream: Feminism, Redemption and Christian Tradition.* London: S. P. C. K.

Hollywood, A. 2002. *Sensible Ecstasy: Mysticism, Sexual Difference, and the Demands of History.* Chicago: University of Chicago Press.

Imbens, A., and I. Jonker. 1992. *Christianity and Incest.* Minneapolis: Fortress Press.

James, W. 1960 [1902]. "Mysticism." In *The Varieties of Religious Experience.* London: Fontana Library, 366–413.

Jantzen, G. 1995. *Power, Gender and Christian Mysticism.* Cambridge: Cambridge University Press.

Kavanaugh, K., O.C.D. 1999. *John of the Cross: Doctor of Light and Love.* New York: Crossroad.

Kavanaugh, K., O.C.D., and O. Rodriguez, O.C.D., eds. and trans. 1980. *The Collected Works of St. Teresa of Avila,* vol. 2: *The Way of Perfection, Meditations on the Song of Songs, The Interior Castle.* Washington, D.C.: I. C. S. Publications.

———. 1987 [1976]. *The Collected Works of St. Teresa of Avila,* vol. 1: *The Book of Her Life, Spiritual Testimonies, Soliloquies.* Washington, D.C.: I. C. S. Publications.

———. 1991 [1979]. *The Collected Works of Saint John of the Cross.* With Revisions and Introductions by K. Kavanaugh, O.C.D. Washington, D.C.: I. C. S. Publications.

Keating, T., O.C.S.O. 1995. *Intimacy with God.* New York: Crossroad.

Kleinman, A. 1988. *The Illness Narratives: Suffering, Healing and the Human Condition.* New York: Basic Books.

Lazar, S. W., G. Bush, R. L. Gollub, G. L. Fricchione, G. Khalsa, and H. Benson. 2000. "Functional Brain Mapping of the Relaxation Response and Meditation." *Neuroreport* 11: 1581–1585.

Litscher, G., G. Wenzel, G. Niederwieser, and G. Schwarz. 2001. "Effects of QiGong on Brain Function." *Neurol. Res.* 23: 501–505.

Lou, H. C., T. W. Kjaer, L. Friberg, G. Wildschiodtz, S. Holm, and M. Nowak. 1999. "A 150-H20 PET Study of Meditation and the Resting State of Normal Consciousness." *Hum. Brain Mapp.* 7: 98–105.

Louth, A. 1983. "Mysticism." In G. S. Wakefield, ed., *A Dictionary of Christian Spirituality.* London: S. C. M., 272–274.

Mitchell, J., and J. Rose. 1985. *Feminine Sexuality: Jacques Lacan and the école freudienne.* New York: W. W. Norton and Co.

Morris, D. 1991. *The Culture of Pain.* Berkeley: University of California Press.

Payne, S., O.C.D. 1990. *John of the Cross and the Cognitive Value of Mysticism.* Boston: Kluwer Academic Publishers.

Peers, E. A. 1943. *Spirit of Flame: A Study of St. John of the Cross.* London: S. C. M.

Perkins, J. 1995. *The Suffering Self: Pain and Narrative Representation in the Early Christian Era.* London: Routledge.

Rodriguez, J. V., ed. 1980. *San Juan de la Cruz: Obras completas.* Madrid: Editorial de Espiritualidad.

Thistlethwaite, S. B. 1989. *Sex, Race and God: Christian Feminism in Black and White.* New York: Crossroad.

Weber, A. 1990. *Teresa of Avila and the Rhetoric of Femininity.* Princeton: Princeton University Press.

Williams, R. 1991. *Teresa of Avila.* London: Geoffrey Chapman.

Wittgenstein, L. 1968 [1953]. *Philosophical Investigations.* Trans. G. E. M. Anscombe. New York: Macmillan.

Pain and the Suffering Consciousness

The Alleviation of Suffering in Buddhist Discourse

Luis O. Gómez

In a touching account of her struggles with chronic arthritis, Darlene Cohen relates a crucial moment in her battle against excruciating pain. Her son and husband had told her how distressing it was for them to hear her walk around the house, moaning, begging for relief. The family devised a strategy to make use of these moments of shared pain. As described by Cohen (2000, 36), the plan worked as follows: "A long moan from me, and then an answering lament from my husband . . . Another deep wail from me . . . A melodramatic drawn-out bawl from my son, wanting to be included. I gladly bellowed back to him, and so it continued down the hall, our entire household erupting in wails and shrieks. By the time I got to the bathroom, my heart was full."

One may understand this ritual as a device for injecting comic relief into an otherwise stark and tormented existence. But Cohen herself understands this family ritual as an example of the way in which pain can reveal its own absurdity and in the process uncover the presence of joy. It is a good example of how pain can be seen as something greater than a localized sensation of hurt. As a sensibility and a state of consciousness that overwhelms the whole person, pain gives the whole person power over the hurt: what one does with pain can affect pain itself. This is at the heart of the techniques that Cohen teaches in her role as massage and movement therapist.

But Cohen also sees her approach to pain as part of a spiritual quest. For her, relieving pain by becoming aware of it is part of her engagement with the Zen Buddhist tradition. What could appear to others as a technique or therapy for the relief of pain is for her an integral part of a religious life. These are not mere therapies of pain but instances of the transformation of pain by accepting it as part of a religious quest and practice.

The humor of the anecdote reported above and the informality of her style disguise the history of the tradition she has embraced as her model. In invoking the Buddhist traditions of mindfulness, she invokes Buddhist conceptions of suffering and the relief of suffering through mental culture.

Tradition has it that during a series of controversies among Buddhists around the beginning of the Common Era, some schools suggested that one could set out on the Path to liberation, or even follow the Path, simply moved by the hearing or uttering of an especially significant word. The most common example offered is that of a monk who enters the Path upon crying out aloud to himself: "Pain, oh pain!" Exactly what this legendary example may mean—and exactly what is meant here with the word "pain"—is problematic.[1] But this tradition brings to mind Cohen's strategy.

The association of Buddhism with concepts of human and animal suffering and with notions of liberation from suffering is undeniable. The literate tradition made the point repeatedly—its definition of what is foundational to Buddhist doctrine and practice more often than not hinged on explanations of suffering, its causes, and the means to overcome it.

It is perhaps equally obvious that suffering was a central concept in the religious and ethical rhetoric of Indian Buddhism, if not of Buddhism in all of Asia. Furthermore, this same religious discourse about pain and suffering is closely connected with general Indian conceptions of moral causation and religious practice as a path of liberation. Such conceptions occupy an important role in most classical modes of theological discourse in India (Potter 1963). In short, pain and its transformation are dominant themes in Indian Buddhism and in other Indian traditions as well.

Suffering and liberation from suffering recur as lead motifs in the canonical literature of Indian Buddhism, reminding the reader that in this essentially monastic genre the Buddha is conceived primarily as the one who reveals the pervasive presence of suffering and the right path out of suffering. Buddhas offer a teaching "that leads to the total calming of suffering" (*Aṅguttara Nikāya* II.52).[2] Those who hear the teaching of the buddhas "see *the impermanent as impermanent, suffering as suffering, no self as no self, the impure as impure.* Possessed of right view, they go beyond all sorrow."

The formula I have italicized in this quotation is that of the four fundamental errors or "distortions" *(viparyāsa).*[3] I shall return to it presently; but arguably the most widespread, if not most influential, conception of the Buddha as a teacher of suffering and its alleviation is the doctrine of the four "Noble Truths." A canonical formulation of these four truths declares that the teachings of the Buddha can be reduced to four statements or "Noble Truths": namely, "This is suffering, this is the origin of suffering, this is the extinction of suffering, this is the path leading to the extinction of suffering" (*Majjhima Nikāya* I: 426–432).

The canonical texts include their own standard definitions of each of the four Truths. An extensive definition of the first Truth, the Truth of Suffering, is found in the so-called First Sermon: "birth is painful, old age is painful, disease is painful, death is painful, encountering what we dislike is painful, losing what we love is painful, not gaining what we want is painful" (*Saṃyutta Nikāya* V: 420–423; cf. *Saṃyutta Nikāya* IV: 329–331; also cf. *Majjhima Nikāya* III: 230–237, *sutta* 139).

This definition, as well as the position of the Truth of Suffering as the first Truth and its location in the mythology of "the first sermon," creates the impression that "suffering" explains all of Buddhism and that Buddhism considers all of existence as suffering. It is common to attempt to epitomize Buddhist doctrine in light of the dogmatic formula of "Four Noble Truths," then proceed to define Buddhism in terms of the first of these truths construed as an unqualified claim that there is nothing but suffering. A recent presentation restates this view. The presentation, which has made its way from the *Encyclopædia Britannica*'s 1981 edition into the *Encyclopædia Britannica Online,* states categorically (emphasis mine): "It may be said that the Buddha based his *entire teaching* on *the fact* of human suffering. *Existence is painful.* The conditions that *make an individual* are precisely those that also give rise to suffering."[4]

These broad generalizations about Buddhism are in good measure based on isolated terms and on a contemporary reader's interpretation of abstract philosophical concepts. A more nuanced summary statement about canonical views on suffering and liberation from suffering can be extracted from a consideration of contexts. One must consider the spectrum of experiences included under the rubric "suffering" *(duḥkha)* and the ways in which a doctrine of the transformation of Buddhism depends on doctrines regarding the relation of pain and suffering to desire and self.

First, the term *duḥkha* includes physical pain as well as psychological anguish and malaise. The possibility of overcoming physical pain is usually considered in mythical and philosophical terms as dependent on (1) control of the awareness of pain and (2) liberation from the cycle of rebirth. Although the two are understood as characteristic accomplishments of the Buddhist saint, the two are not necessarily interdependent—one is possible without the other. In this context, it is difficult to separate Buddhist conceptions of *duḥkha* as physical pain from *duḥkha* as anguish, sorrow, and suffering.[5]

In addition to the broad extensional definition of *duḥkha* as states of bodily and mental pain, Indian Buddhist texts propose two other kinds of suffering (Schmithausen 1977), thus suggesting three levels of suffering. First, pain qua pain is the experience of hurting, the present state and the awareness of being in pain. This is the actual state of feeling hurt, or of lamentation or grief resulting from the loss of what one desires or the meeting with the undesirable. But pain also results from the expectation of such outcomes. This second form of suffering may be termed consequential suffering *(pariṇāma-duḥkhatā)*. Suffering is not only a present conscious state; it is also an expectation of frustration that can taint pleasure itself.

The Buddhist texts also claim there is a third type of suffering: suffering takes a third form in the subtle, preconscious condition of malaise or dissatisfaction. To the wise the very state of conditioned existence is unsatisfactory *(saṃskāra-duḥkhatā)*. It is this third type of suffering that is sometimes misconstrued as universal suffering. This "inherent pain" is not the awareness that there is no pleasure or release from pain but rather the knowledge that pleasure never meets the expectations of desire.

This scholastic view of what constitutes the full range of suffering is summarized in the words of the fourth-century South Indian scholar Buddhaghosa:

> There are many kinds of suffering *(duḥkha)*. There is, for instance, the suffering of experiencing pain, suffering arising from changes in what is not painful, and the suffering intrinsic to all experiences. . . . Among these it is the painful sensations of body and mind that are called the suffering of experiencing pain, because of their inherent painfulness, their nature and the way we speak of them. Pleasurable feelings and sensations are called suffering from change when they change, because they then become the basis for the arising of pain. Neutral feelings and sensations, as well as all other conditioned states in all three worldly realms are called intrinsic suffering because the natural rise and fall of existence causes distress [even as one abides] in such [neutral] states and sensations.[6]

This short analysis also applies of course to all the other human experiences listed in the previous extensional definition of suffering (old age, disease, death, etc.). Notice that the point is not that all existence is suffering but that both pleasure and suffering can be deceptive. Suffering can be the consequence of pleasure, or it can inhere in the desire that demands the pleasure. Suffering also reflects the inherent shortcomings of anything that is dependent and by necessity subject to the laws of rise and fall, coming to be and ceasing to be.

Although this may be read to mean that happiness is impossible, it can also be understood to mean that release from suffering can be achieved by transforming one's "attitudinal frame" (cognitive, affective, behavioral) with respect to pain and pleasure and what causes them. Predictably, this understanding of the Noble Truths is especially attractive to contemporary readers. It has, nevertheless, a long pedigree in Asia, in some forms of Mahāyāna in India, and in East Asian forms of Buddhism (see, e.g., Sheng-yeng 2000).

Kornfield (1996) describes the teachings of Thai meditation Master Achaan Naeb, who asks her disciples to sit still so that they may experience the natural arising of discomfort. Throughout the day, she observes, we keep changing our activities in order to avoid or outrun discomfort and pain. In Kornfield's words, she teaches that "each movement, each action, is not to bring happiness but to ease the inevitable suffering that comes from being born with a body" (131–132). Most Buddhists would add "and with a mind."[7] Whatever the explanation as to the origin or location of suffering, the point is that suffering is inevitable. The doctrine does not propose that all existence is suffering but that suffering is the inevitable outcome of existence.

However, the attribution to Buddhism of a vision of the world as "nothing but suffering" *(duḥkha)* also has sources within the tradition itself. It is in part reinforced by the ascetic rhetoric that permeates much of the canonical literature of Indian Buddhism. This rhetoric often defines the content, vocabulary, tone, and structure of the canonical writings. It is also central to many canonical formulations of the behaviors that are supposed to lead to the relief of suffering ("the path that leads out of or away from suffering"). An ascetic worldview is linked, for instance, to the notion that suffering is somehow intrinsic to desire, whereas pleasure is extrinsic—or, one may say, desire presupposes the incompleteness of pleasure and hence implies a state of discomfort. This doctrine is explained masterfully in the classical Indian treatise *Catuḥśataka* by Āryadeva and in its commentary by Candrakīrti.[8]

Moreover, whatever may be the preferred ontology of suffering, its etiology is linked to pleasure. The path is usually seen as a derivative of the second Noble Truth: that the cause of suffering is human craving. The path is then in good measure an antidote to craving, and hence it pursues an ideal of restraint and abstention. Although this path is considered a middle way between the extremes of self-mortification and self-indulgence, it entails what is by modern standards an ascetic practice. When conceived in terms of this derivation, a Buddhist ascetic rhetoric or doctrine of world renunciation is seen as an expansion of the presumed core of the Buddhist transformation of suffering: suffering is changed by the abandonment of an underlying attachment.

A formulaic definition of *duḥkha* found in the *Saṃyutta Nikāya* collection suggests this dichotomous view of suffering and its abandonment.[9] The passage raises the question: "One repeatedly hears . . . - 'suffering, suffering.' What is then this suffering?" To this question the Buddha is supposed to have answered in stereotypical fashion:

> The body is suffering. Feelings and sensations are suffering; conceptions are suffering, habits and propensities are suffering, consciousness is suffering.[10] The learned noble disciple who sees things this way draws away from the body, draws away from feelings and sensations; draws away from conceptions; draws away from habits and propensities; draws away from consciousness. When he draws away, he becomes dispassionate; because he is dispassionate he becomes free. When he is free he knows that he is free. He discerns clearly that rebirth has been exhausted, that the holy life has been lived fully, that he has completed the task he had to accomplish, that there is no beyond the here and now.

Expressions like "[w]hen he draws away, he becomes dispassionate," "rebirth has been exhausted," and "there is no beyond the here and now" lend themselves to the sort of interpretation that assumes only one possible reading of the doctrine of suffering and its transformation: suffering is everywhere and can be overcome or transcended only by leaving the world of suffering. These expressions are part of the ascetic rhetoric I have mentioned above. One may also speak of a rhetoric of abandonment or renunciation. But this renouncing is supposed to result in an ultimate state that is somehow beyond suffering.

Thus, the third Noble Truth, the truth of the extinction of suffering, also signifies freedom from rebirth, freedom from all possibility of future suffering. When so conceived, the extinction of suffering is the contrary of universal suffering—hence, relief from suffering can only occur outside of existence.

All of this suggests that the alternative to suffering is the total absence of suffering, that is, not a transformation but an abandonment. The texts, however, offer alternative views of the process and may even propose alternative interpretations of how suffering is abandoned and how this abandonment leads to liberation.

We must ask, then, how the transformation of suffering by detachment, or by other means, is possible according to the literature I am considering in this chapter. First, by way of introduction to this topic, I would like to consider a conception of "liberation" in which the good to be attained is a state of restored health *(kuśala)*. This is a conception of religion as medicine, as it were.[11] One such conception of healing medicine in Buddhism views healing as the application of allopathic means for the relief of pain. The medical metaphor is explicitly formulated in a sutra titled "The Monarch of All Great Physicians." The sutra states:

> A person who has complete mastery of four principles, is called The Monarch of Great Physicians. . . . First, he understands fully the disease. Second, he understands fully the causes of the disease. Third, he understands fully how the disease is to be treated. Fourth, he understands fully the right treatment; so that, once treated the disease will not arise again.[12]

The sutra then matches each of these abstract formulations with one of the Four Noble Truths. But it leaves us nevertheless wondering what the physician's understanding of these Truths might be. The sutra makes at least two points clear: the remedy is allopathic, and the remedy is total and permanent. Thus, the text states:

> What do we mean when we say that the good physician understands fully how the disease is to be treated? This means that the good physician understands fully that this type of disease is best treated with this herbal balsam, this emetic, or this purgative, this inhalant, this fumigation, or this sudorific.
>
> What do we mean when we say that the good physician, once he has understood fully the treatment, prevents this disease from arising ever again? This means that the good physician treats a disease of this or that kind so that it is cured and never occurs again.

Still, one must wonder, what is the nature of this remedy that is so comprehensive and radical? What is the cessation of suffering, which the Third Noble Truth defines as "the complete cessation of that very same thirst, leaving no remainder"? Perhaps a hint of one (among many) ways of looking at this is in the concluding phrase of the same Noble Truth: "giving up this thirst, discarding it, becoming free from it, no longer dwelling on it."

It is true that at least in the texts that expound the Noble Truths, the Fourth Noble Truth, the Truth of the Path Leading to the End of Suffering, is believed to take care of our question. But the definition of the Path, like so many other formulas in the canonical literature, only offers an outline; it gives us a glimpse, perhaps an insight, but not a complete answer.

> This Fourth Truth is the same as the Noble Eightfold Path, that is to say: the right view, the right intention, the right speech, the right action, the right means of livelihood, the right effort, the right mindfulness, the right concentration. . . . The middle way to which the Tathāgata awoke, [a path that] generates insight, generates knowledge, leads to realization, full understanding, full awakening, and nirvana.[13]

As most textbooks and surveys will note, this is a path of self-cultivation, in many ways a path of moral and contemplative cultivation but also a path of awareness or changed consciousness. But how is this cultivation related to this new consciousness, and how is it related to the notions of relinquishing, abandoning, detachment?

To understand these connections, or at least one alternative way of understanding them, one must review once more some of the ways in which different elements of canonical doctrine have been integrated into various systems of doctrine and practice.

For instance, it is common to assume that the main consequence of following the path is freedom from rebirth and hence an escape from the locus of suffering. This is in fact an important element of Buddhist traditional doctrines, but it is not the only way to understand the process. One may also imagine that the practice of the path is a method for silencing suffering, as it were. One is able to muffle pain and eventually transform its experience into a liberating experience.

Alternative interpretations exist, however, and occur not only in other historical and literary manifestations of Buddhism but within the canonical literature itself. For instance, it is clear that in most passages that address the issue, "no self" is a characteristic of both the state of suffering and the state of liberation; awareness of no self is therefore not a desensitization but a heightened awareness of a reality that, unseen, underlies suffering but properly grasped holds the key to liberation. Complete health is paradoxically a health that is not mine—and one that derives from an awareness that suffering is not mine, either.[14]

This may become more clear if we take a short sidetrack back to some additional passages that undermine the notion that the canon speaks of universal suffering. For instance, our textbooks and surveys still speak of a doctrine of the "three marks of existence." According to a common assumption expressed in modern writings on Buddhism, one of the fundamental "teachings of the Buddha" was the "three marks of existence"—namely, that "all things are impermanent, suffering, and without a self."[15] These sweeping statements about all of reality are not attested anywhere in Buddhist canonical literature.[16] The idea that impermanence, sorrow, and no self are the marks of all entities or of all of human existence appears to be due to a confusion in early Western writings on Buddhism between two distinct doctrines. On the one hand, the Abhidharma of the Sarvāstivādins proposed that the process of becoming had three phases or distinguishing marks *(lakṣaṇa),* hence "three marks of existence": namely, arising, duration, decay. On the other hand, the canonical literature often presented as key concepts of Buddhism three "seals" that guarantee a doctrine as Buddhist: namely, the notions of impermanence, suffering, and no self. The two doctrines are distinct but may have been conflated in the mind of some students of Buddhism.

The oldest formulation may be a stock formulaic fragment incorporated in a variety of contexts, including the "second sermon" of the Buddha, his sermon on "the mark of no self" (Pāli: *anattalakkhaṇa-sutta*). However, in these passages, as well as elsewhere in the canonical literature, the doctrine in question is not that "all things" are characterized by three marks. No expression similar or equivalent to the common English "three marks of existence" is ever used in the canonical literature to refer to the "marks" or characteristics of impermanence, suffering, and no self. Rather, the Buddhist texts speak of several (sometimes three, sometimes four) "indicators" or "seals" of the Buddhist teaching.

In the Pāli texts these seals are impermanence, suffering, and no self. But the tradition of the Sarvāstivādin school identifies impermanence, no self, and the peace of nirvana as the three seals of the Buddha's Dharma. Here nirvana appears to be the contradictory or the counterpart of *duḥkha.* Implicit in the Truth of Suffering is the truth of liberation. A famous scholastic formulation summarizes the Sarvāstivādin version of the three seals:[17]

> The Dharma is [a law] present in everything, without impediment or exception. If one possesses the seal of the Buddha's Dharma, one penetrates [the reality of] all things. . . . There are three seals or marks of the Dharma of the Buddha. First, all conditioned dharmas arise and cease in every instant, so that they are all impermanent. Second, all dharmas are without a self. Third, perfect peace is nirvana.
>
> This triple world is all [made of] conditioned things [that must] arise and cease. . . . This is the mark of impermanence of all constructed things.
>
> [Now, as to] all things lacking a self, [this means that one cannot find] within any thing a master, an agent, a knower, a perceiver, a kernel of a living being *(jīva)*, or an [Now, as to perfect] calm, it is nirvana; because in nirvana one extinguishes the fire of the three poisons and the three afflictions.[18] Therefore nirvana is the seal of calm.
>
> Why is the [designation] "seal of calm" only applicable to nirvana, and not to any other thing? With the first seal, one is speaking of the five aggregates *(skandhas)*.[19] With the second one is speaking of all things *(dharmas)*, all of which are regarded as no self. With the third seal one is speaking only of the fruit of the first two, that is to say, nirvana, which is called the seal of calm.

This second seal, the seal of no self, has had as much to do with our perception of Buddhism as a religion of nothingness as the seal of suffering has had to do with our perception of Buddhism as a religion of suffering. However, the connection between no self and liberation from suffering calls into question any simplistic notion of a choice between affirmation and nihilism.

> The yogi knows that all things are without a self. . . . When he recognizes this, the yogi no longer engages in the diffuse mental chatter *(prapañca)* [of common men]; then he has nowhere else to

go for a point of reliance, so he only takes as his refuge the calming [of all suffering]. This is why one speaks of a third mark that says that nirvana is peace.

With this we return to the notion of a state beyond suffering. If we ask what sort of peace is here called nirvana, we will meet many different answers. Even the idea of being beyond sufferings admits of more than one interpretation. I have suggested that there may be more than one way to read the expression "that there is no beyond the here and now" in the passage quoted earlier.

Still another way of conceiving the state of freedom from suffering is expressed by means of yet another standard canonical formula. Four short Pāli texts describe the classical four stages of contemplation by telling of an encounter between the young Ānanda and the elder Sāriputta.[20] Sāriputta has been meditating in solitude, and as he returns from his meditation, Ānanda, noting his changed appearance, remarks: "Your faculties appear serene, your complexion appears purified, cleansed. In which abode has the reverend Sāriputta dwelt today?"[21] To this, Sāriputta replies,

> I here dwell having attained the first state of contemplation, which follows detachment from desire, detachment from negative actions and states of mind, which is discursive and analytical, and encompasses the joy and happiness that arises from detachment.[22] This thought does not occur to me, venerable: "I am entering the first stage of contemplation, I have entered the first stage, I have arisen from the first stage."

And then, speaking in the third person (whether for Sāriputta or the narrator one cannot tell), the *sutta* adds:

> This is because long ago the venerable Sāriputta uprooted the conscious thought and the propensity to think of "me" and "mine." Therefore, this thought does not occur to the venerable Sāriputta: "I am entering the first stage of contemplation, I have entered the first stage, I have arisen from the first stage."

This passage is followed by a series of variants with the same narrative frame, each one responding in a parallel fashion to Sāriputta's experience of each of the other three stages of contemplation. The stages are characterized, predictably, according to the consecrated formulas that we find repeated throughout the canonical and scholastic literature.

The second, third, and fourth stages of contemplation are treated in a similar manner in the *sutta*s immediately following the above. The only difference is the brief and stereotypical definition of each stage. Thus, the second contemplation is "the inner calming that follows the calming of discourse and reflection, the onepointedness of mind, free from discursive thought and mental consideration, born of concentration, joyful and pleasing."[23]

This is, of course, a transformation of both desire and pain, but even the resulting joy must be transformed. This is shown in the definition of the third contemplation: "by becoming detached from this joy, I dwell evenminded, mindful, attentive, experiencing bodily pleasure, in that stage that the noble ones characterize as 'dwelling in evenminded, mindful bliss.'"[24]

Finally, in the fourth contemplation, evenmindedness *(upekkhā)* dominates:[25]

> When I abandoned pleasure and pain, and when all former states of elation and dejection had set like the evening sun, I dwelt in the fourth stage of contemplation, which is free from both pleasure and pain, and in which evenmindedness and mindfulness are pure.

This process of gradual removal of pleasure and pain is of some interest, but in the present context I want to highlight the common theme of these four short *sutta*s. In all four Sāriputta explains his changed demeanor and appearance in a similar manner, denying his awareness of being in such a state as a causal agent or as an experiencing subject separate from the experience itself. It is not clear that his response describes the experience of these four stages or aspects of meditation. His words seems to be more a commentary on his attitude toward such experiences or a description of a state of consciousness.

His statement is reminiscent of a number of passages in which the elimination or transformation of suffering is understood as a transformation of consciousness. This is a family of passages that seem to focus on meditation. One could see these practices as examples of the technical facilitation of religious experiences (Hood 1995). Nevertheless, the ideal of experiencing without preconceptions, or even without concept and judgment, is an idea that is broader than the practice of meditation in its most technical meanings and broader than notions of "religious experience." For instance, in another passage on liberation from suffering by the transformation of experience, the canonical writings attribute to the Buddha a doctrine that is, strictly speaking, not one of abandonment or cessation but one of transformed awareness (*Udāna,* 8, *i.*10). The ascetic Bāhiya asks for instruction, "so that it may benefit me and give me happiness for a long time to come." The Buddha replies:

> You should train yourself as follows: When you see, you should only see. When you hear, you should only hear. When you think, you should only think. When you are aware, you should only be aware. In this way you should train yourself, because then, if you only see when you see, only hear when you hear, only think when you think, only remain aware when you are aware, then there will be for you no "there." And when there is for you no "there," there is for you neither a here nor a beyond, nor a middle place in between. This alone is the end of suffering.

In this passage we find the outlines of a theory of relief from suffering that implies a therapy of memory and self-awareness. I would argue that this is a variant of the shift in consciousness expressed by Sāriputta's insistence that he does not think of himself as in meditation. This is thus one alternative to the simple statement that universal suffering is abandoned by some sort of metaphysical escape. It is not necessarily an alternative that excludes the others, but it does confirm the obvious that there are many ways of interpreting the Noble Truths.

It is also a view of suffering different from the notion that suffering itself may be a source of insight, inspiration, or deliverance. This conception is not absent from the canonical literature, the scholastic literature, or contemporary Western readings of Buddhism (Young-Eisendrath 1996, 1998). It is nevertheless a different conception of what one is to do about suffering, if not "with suffering."

Pain is thus intertwined with suffering, and suffering with one's sense of self and the sense of time implicit in the assumption that things are permanent, despite their obvious nonselfhood and impermanence. One may be tempted to dismiss some of the Buddhist reflections on pain as overlooking the apparently fundamental difference between pain and suffering, but one may also propose that the averred confusion is in fact a statement regarding the role of suffering in the processing of pain.

It is not at all self-evident that within the normal range of human experience one can be totally free of pain and suffering, as the Buddhists claim is the case with the enlightened. But I see no reason to quarrel with the fundamental intuitions I have outlined so far: that pain is inseparable from our ideas about suffering and the self that possesses that suffering. Research in the conditioning of pain by mood and expectation suggests that pain is, at least in certain circumstances, virtual pain (Fields 2000). Biofeedback also suggests that pain is modulated by awareness and by our sense of its location (Benson and Klipper 1975; Shapiro 1982).

It is by now common wisdom that a person's understanding of what pain is, how it comes about, and its end and consequence affect that person's experience of pain. And this appears to be true of physical pain as well as of psychic pain (Fields and Besson 1988; Frank and Frank 1991). It is also perhaps trite to say that religious traditions, understood broadly, often play an important role in the manipulation and hence the experience of pain and that this is done mostly through the tradition's definitions of pain and its meanings.

The one variant I have highlighted in this chapter can be read as a technology of self that proposes the transformation of memory, attention, and awareness as a means to transform or transcend suffering (Martin, Gurman, and Hutton 1988). Technologies of this sort cannot be separated from the practice of meditation, a context in which, as suggested by Padmal de Silva (1984, 1985, 1990), such religious practices and ideologies have much in common with contemporary secular cognitive behavioral therapies. Other Buddhist techniques have clear affinities to relaxation therapies, biofeedback, and guided imaging and bring to mind the concept of the relaxation response (Benson and Klipper 1975; Shapiro 1982). But one would do well to consider also what is *different* in these therapeutic manipulations of cognition and affect.

Of course, a psychological reading of Buddhist doctrine and practice is not the only possible reading.[26] The tradition offers more than one alternative, and explanations that are not psychological, at least not in the contemporary sense in which this word is used today, are often as common as psychological ones.

This brief incursion into Indian Buddhist canonical texts suggests that already in India and at the stage of canon formation there was more than one Buddhist notion of how suffering is overcome—or, if you will, of how pain is transformed. This is, of course, not surprising; but it is one of those obvious facts that continue to be ignored in writings about Buddhism.

An excursion further into the literature of other Buddhist cultures and other Buddhist denominational developments would show that Buddhist voices on pain and suffering continued to multiply as Buddhism adapted and struggled in other settings. A wide spectrum of practices and doctrines would appear before us, further showing the degree to which statements that Buddhism is about universal suffering are not very useful. This spread would also reveal commonalties between Buddhism and other types of religious healing not mentioned in this chapter—and, needless to say, would show as well that much of Buddhism is not about pain and suffering but about other dimensions of religiosity.

This is not to say that there are no common themes within Buddhism, but the continued heterogeneity of Buddhist views is something that should be borne in mind when speaking about its traditions. This is desirable not only for scientific purposes of historical accuracy but also as a check on the frequent quasi-religious use of discourse about religion, a practice that often hides surreptitious claims of theological authority.

Notes

1. The dispute is summarized in the *Kathāvatthu* II.5–6 and XI.4; also compare IX.1. The word translated here as "pain," and variously translated as pain, sorrow, suffering, or ill, is *dukkha* in Pāli, the original language of this text, and *duḥkha* in Sanskrit.
2. All references to the Pāli scriptural *(sutta)* texts are to the volume and page in the editions of the Pali Text Society of London.
3. Early translators rendered the technical term for these four, *viparyāsa* (Pāli *vipallāsa*), with the English expression "perverted view." This was an

unfortunate choice of words, given the connotations of "perverted" and "perversion" in contemporary English. A *viparyāsa* is not a perverted view but an "inverted" view. In other words, it is not a corruption or an intentional distortion of knowledge but an inversion of reality, a view that is contrary to fact, mistaken, or erroneous and conceives of something as its opposite (e.g., imagines suffering as pleasure).

4. From the article "Buddhism" in the *Encyclopæadia Britannica Online* at www.eb.com/. This article appears to use materials by various authors: Hajime Nakamura, Frank E. Reynolds, and Giuseppe Tucci. Also see the articles on *dukkha* and "Four Noble Truths" in the same encyclopedia. The latter restates several common confusions of normative tradition with historical fact, for instance, that the Four Noble Truths are "the essence of Buddhist religious doctrine, expounded by Gautama Buddha in his first sermon" and that the first Truth states "that existence is suffering." The claim that "these four truths are universally recognized by Buddhist schools" can also be misleading.
5. Whatever one may think about the rationality of mixing the moral, the psychological, and the physical dimensions of pain, the blurring of these distinctions is common in many religious traditions, and Buddhism is no exception. Some of this blurring of conceptual boundaries may reflect the experience of pain itself. See Hirschfield 2000.
6. *Visuddhimagga of Buddhaghosācariya* XVI.34–35, 424 ff. See also *Majjhima Nikāya* I: 30; *Saṃyutta Nikāya* IV: 59; Schmithausen 1969.
7. Here Kornfield may have unwittingly followed his Western presuppositions, but it might just as well be the Achaan Naeb has an unusual view of things. The most common Buddhist view is that suffering is both mental and bodily but mostly caused by desire and error and hence derived from mental states and contents. The issue is not moot; see, for instance, stanzas 33–34 in Āryadeva's text (Lang 1986, 35).
8. Chapter II of Āryadeva's text, stanzas 26–50 (Lang 1986, 33–39).
9. Dukkhaṃ suttaṃ, *Saṃyutta Nikāya* III: 196.
10. The particular phenomena that are declared to be suffering in these two sentences are the five *skandhas:* (1) body, (2) feelings and sensations, (3) conceptions, (4) habits and propensities, and (5) consciousness. These five are supposed to describe the set of all the phenomena we associate to or presume to underlie the notion of "self."
11. Halbfass (1991) questions the association of this concept to *actual* medical theory and practice in ancient India. Be that as it may, at least some Buddhists believed there was such a connection. Of course, the notion of the Buddhist religious path as "therapy" is naturally attractive to contemporary Western culture and to contemporary Buddhists. See Rieff 1966; Fisher and Francis 1999; Simpkinson 2000.

12. The sutra is found only in Chinese translations of the Indian Buddhist *āgamas*. It is part of the *Samyuktāgama* or *Za-ahan jing*, preserved in the Japanese edition of the Taisho Era (*Taishō Daizōkyō* ii, #99 (389), 105a24–b20, and also appears as an independent text in iv, #219. References to the *Taishō Daizōkyō* are by volume, work number, page, section, and line.
13. Summary explanation by Wayman in Bleeker and Widengren 1969, vol. II, 438–439. Buddhaghosa's classical explanation is found in *Visuddhimagga* XVI.75–83, 95–101, 433–432, 436–438.
14. On this concept, see Schmithausen 1969, Norman 1981, Gómez 1999, and the bibliography in these three articles.
15. The standard reading of this doctrine among English-speaking interpreters is illustrated by Nyanaponika 1973a, 1973b, 1974.
16. Note also how the *Encyclopædia Britannica* defines *dukkha,* the Pāli form of Sanskrit *duḥkha* (again, emphasis is mine): "('sorrow,' 'suffering,' 'imperfection,' or 'spiritual anguish'), in Buddhist thought, the *true nature* of *all* existence. *The whole* of Buddhist doctrine is based on *the fact of suffering*. . . . Recognition of the fact of suffering as one of three *basic characteristics of existence*—along with impermanence *(anicca)* and the absence of a self *(anatta)*—constitutes the 'right knowledge' that is the first step along the course of spiritual development known as the Eightfold Path that leads ultimately to enlightenment (nirvana) [*sic*]." From the article "dukkha," *Encyclopæadia Britannica Online* at www.eb.com/.
17. This work is preserved only in a single Chinese translation: *Dazhidu lun* (*Taishō Daizōkyō xxv*, #1509). The quotation is from p. 222a28–c6.
18. Craving, hatred, and stupidity.
19. See note 10.
20. Sāriputtavaggo, *Saṃyutta Nikāya* III: 235–237. The name Sāriputta is, of course, the Pāli form of Sanskrit Íāriputra. The four stages of contemplation *(dhyāna)* are simply known as the first, second, third, and fourth *dhyānas*. They are similarly defined, with minor variants, in the scholastic literature of all schools.
21. This phrase is the stereotypical form for addressing a person who has achieved insight or who has just arisen from a state of deep concentration or contemplation.
22. This is the standard, canonical and scholastic, definition of the first contemplation *(dhyāna)*.
23. Avitakka suttaṃ, *Saṃyutta Nikāya* III: 235–236.
24. Pīti suttaṃ, *Saṃyutta Nikāya* III: 236–237.
25. Upekkhā suttaṃ, *Saṃyutta Nikāya* III: 237.
26. For a contemporary Buddhist reading that takes into account other canonical texts and adopts a psychological-cognitive interpretation, see Ñāṇananda 1971, 1974.

References

Aṅguttara Nikāya. 1885–1910. 6 vols. Ed. R. Morris and E. Hardy. London: H. Frowde for the Pali Text Society. (2nd ed., 1961–1981. London: Luzac and Co., for the Pali Text Society, 1955–1961.)

Benson, H., and M. Z. Klipper. 1975. *The Relaxation Response.* New York: Avon Books.

Bleeker, C. J., and G. Widengren, eds. 1969–1971. *Historia religionum: Handbook for the History of Religions.* 2 vols. Leiden: E. J. Brill.

Cohen, D. 2000. *Finding a Joyful Life in the Heart of Pain.* Boston: Shambhala Publications.

de Silva, P. 1984. "Buddhism and Behaviour Modification." *Behaviour Research and Therapy* 22(6): 661–678.

———. 1985. "Early Buddhist and Modern Behavioral Strategies for the Control of Unwanted Intrusive Cognitions." *Psychological Record* 35(4): 437–443.

———. 1990. "Buddhist Psychology: A Review of Theory and Practice." *Current Psychology: Research and Reviews* 9(3): 236–254.

Fields, H. L. 2000. "Pain Modulation: Expectation, Opioid Analgesia and Virtual Pain." *Progress in Brain Research* 122: 245–253.

Fields, H. L., and J. M. Besson, eds. 1988. *Pain Modulation.* Progress in Brain Research, vol. 77. New York: Elsevier.

Fisher, M., and Brother Francis, O.S.B. 1999. "Soul Pain and the Therapeutic Use of Ritual." *Psychodynamic Counseling* 5(1): 53–72.

Frank, J. D., and J. B. Frank. 1991. *Persuasion and Healing: A Comparative Study of Psychotherapy.* 3rd ed. Baltimore: Johns Hopkins University Press.

Gómez, L. O. 1999. "The Elusive Buddhist Self: Preliminary Reflections on Its Denial." *Communication and Cognition* 32(1–2): 21–51.

Halbfass, W. 1991. *Tradition and Reflection: Explorations in Indian Thought.* Albany: State University of New York Press.

Hirschfield, R. 2000. "In the Land of the First Noble Truth." *Tricycle* (Summer): 56–58.

Hood, R. W., Jr. 1995. "The Facilitation of Religious Experience." In R. W. Hood, Jr., ed., *Handbook of Religious Experience.* Birmingham: Religious Education Press, 568–597.

Kathāvatthu. 1894–1897. Ed. A. Taylor. London: Pali Text Society. (Repr. 1979.)

Kornfield, J. 1996. *Living Dharma: Teachings of Twelve Buddhist Masters.* 1st Shambhala ed. Boston: Shambhala. (This is essentially the same work that appeared in 1977 under the title *Living Buddhist Masters.* Santa Cruz, CA: Unity Press.)

Lang, K., ed. and trans. 1986. "Āryadeva's Catuḥśataka: On the Bodhisattva's Cultivation of Merit and Knowledge." *Indiske Studier* 7. Copenhagen: Akademisk Forlag.

Majjhima Nikāya. 1888–1925. 4 vols. Ed. V. Trenckner and R. Chalmers. London: H. Frowde for the Pali Text Society.

Martin, L. H., H. Gurman, and P. H. Hutton, eds. 1988. *Technologies of the Self: A Seminar with Michel Foucault*. Amherst: University of Massachusetts Press.

Ñāṇananda, Bhikku. 1971. *Concept and Reality in Early Buddhist Thought*. Kandy, Sri Lanka: Buddhist Publication Society.

———. 1974. *The Magic of the Mind in Buddhist Perspective: An Exposition of the Kālakārāma Sutta*. Kandy, Sri Lanka: Buddhist Publication Society.

Norman, K. R. 1981. "A Note on Attā in the *Alagaddūpama-sutta*." *Studies in Indian Philosophy. Memorial Volume for Pandit Sukhlalji Sanghvi* (Lalbhai Dalpatbhai D. series, 84. Ahmedabad: Lalbhai Dalpatbhai Institute of Indology), 19–29. (Repr. in Norman 1990–1994, vol. II [1991], 200–209.)

———. 1990–1994. *Collected Papers*. 5 vols. Oxford: Pali Text Society, distributed by Lavis Marketing.

Nyanaponika, T. 1959. *Anatta and Nibbana: Egolessness and Deliverance*. The Wheel Publications, 11. Kandy: Buddhist Publication Society.

———, ed. 1973a. *The Three Basic Facts of Existence. I, Impermanence (Anicca). Collected Essays*. The Wheel Publications. Kandy: Buddhist Publication Society, 186–187.

———, ed. 1973b. *The Three Basic Facts of Existence. II, Suffering (Dukkha). Collected Essays*. The Wheel Publications. Kandy: Buddhist Publication Society.

———, ed. 1974. *The Three Basic Facts of Existence. III, Egolessness (Anattā). Collected Essays*. The Wheel Publications. Kandy: Buddhist Publication Society.

Potter, K. H. 1963. *Presuppositions of India's Philosophies*. Englewood Cliffs, N.J.: Prentice-Hall.

Rieff, P. 1966. *The Triumph of the Therapeutic: Uses of Faith after Freud*. Chicago: University of Chicago Press.

Saṃyutta Nikāya. 1884–1904. 6 vols. Ed. L. Feer. London: H. Frowde for the Pali Text Society.

Schmithausen, L. 1969. "Ich und Erlösung im Buddhismus." *Zeitschrift für Missionswissenschaft und Religionswissenschaft* 53: 157–170.

———. 1977. "Zur buddhistischen Lehre von der dreifachen Leidhaftigkeit." *Zeitschrift der Deutschen Morgenländischen Gesellschaft. Supplement III.2*, Vorträge des XIX. Deutschen Orientalistentages in Freiburg, Wiesbaden, 918–931.

Shapiro, D. H. 1982. "A Clinical and Physiological Comparison of Meditation with Other Self-Control Strategies—Biofeedback, Hypnosis, Progressive

Relaxation. A Review of the Literature." *American Journal of Psychiatry* 139(3): 267–274.

Sheng-yeng, (Venerable/Master). 2000. "The Four Noble Truths." *Ch'an Magazine* 18(2): 16–25. (Running footer reads, erroneously, "Winter 2000"—this is the Spring number.)

Simpkinson, A. A. 2000. "Riding Two Horses." *Tricycle* (Summer): 59–61, 112–117.

Taishō Daizōkyō. 1925–1935. 100 vols. By J. Takakusu, J. Watanabe et al. Tokyo: Taishō Issaikyō Kankōkai.

Udāna. 1885. Ed. Paul Steinthal. London: H. Frowde for the Pali Text Society. (Repr. 1948. London: G. Cumberlege, Oxford University Press.)

Visuddhimagga of Buddhaghosācariya. 1950. Ed. H. C. Warren and D. Kosambi. Harvard Oriental Series, vol. 41. Cambridge, Mass.: Harvard University Press.

Young-Eisendrath, P. 1996. *The Gifts of Suffering: Finding Insight, Compassion, and Renewal*. Reading, Mass.: Addison-Wesley. (Repr. 2000 as *The Resilient Spirit: Transforming Suffering into Meaning and Purpose*. Reading, Mass.: Perseus.)

———. 1998. "What Suffering Teaches." In A. Molino, ed., *The Couch and the Tree: Dialogues in Psychoanalysis and Buddhism*. New York: North Point Press, 344–353.

Response:
The Incommensurable Richness of "Experience"

Arthur Kleinman

It has been said that we are now in an age of the tyranny of health and healing in which the healthy body, not the sick soul or the sick self, is the salvific project and in which the tie between affect and value has changed, not only in content but perhaps even in form. In its very concreteness, the argument that Sarah Coakley has made about contextual specificity in the Christian tradition of sixteenth-century saints' devotional practices challenges an interesting idea of our time. She identified that idea with Herbert Benson, though it could be associated with many other people.

As I hear it, she makes the argument that, for Teresa, prayer intensified rather than relieved or dampened pain, at least in a central part of the experience. That intensification gave rise to a transformation whose contextual specificity is crucial to understanding what it meant both for the individual and for the collective.

I see this pointing to a tension between the humanities and social sciences on the one side and biology on the other. The social sciences and the humanities demand a contextuality of detail that makes it difficult for biologists concerned with mechanism and its universal implications to accommodate to easily. And I want to argue for the importance of there *being* no easy accommodations. It's not just a representation of the self or the body or experience that is distinctive in the social sciences and the humanities but the lived experience of the self, of the body, of "experience." We are not the same selves our great-grandfathers and great-grandmothers were, and our great-grandchildren-to-be will not be the same selves that we are. The very process of affect is changing—the way affect is made meaningful and tied to values in the world. It's not just the content of that meaning but the processes that link the meaning together.

William James argued in the *The Varieties of Religious Experience*, and in other works, for a "moreness" in experience, which he saw as definitive of the human condition (see James 1985 [1902]). The "moreness" couldn't be explicated by reductionism. It was the complexity and density of connections, the "something more," that defined what it was to be human.

It seems to me that this is the great tension in our period. We are obviously living in the great age of molecular biology; we already heard a brilliant presentation about that by Clifford Woolf. This kind of biology is very different from the biology dominated by physiology, which was an important part of intellectual life of the first half of the twentieth century, even up until the time that some of us trained in medicine. That physiological approach, which dealt with levels of integration, could accommodate context much more easily than the search for molecular mechanism can.

From Woolf we heard very explicitly that molecular biologists are defining pathways, receptors, and molecules that will separate the "pain" from the "suffering." It's important to recognize that, from the perspective of social science, that would transmute the subject into something radically different from "experience." When we obtain knowledge like that, what kind of knowledge will we have? We'll have a knowledge of mechanism that's extraordinarily powerful and may lead to a new generation of drugs that will change the nature of the human condition vis-à-vis pain. At the same time we are going to continue to have human experiences that simply don't accommodate themselves to that sort of separation into suffering and pain as two distinctive things.

Coakley also alluded to the fact that in the sixteenth century a larger space in social life in the West was occupied by religious experience than is occupied today. Certainly on the level of public discourse, we live in a time in which legal procedure, policy, science, and technology form the dominant public discourse of our time. Moral and religious discourse are important, but they occupy a different and distinctive space, and usually (especially in the United States) a separation is made between the strategic talk of the legal, technical, and scientific worlds and the value-oriented talk of the moral and religious worlds. It's not very clear to us what kind of bridging terms or "strategies," to use Anne Harrington's words, will pull these things together.

Part of the issue is that the presentations we heard today can be easily bypassed by biological research, which will not trouble itself with the difficulty I just presented: that in lived "experience," pain and suffering may be impossible to disarticulate. We will have a kind of knowledge production that increasingly lacks commensurability. That absence of commensurability will lead to different domains and different uses of this knowledge. There won't be a single domain of knowledge production in which we bring these things together. We might say, stepping back, that there is seemingly no means of crossing from the biological knowledge we heard of from Woolf to the knowledge of today's presentations. Those people who've so far tried to do so have made changes that are problematic on both sides.

I'll use Herbert Benson as an example. He has worked so hard to develop therapeutic techniques that cross these domains. As we've just heard, both in the Christian tradition and in the Buddhist tradition context is critical to understanding what those traditions are saying. Neither tradition is easily reducible to the idea of "relaxation" (see Benson and Klipper 1975); both are about something else. At the same time Herb has to meet completely different objections from the biomedical side—and in this he's been a fine example of a long-distance runner. He can't talk to us about things that sound too specific or too particular, because we want universal mechanisms and we want them specified on the molecular plane, not just the physiological.

So my first point, and the important one, is this incommensurability. The second point, which is embedded in the first, is the difficulty of moving from representation to experience. What do we mean by experience? Obviously it would be nonsense to think of experience taken neat, separate from meaning, but on the other hand we know that the lived engagement of everyday life is a different thing from representations in myth, in texts, and in statues. What does the shift to a concern with experience have to do with the two kinds of knowledge that we see? Is focusing on experience a way of crossing domains? That's what

I heard Luis Gómez attempt to do in his presentation. He suggested that a stereotypical view of the Buddhist tradition in representational terms changes if one begins to look at the techniques of experiential transformation. It becomes more complicated and less easily polarized.

Let me just give one example of a way of pulling things together. The example is not from a domain I know much about, so if there are any cognitive neuroscientists in the room, please correct me. It seems to me that Michael Posner's division (Posner et al. 1988) of the system of awareness into two components, a frontally based cortical component related to vigilance and a posterior component that has to do with targeting, is an intriguing way to think about what we heard from Sarah Coakley and Luis Gómez concerning the experience of intensification of suffering to produce union and the Buddhist techniques of transforming suffering through transformations of the self and awareness. Posner's idea suggests a research project: In states of calmness and peace, is there a relaxation of vigilance or a change in the content of vigilance? Has targeting disappeared, or has targeting changed? I think this is an example where cognitive neuroscience and physiology allow for a language that can cross domains. There is potential for questions from both sides to be examined together, without giving up the richness of context for the simplicity of mechanism.

References

Benson, H., and M. Z. Klipper. 1975. *The Relaxation Response*. New York: Avon Books.

James, W. 1985 [1902]. *The Varieties of Religious Experience*. Cambridge, Mass.: Harvard University Press.

Posner, M. I., S. E. Petersen, P. T. Fox, and M. E. Raichle. 1988. "Localization of Cognitive Operations in the Human Brain." *Science* 240: 1627–1631.

Response:
The Theology of Pain and Suffering in the Jewish Tradition

Jon D. Levenson

I have learned a great deal from the essays on Christian contemplation and Buddhist meditation; and I was interested particularly in a theme that Professors Sarah Coakley and Luis Gómez both touched upon: pain as a means of spiritual transformation, as Sarah put it, or as Luis put it, pain as the path of transformation. That there is more than one Buddhist approach on this is no surprise to me, for this is also very much the case with the Jewish materials. In Israel, there is an old quip that if you put two Jews in a room, you get three political parties. The same phenomenon can be observed, mutatis mutandis, in Jewish theology as well.

Still, one can speak about a common dimension of a number of Jewish approaches to pain in which pain is seen as transformative, and it is this dimension that I shall highlight. Along the way, I also hope to say something about the instrumental use of religious practice—the attempt to separate religious practices from the larger theological conceptions and matrices in which they are embedded. As you will see, the Jewish materials (again, I suspect, like the Christian and the Buddhist materials, for all the obvious differences) cast doubt on attempts to convert the practices into therapeutic techniques in and of themselves that make no encompassing claim upon those who use them.

One of the most obvious ways to make sense of pain in a theistic universe, one in which a God governs history and exercises providential sovereignty, is to interpret pain as punitive. This has, to be sure, generated much of the negative view of traditional religion in the modern world, some of it doubtless justified. But we must not forget, as many modern critics tend to do, that within the perspective of the Hebrew Bible and Rabbinic Judaism punishment is usually a preface. When pain is punitive, its purpose is to bring about a positive result, an inner transformation. It is, so to speak, a wake-up call that results (ideally) in a reconciliation between God and the ones punished, whether the people Israel or the nations. The structure of a number of the larger prophetic anthologies in the Hebrew Bible gives abundant evidence of this. These books often begin with oracles of judgment against the people Israel, but oracles of judgment against the nations then ensue, followed, in turn, by oracles of restoration—at least the restoration of Israel and often the restoration of the whole world, now reconciled with its creator and judge.

The assumption here seems to be that the punishment is necessary to get communities into, or back into, the right relationship with God. Here, punishment is a carrot and not just a stick. Underlying this is a rather pessimistic—or, as I would prefer to say, highly realistic—view of human nature. In our natural state—our instinctive, nonreflective state—we are in desperate need of guidance, feedback, a wake-up call. Simply behaving in accordance to our own unformed, untutored lights, we are not likely to act in a way that brings pleasure to God or credit to the image of God in which we have been created.

Rabbinic literature talks about two urges in the human heart, a *yetzer ha-ra'*, an evil inclination, and a *yetzer ha-tov,* a good inclination. In modern times, Jewish apologists have sometimes cited this idea to show how wonderfully optimistic Judaism is, as opposed to Christianity, with its doctrine of Original Sin, which views human beings as inherently depraved and unable to do the right thing apart from God's special intervention. There is a grain of truth in this rather self-serving contrast, to be sure, but we must not miss the crucial fact that Rabbinic Judaism, like its biblical predecessors, is anything but optimistic about the human possibility of doing good. An early work of midrash (rabbinic interpretation of the Bible), for example, likens the *yetzer ha-tov,* the good inclination, inside the human body, to a prisoner, presumably awaiting the next beating from his jailer (*Avot de-Rabbi Nathan* A 16). This is not a terribly optimistic view of what it is like for us humans to combine an embodied existence with an aspiration toward the good. The guiding concept here is that human goodness is indeed possible, but fragile, and not the sole or most potent tropism of our nature. To emerge and be sustained, it requires much struggle, a great deal of adversity, some of it highly painful, not to mention a large dose of divine grace. To cite another rabbinic metaphor (e.g., *Numbers Rabbah* 15:16), the righteous must fight against their *yetzer ha-ra'* in this world if they expect to have peace and tranquility in the world to come. If so, then punishment is not quite so sadistic or mindless as it seems to people with a more optimistic view of human nature. Accepted in wisdom and faith and under the guidance of the Torah, it can lead to a higher spiritual awareness and a deep inner transformation for the individual and the nation alike.

Alongside the familiar notion of pain as punishment, rabbinic theology also displays a belief in redemptive pain. This is closer to the sort of theology that Professor Coakley has elucidated in connection with John of the Cross and Teresa of Ávila, a theology in which pain can yield a greater closeness to God. Here, of course, the great question of theodicy looms large: how shall we explain the fact that righteous persons experience adversity, or that evildoers experience prosperity—a matter, needless to say, of profound concern in traditional Jewish literature? One answer (of many that are given) relies upon a sacrificial theology that is very difficult for moderns to grasp, myself certainly included: the pain, suffering, or death of the righteous effects atonement. Lest one suspect that this positive evaluation of pain and suffering is really a license for sadism, divine or other, I must point out that the ethic with which it is associated demands that we do all we can to alleviate the undeserved pain of others and to avoid the hubris of pronouncing it to be in accordance with God's will. Nor should any Jew regard himself or herself as one of the righteous few whose suffering effects atonement and allows the world to endure. When we experience that temptation, much Jewish ethical literature advises us to consider that our pain may instead be a signal to repent and amend our ways.

We must also mention the important rabbinic idea (again with biblical precedents) that God himself is involved with pain, for example, the pain of the Jewish people in exile. That sort of theology connects closely with some of the themes Professor Coakley was talking about, such as the internalization of Christ's wounds and passion in certain forms of

Spanish Christian mysticism. It is, of course, ostensibly very much at odds with Aristotelian notions of divine impassability, which become important in medieval philosophy, including Jewish philosophy.

Some rabbinic literature speaks about the possibility of happiness even in pain. The classic examples are martyrs, people, that is, who have died a voluntary death because of a refusal to renounce their deepest Jewish convictions and to abandon their observance of Torah. The martyrs are able to experience torture and a grisly death with an equanimity that characterizes a very high spiritual level. *Shabbat,* the Talmud tractate dealing mostly with the laws of the Sabbath, records this early rabbinic statement: "Those who are insulted and do not insult back, those who hear their own abuse but do not reply in kind, those who perform (religious acts/religious duties) out of love and rejoice in chastisements/suffering/adversity are like the sun when it goes forth in its strength—of them Scripture says, 'Those who love Him are like the sun rising in its might' " (*b.Shabbat* 88a, quoting Judges 5:31). In other words, if we can resist the temptation to respond in kind to experiences of adversity and weakness (including those that seem to come from God himself), we can transform our ostensible weakness into great strength and a demonstration of our love for God. Of course, this is connected to an ethic that urges people not to insult, abuse, or inflict suffering to begin with. But given the ubiquitous evidence for the frailty of human goodness, we should not be surprised when we experience so much insult and abuse, not to mention the absence of worldly rewards for faithful religious observance. The statement in *Shabbat* quoted above alerts us that lurking in all this pain is a precious opportunity to reach a higher spiritual level.

Closely associated with the experience of suffering in the Jewish tradition lies that great question of theodicy that I mentioned a moment ago, a pressing question for Jews long before the Holocaust, I might add. Why do the innocent suffer in a world in which a good and omniscient God is the sole and absolute ruler? I hope no one here will be disappointed if I abstain from the Miltonic task of justifying the ways of God to man. But one of the things that is often missed is that the Jewish tradition by and large maintains that the world is not yet at that stage in which God's will is absolute and unchallenged. Reality has not yet gotten to the point when the universe is simply governed by a good, omniscient, omnipotent, and unchallenged deity. In my book *Creation and the Persistence of Evil* (Levenson 1988), I have tried to show that, in the Hebrew Bible, the omnipotence of God is a dynamic and enacted omnipotence that is oriented to the future. The victory of God that is described in creation is not something that happened only in the past; it is also a proleptic glimpse of ultimate reality, yet to happen in the eschatological fulfillment, the end of time. This understanding of omnipotence—altogether different from Aristotelian notions of divine immutability—remained very much alive in Rabbinic Judaism as well and is highly prominent in the Jewish liturgy to this day.

This diachronic dimension is often the first casualty when such theological affirmations, based in mythic language and nourished in liturgy, are demythologized and then reencoded as philosophical propositions about an unchanging deity with an invariable attitude toward his world. It is essential to recognize that whatever the answer may be to the pressing question of God's justice, this biblical and rabbinic literature acknowledges that the world is not currently governed by a deity who has actualized all his potentialities and thus blasted evil and the suffering it produces from his world. And yet that deity has solemnly pledged that such a world will come into existence and has given human beings a key role in bringing that future about.

Finally, I must also not neglect the idea in rabbinic literature that being happy in this world is not necessarily a good sign. If one is happy with the world as it is, he or she may have lost sight of that promise of an eschatological transformation and mistakenly taken the current order of things for the Kingdom of Heaven—and his own flawed nature for the best he or she can ever be. One has, in short, taken an untransformed reality and an untransformed self as ultimate, giving up on the all-important messianic hope and the all-important task of self-transformation with which it is often associated.

In an illuminating midrash, God poses this question to the wicked who expect to be happy: "The righteous were not happy in My world, yet *you* seek to be happy in My world?" The text then lists Adam, Abraham, Isaac, and Israel (Jacob) and gives textual evidence for the unhappiness of each. But this is not the end of the story, for quoting Psalm 149:2, it assures the readers that "Israel will rejoice in its Maker"—that is, in the things that God makes/does (the same word in

Hebrew) in the eschatological future. Indeed, the midrash goes on to say, God himself, as it were, has not rejoiced in his world but will do so. Here the proof text is Psalm 104:31, which the midrashist understands to mean, "The LORD *will* rejoice in His deeds"—in the deeds of the righteous in the world-to-come" (*Leviticus Rabbah* 20:2). The world without pain and suffering—what one might think the world ought to be like now, given its governance by a totally just, good, and omnipotent deity—has not yet come into existence. Those who expect to live as if it has indeed come into existence are making a fundamental mistake. In that sense, relaxation and contentment in the world may be signs not of spiritual discipline but of its opposite, moral and spiritual failure. There is a superficial happiness that comes from giving up the struggle against evil, especially the evil within human nature, and abandoning faith in the God who transforms the world. This is not the happiness of which the rabbis speak, which is a deeper felicity rooted in a vibrant and obedient faith in the God of Israel, a felicity that arises, to some degree, through and not despite pain.

In discussing the rabbinic view of pain, we must not miss the important interaction between the two worlds, the painful and uncertain world in which we live and the (potentially) blissful world to come. Moderns often think of the latter as pie in the sky, a crude consolation prize, rather like the candy bars that were dropped on a village during the Vietnam War after it was learned that the wrong site had been bombed. In fact, the interaction of the two worlds in the Hebrew Bible and rabbinic literature is much more complex than that. The *Mishnah*, the earliest surviving law code of Rabbinic Judaism, includes this statement in the name of a sage of the second century CE: "Better one hour of repentance and good deeds in this world"—one hour of returning to God in a radical self-transformation—"than the entire life of the world-to-come; and better one hour of spiritual bliss in the world-to-come than the entire life of this world" (*Avot* 4:17). The process of inner transformation may itself produce a state of spiritual bliss that surpasses even the spiritual bliss of the life without struggle and pain in the world to come. The two worlds are not detached one from the other, with the second simply a compensation for the pains of the first. Rather, they are inextricably linked in ways that have major implications for behavior. This world is a testing chamber for the future world, a place where it can to some degree be rendered immanent, and with God's help, we can make ourselves worthy of it to some degree.

There is, of course, something here similar to the Western perception of Buddhist pessimism of which Professor Gómez spoke, but there is also an optimism that the pain and struggle will eventuate in a higher mode of existence. It is both a spatial model, overcoming pain through embracing it and learning from it in this world, and a temporal model, enduring our own pain and alleviating that of others as efficacious elements in bringing about the future world.

In the regimen of Jewish observance that the classical rabbinic texts detail and assume, a number of practices are designated as affording access to that future higher blissful world. In this sense, too, the world to come is not only future but also contemporaneous, a mode of existence that is possible at moments even now, though it will be sustainable and total only in the world to come. Particularly noteworthy among such practices are the study of Torah and the observance of the Sabbath. But a Jew who would adopt these practices primarily for the contentment or relaxation they bring and not in order to serve God (thus avoiding the lifelong program of inner struggle and self-transformation) would be badly missing the point. For it is not the reward but the service that counts most. That is itself a major aspect of the Jewish theology of pain and suffering.

Reference

Levenson, J. D. 1988. *Creation and the Persistence of Evil: The Jewish Drama of Divine Omnipotence.* San Francisco: Harper & Row.

Discussion:

The "Relaxation Response"—Can It Explain Religious Transformation?

SARAH COAKLEY: Professor Benson, your theory about the "relaxation response," and its capacity to ameliorate pain, has been mentioned more than once already in this discussion. Before we go further, perhaps you would explain for yourself what it is?

HERBERT BENSON: Certainly. Basically, the relaxation response is evoked by two steps. One is the repetition of a word, a sound, a prayer, a phrase, or even a repetitive muscular activity. The second is that when other thoughts come to mind, you passively disregard them and come back to the repetition. (I believe that some forms of Buddhism use the pain itself as the focus of the repetition, to break the train of everyday thought and therefore neutralize the pain.) When a person practices these two steps, there are a set of physiologic changes that occur: decreased metabolism, heart rate, blood pressure, and rate of breathing and distinctive brain waves. The physiologic changes are consistent with decreased sympathetic nervous system activity, which has led to the application of the relaxation response in states of increased sympathetic activity, namely, that of stress (see Benson 1975, 1984).

A paper was published in *NeuroReport* by Sara Lazar (Lazar et al. 2000), from our group, reporting on a collaborative effort by the Massachusetts General Hospital, Beth Israel Deaconess Medical Center, and Brigham and Women's Hospital. She reports on the fMRI of what occurs when one goes through these two basic steps of repetition and the disregard of everyday thoughts. In this case the repetition was the word *satnām,* as we were working with a group of Sikh individuals. What we found were highly significant changes in brain wave activity comparing this state with the control state, where the subject was thinking of animals: dog, cat, bird, what have you. First of all, there was a quietude of the entire brain that came about with P values of ten to the minus thirty. These are highly significant, unbelievable changes. Following that period of quietude came activity with P values of ten to the minus seven, and then to the minus thirteen, in the brain areas of the limbic system that control the autonomic nervous system. These lit up, as did areas of the brain that control attention and emotion.

I do believe that these experiments are very important. They may not be what Anne Harrington is speaking to in terms of bridging, or what Arthur Kleinman calls crossing domains. But perhaps these experiments will do away with the mind/body dichotomy, where the laws of causality hold that something nonspecific and ill-defined, such as mind, cannot affect something specific and defined, such as body. I do believe these experiments show that here the ill-defined thoughts, the repetition of *satnām,* led to physiologic changes in the brain, which then explain the physiologic changes in the body.

I think the reductionist approach, exemplified here by fMRI, is a bridge that can bring these worlds together. Does that mean that one can ultimately explain all religious beliefs as an evolutionary strategy for quieting the pain of existence? I don't think so, because ultimately we don't know the origin of such brain mechanisms. One could easily argue that they come either for evolutionary reasons, reductionistically, or from God.

But at any rate, immediately after these quieting thoughts, the mind is more open. That's when the visualizations of the various religious traditions come in, particularly in Buddhism, and then the physiology changes. As Howard Fields showed in his marvelous work on the placebo effect (Fields and Price 1997), perhaps this is an entry point for belief to come in and for other physiologic mechanisms to be manifest.

COAKLEY: I am fascinated by a variable that I don't know whether you have explicitly tested. Are you attributing to the particular mantra, *satnām,* the capacity for this deeper transformation?

Or is it that what matters more is the length of time and the dedication of the *practice?* By and large, as I understand it, the people you choose to test out in hospitals don't already have established religious practices associated with their beliefs; then they do some of this practice of "relaxation"—and, presto, it's not at all surprising to me that they start having beliefs. It's as if untaught bodies can't believe.

But there is another set of people, surely, who have a lifetime of practice before they confront a serious or final illness? I'm interested in what the difference would be if you could test the fMRI of those people's physiologic response. Could you answer that?

BENSON: We can invoke the relaxation response using any term. There is a common physiology regardless of the word, sound, prayer, phrase. It doesn't matter whether it's *om mani padme hum* or *Hail Mary full of grace*, we get the same physiologic changes. Or it could be the number one, the word *peace,* the word *love.* The purpose is to break the train of everyday thought. But we have found, through the work of Jerrod Kass (Kass et al. 1991), that when one regularly evokes the relaxation response, one feels more spiritual. People define that spirituality as feeling the presence of a power, force, energy, God, if you will, and secondarily, they feel it is close to them.

Belief is important up front in choosing for the patient, or the patient choosing for herself or himself, a secular or religious term that conforms to his or her own belief system. The quality of belief system is a whole other discussion, but the point is that when the mind opens, then the belief system kicks in.

COAKLEY: But you do admit in your fascinating discussion of Tibetan Buddhists (see Benson 1984, 1987, 1996) that they were able to lower their metabolic rate to a fantastic level that no one in your hospital would be able to reach through the "relaxation response"?

BENSON: It's true. But is it a question of practice or of the words themselves? They took several years to be able to decrease their metabolism 64 percent and reduce their breathing to five or six breaths per minute for hours on end. Can any of us do this? I believe so, in principle. But ultimately, the belief system may bring in another dimension that is far beyond what we can discuss today.

LUIS GÓMEZ: I'm not surprised that many words work, given the fact that within Buddhism there are so many different practices that presumably "work." I don't think that diminishes in any way the value of the practice. (I'm also sure there are certain words that *wouldn't* work, like *pizza* or *Coke,* but who knows?) Whether the relaxation response explains religion is, of course, the big question. I'm inclined to say no, it doesn't. Religion is a lot more than just relaxation: a lot, lot more. It includes a lot of things that are not as nice as relaxation, such as a negative definition of oneself, and opposition to other people, which of course leads to many problems that we have experienced in history.

I also think that a reduced metabolism itself does not explain the experience of serenity or calm that is described in the literature. That experience has all sorts of moral connotations that need to be explained, and I'm not sure they can be explained merely physiologically.

Last but not least, we have to remember the fact that we are all to some extent culturally determined. "Spirituality" is a term that is as culturally specific as they come. It starts to rear regularly for the first time, I think, in the early modern period in Europe, and even then it doesn't quite have the meaning it has today. When people say that they feel more "spiritual," I would take that with a grain of salt. I'm not sure what they're actually referring to. I know the context in which people use that word, but I'm not too sure what it means.

COAKLEY: No one can deny the extraordinary efficacy of what Professor Benson has discussed in the "relaxation response" and the relief it has accorded to so many patients. What fascinates this particular group of specialists, however, is whether the neurobiological experiments in this area could be refined and complexified to account for such variables as (1) the *specific* content of the different metaphysical beliefs accompanying such practice or (2) the *changes* that might come about through many years of practice (since the "relaxation response" is apparently almost instantaneous)—or (3) whether lengthy practice over years could actually *intensify* various sorts of pain (especially the "pain" of compassion) in addition to, or instead of, alleviating it. Presumably these are investigations that could lie before us.

References

Benson, H. 1975. *The Relaxation Response*. New York: Morrow.

———. 1984. *Beyond the Relaxation Response: How to Harness the Power of Your Personal Beliefs*. With W. Proctor. New York: Times Books.

———. 1987. *Your Maximum Mind*. With W. Proctor. New York: Times Books.

———. 1996. *Timeless Healing: The Power and Biology of Belief*. With M. Stark. New York: Scribner.

Fields, H., and D. D. Price. 1997. "Toward a Neurobiology of Placebo Analgesia" and "The Contribution of Desire and Expectation to Placebo Analgesia: Implications for New Research Strategies." In A. Harrington, ed., *The Placebo Effect*. Cambridge, Mass.: Harvard University Press, 93–116, 117–137.

Kass, J. D., R. Friedman, J. Leserman, P. C. Zuttermeister, and H. Benson. 1991. "Health Outcome and a New Index of Spiritual Experience." *J. Sci. Stud. Religion* 30: 203–211.

Lazar, S. W., G. Bush, R. L. Gollub, G. L. Fricchione, G. Khalsa, and H. Benson. 2000. "Functional Brain Mapping of the Relaxation Response and Meditation." *NeuroReport* 11: 1581–1585.

Discussion:

Reductionism and the Separation of "Suffering" and "Pain"

ELAINE SCARRY: I was puzzled over exactly how one would want biology and biochemistry to cease being "reductionist."

Admittedly, I am wholly sympathetic with the worry that we are, at least for middle economic groups in the United States, overdrugged for things like depression. The number of drugs given to children is astonishing.

I recently had a friend whose mother died. Shortly before, people wanted to give her mother a drug because they said she had pathological levels of fear. What she was afraid of was dying. As her son pointed out, that doesn't seem so "pathological," since she was two days away from dying.

So I accept the general framework that we should not assume that suffering is something that automatically needs to be completely eliminated. But I want to ask if that framework should be decoupled from biological studies of pain and of painkillers. First of all, just one detail: I think what Arthur Kleinman said about separating out the minutiae does not have to mean separating pain from suffering altogether but could involve damping down the pain while not damping down other sensory experience, like the feeling of touch and so forth. It seems to me that the *biological* models of pain and painkillers already often allow for some of these complexities. They certainly allow for the possibility that if you can restore enough ground to somebody in acute physical pain so that they can begin to think of something other than the pain that is appropriating all their attention, they can take a step forward to the world-building acts that are described in both Teresa's and John's accounts and also by the Buddhist experts of whom we have heard. Even to have enough license over your own thoughts to begin to carry out the Buddhist practice of eliminating the self requires not having a *coercive* invasion of pain.

Thus my one main worry, which Sarah Coakley embedded in her talk and which feminist critics share, is a view that might seem to license the infliction of pain, what Jon Levenson called a license for sadism. On the one hand, we have to remember how a shaman can willfully take on pain and actually bring about amazing world-transforming effects through his own meditations on it. On the other hand, there is the kind of pain that a person has no say over, did not authorize, and does not have the option of expressing in Teresa's or John's beautiful language.

I realize that tonally and thematically there are vast differences, but it could be argued that any talk from the medical world that tells people with terrible pain who aren't, for example, being given opiates about secondary gains that the person might get from pain is a horribly crude way of saying: "It's okay that you're in pain. There is great meaning to be built from this, so live with it." The medical establishment's worst offense toward people in pain has been in not trying to understand it, not building careful biological models of what's going on.

ARTHUR KLEINMAN: I agree very much with the last point you made, and it's very important to understand that. It's like Tolstoy's argument in *The Death of Ivan Ilyich* (1994), that medicine takes away something important from suffering that it shouldn't, and that people should suffer. Yet there is a horrible dimension to that. It's been said that it sounds like Frederick the Great yelling after his troops after they were routed in battle, "You dogs, would you live forever?"

On the first point, there is no way of stopping reductionism. Reductionism is the dominant form of biological work today. It's incredibly successful, and we all benefit enormously from it. Anyone who has cancer or heart disease (or, for that matter, depression) recognizes the incredible importance of such biological reductionism, even in psychiatry. But as a form of knowledge, it will require rebuilding in order to accomplish the bridging that we're talking about here. That rebuilding has to happen through the work of biologists like Howard Fields, who take not just physiological knowledge but molecular knowledge and rebuild it into physiological systems. We need a recrudescence of physiologic thinking, which right now I don't see happening. We need to have the biological knowledge placed in formats that will allow for its connection with the social world, as an earlier generation of biologists systematically tried to do.

We've lost something in that domain even as we've gained a great deal through reductionism. But I'm sure that as biology develops, we will see this happen. A very good example of this approach appears in Richard Lewontin's book *Biology as Ideology: The Doctrine of DNA* (1992). For Lewontin, who is a fine population geneticist, DNA is as real as this table in front of me. But then he shows how DNA is commodified, socially constructed, and organized in ways that change our world at the ideological level. That kind of integration is what we need to see from biologists, not just from people in the social sciences.

References

Lewontin, R. 1992. *Biology as Ideology: The Doctrine of DNA*. New York: HarperPerennial.

Tolstoy, L. 1994. *The Death of Ivan Ilyich and Other Stories*. New York: Signet Classics.

Discussion:

The Instrumentality of Pain in Christianity and Buddhism

STANLEY TAMBIAH: I'd like to ask Sarah Coakley and Luis Gómez whether there is a difference between the Buddhist and Christian conceptions of liberation or salvation. The deep sense of Christian suffering, which is very moving, seems to involve a purgation of bodily and spiritual suffering through union with God. In other words, Christ on the cross becomes what you appropriate for yourself, and his suffering is redemption for mankind. The Buddhist notion of *duḥka* and its origin, and the process by which you liberate yourself, does not simply start with suffering as we know it in everyday language. *Duḥka* comes from every use of the senses, including attachment and happiness. How you transform yourself, liberate yourself from attachments and from the process of the becoming and passing away of things in impermanence, how you dissolve your inner sense of self and make the final ascent to liberation, seems a different goal from the Christian one.

LUIS GÓMEZ: Anybody who does Buddhist studies lives under a curse. Any time you have to talk about Buddhism to a group like this—in other words, when you're not speaking to the twenty other specialists in the world who share your own interest—it's as if Sarah had stood up and said, "I'm going to tell you something about Christianity." Instead she talked, quite specifically, about the Carmelites.

So the first problem is that there are many kinds of Buddhism. I know many, many Buddhists who never use the word *duḥka* or its translations. Another problem is that sometimes Christianity comes very close to Buddhism. For example, hesychastic Orthodox Christianity (involving a long-term practice of the "Jesus prayer") actually has a lot of resonance with some kinds of Buddhism. Pure Land Buddhism is also resonant with some kinds of Christianity. It's extremely complicated. I think the real issue is not how Christianity and Buddhism are different but how are *specific* communities and individuals different?

CHARLES HALLISEY: Something struck me listening to Luis Gómez and Howard Fields, that pain was one of the ways we interact with the environment that makes it *less* dangerous to us. You could say that in Buddhism suffering is the way that we interact with the world, especially the world of other people. It's almost the reverse notion: rather than making other people or the environment less dangerous to us, suffering makes *us* less dangerous to other people.

Something about the connection we have to other people in suffering transforms our selves and how we relate to them. I thought Luis was quite good at exploding the conventional modern way of seeing suffering as something to escape. It's something to escape, but it's also a real benefit to our moral sensibilities because of how it affects the way we receive other people. There are points of contact in that to what Sarah was talking about, even as we're profoundly aware of the differences.

LAURENCE KIRMAYER: I want to suggest, in a moment of boundless optimism, that we are actually talking a lot about very meaningful mediating structures. The point at which things become problematic is in how people make *use* of those structures. Earlier, in our presentation in this conference, we saw the image of the anterior cingulate gyrus lighting up, representing a locus of affective elaboration and meaning and attentional control through the frontal lobe. That's an example from the physical arena of mediation of attentional processes.

Where we run into differences among us is in the kind of *instrumentality* that is given to pain. Is pain a signal to avoid problems in the outer world that should be eliminated when it is gratuitous? That leads us to the whole reductionist project of how to control or reduce pain. Or does it have a moral meaning that moves outward into the world and has other implications? Maybe some of the friction that arises when bridges seem to be missing has to do with those two different uses of pain, the two different directions in which our theories go. They are not incompatible; they are about different dimensions of a process that nevertheless interact. If we medicate ourselves, that is a social fact, a political fact, and an economic fact that also changes our biology. There is a circularity in the whole process: the discovery of new ways of making certain kinds of pain go away will have consequences for the moral landscape. It's the weaving together of these dimensions that has to be thought through.

It seems the mediating arena is opening up to us. We have images; we have notions of the processes involved. The contention is not about that but about the uses to be made of these things and the direction we should look. Do we look from the top down and make bodily pain go away because it afflicts people, or do we look outward at how a person navigates a social world with this information and what implications it has for one's life, for one's actions with other people? These are very much complementary things that interdigitate rather than things that are totally incommensurable.

JEAN JACKSON: There is a definition of pain from John Loesser (1996), a pain specialist, that I think is very useful. It complicates the matter, but I think that's the direction to go in. He says that pain is not a thing but a set of observations we make about ourselves and other people. We reify pain because the English language pushes us in that direction. I think it's a good idea to keep that in mind in this interdisciplinary discourse.

NICHOLAS WOLTERSTORFF: A challenge that emerged from Sarah Coakley's wonderful description of Teresa and John was that we see in them a certain valorization of pain as a means of spiritual transformation. The question that really intrigues me is whether we find in them, and in Buddhism, the more radical view that pain itself is to be somehow *transformed,* rather than used, as a means toward spiritual transformation. Do you see what I mean by that distinction? It's certainly true that pain can serve an instrumental good and become redemptive. But the Christian mystics and martyrs sometimes seem to hint at a much more haunting and difficult thought, that the pain itself can be transformed somehow, so that it becomes an intrinsic good and not just an instrumental good. I find that systematically and historically mystifying.

SARAH COAKLEY: It's an excellent distinction. The trouble is that when we apply it to the Carmelites, I think we find we have to complexify the distinction yet further. Let's take the idea of "pain" as an "instrumental good" first. That might be construed manipulatively, as if one could *force* the effects of spiritual transformation out of a deliberately applied pain event, but we've seen that the Carmelites are quite suspicious of such a self-induced approach. Nonetheless, for them the idea of pain as an "instrumental good" does still apply, but only I think in a subtler sense: trials and sufferings and physical pains that we have not ourselves asked for can nonetheless be used by God as a means of purgation and of bringing us nearer to Christ.

Now take your second idea—of pain as an "intrinsic good." Again, I'd want to generate another subdistinction. One could indeed take this idea, first, as a valorization of *pain for pain's sake,* and I do not myself find this thought in the Carmelites' repertoire—even though I admit it has made its regrettable appearance at times in the Christian tradition. But one could also see the "intrinsic good" as lying not in the pain per se but in the "union" that accompanies it and so also completely transforms it. Here Christological identification becomes central: the pain is not any old pain, one might say, but a particularly unique form of pain that accompanies this intense closeness to God.

GÓMEZ: I cannot think of any example of the latter position in Buddhism, that is, of pain as an "intrinsic good." The pain is usually instrumental, sometimes in a very proactive sense. In other words, it's not just a question of getting away from pain but actually using pain as a teacher or using the stress of pain as the basis for action. The only thing that comes close to what you've mentioned, although it might be different, would be in Tantric Buddhism where you can use pain as an inherent manifestation of Buddhahood. But I'm not sure even that comes anywhere close to what Sarah is describing.

Reference

Loesser, J. D. 1996. "Mitigating the Dangers of Pursuing Care." In M. J. M. Cohen and J. N. Campbell, eds., *Pain Treatment Centers at a Crossroads: A Practical and Conceptual Reappraisal.* Seattle: IASP Press, 101–108.

Grief and Pain

The Mediation of Pain in Music

Voice, Metaphysics, and Community

Pain and Transformation in the Finnish-Karelian Ritual Lament

7

Elizabeth Tolbert

The Voice of Lament

What is the relationship between voice, self, and other, and how does it inform musical and emotional experience?[1] This question will be explored from the perspective of the Finnish-Karelian *itkuvirsi,* or ritual lament, a beautiful and moving genre performed only by women and one in which the embodiment of emotional pain is particularly prominent.[2]

The Karelians are a small minority people closely related to the Finns in both language and culture, living along the border area between Finland and Russia. Prior to World War II, the *itkuvirsi* was an integral part of the non-Christian rituals of ancestor worship in the traditional death and wedding ceremonies of peasant village life. In Finland today, laments are usually performed to mourn the forced relocation of the Karelians to Finland after the war. As the lament once helped to ease the transition from this world to the next, it now serves to mediate between the world of the past and the world of the present. When Karelian lamenters mourn for their past, their lost culture, and their former homeland, they counteract their loss by lament performance, performance that not only helps to sustain the tradition but contributes to the ongoing re-creation of Karelian identity in new and evolving contexts.

The *itkuvirsi* is performed in an ecstatic style reminiscent of a shamanistic trance, showing influences from indigenous religious traditions in addition to Eastern Orthodox Christianity. Lamenters emphasize that their performance is a serious duty, not to be taken lightly; each lament is a "work of sorrow," improvised anew for each particular occasion. The prototypal context is death, where the lamenter serves as a conduit to Tuonela, the Finnish-Karelian land of the dead. She is a powerful magicoreligious practitioner, leading the souls of the deceased to Tuonela and bringing messages back and forth from between the living and the dead. She guides the soul by "finding the words," *löytää sanoja,* words that gain power by being "cried" in performance. Performed in a manner that mixes ritual text, stylized crying, and a sighlike melody, the lamenter "cries with words," as opposed to ordinary crying, or "crying with the eyes." She not only gives vent to her own feelings, but through the projection of her individual experience of grief, she helps the society as a whole to mourn, preserving the balance between this world and the next.

Poised at the nexus between voice and body, self and other, the lamenter creates an intersubjective understanding of emotional pain by expressing the inexpressible, by rendering the isolation of individual mourning into an intensely communal experience. In the following refugee lament to her deceased mother, Alina Repo grieves for the loss of her home in Karelia, which was ceded to the Soviets after World War II. She wistfully remembers her large family farm of "300 hectares without stones," where the land was farther south than her present home in Finland and the growing season longer. Alina alternates references to the "terrible winter" of her own life experiences with the common Karelian experience of losing one's homeland. She sprinkles her lament with particulars, the particulars of her own life along with the particulars of the past, images that are personal yet also communicate a lifestyle known to all Karelians. Alina evokes the common experience of the "bad days, the times [that] had all kinds of crying and sadness," despairing that "the home lanes have been given to strangers." She names the place Sinisokola and situates especially poignant feelings in her own "home lanes" and her own "fields." She longingly remembers the "window sill that father made" and "playing in the waters off our own Karelian shores." Alina expresses her grief in the linguistic and musical conventions of the lament form, thus exhibiting an essential feature of lament performance—the "dynamic interplay of individual expression and collective forms and sentiments" (Feld 1990, 241). By "crying with words," she both enacts her grief and tells the story behind her tears, thereby denying the inexpressibility of individual grief by bringing its interpretation into the social realm.

Alina's personal experience of pain is highlighted when she cries to her mother, "[D]on't forsake me, the lonely one," prefacing her pleas with traditional modes of address such as "my dear bearer" or "my dear golden sunshine." Crying "if only I had been left to the orphan's fate," she uses traditional formulations for the deeply personal sentiment of unallayed loss. When she prays to the saints to "protect the small ones of Sinisokola, covered with wings in the nest," and to "bless all people that they live in harmony," Alina underscores the plight of the Karelian refugees while using traditional phrases from wedding and funeral laments. In this way, her individual experience of grief gains multiple voices in performance and is used to negotiate between individual meanings and the social goals of catharsis, the regulated expression of grief, anger, and sorrow, and in the case of the refugee lament, the ongoing creation of a Karelian past.

Alina begins her lament with the traditional muffled sobbing, covering her face with the *itkuliina*, or "crying cloth," so that the evil spirits will not enter her mouth. Shielding her eyes with her hands, she sways gently in a circle and starts to lament, employing stylized crying, the special lament words, and the sighlike melody to contact her mother in Tuonela. As she begins to "find the words," the melody descends in an unadorned manner, interspersed with sporadic, forced crying. As the performance develops, the melody becomes more elaborated, more text is inserted into each sighlike melodic phrase, and the stylized crying intensifies and gains momentum. Each of these formal intensifications in turn generates an increase in micromodulations of pitch and rhythm, a sign not only of emotional intensity but of spiritual presence, an indication that the lamenter is entering a trancelike state to communicate with her mother in Tuonela.

Alina Repo, Juuka, Finland, August 1985
Refugee Lament

1 Kuule kuldaine kukad (i) päiväizeñi.
Listen my dear flower sunshine.

2 Kallejen malittuizeñi majitciaizeñi.
My dear bearer, my mother

3 Emozeñi kallis kandajaizeñi.
My mother, my dear bearer.

4 Kui jo liennet piässy igävie päiväizil (i) piälici.
I wonder how you passed the bad days.

5 Oli ai katalaizel laizel kaiken (i) moized (i) igäväized da itkuized.
The times had all kinds of sadness and crying.

6 O kallis kandajaizeñi.
Oh my dear bearer.

7 Kui oli iliman suuruized igäväized.
It was such great unhappiness.

8 Kui ai emmo voinnu ihastellakse izäizie laittuloiz (i) ikkunpiälyziz.
Because we couldn't enjoy the window sill that father made.

9 Emogo voinu veseldelläkse omis Karjalan vesirandaiziz veseldelläkse.
And we couldn't play in the waters off of our own Karelian shores.

10 Aa näin elee kaiken (i) moized (i) katalaizill laizil.
So, one lives in all kinds of unhappiness.

11 Pidän ylästä (i) ylen suured (i) igävïzed.
In very great unhappiness.

12 Kui jo ollygö kotikujoized
Because the home lanes have

13 kummalle kuksistuttu.
been given to strangers

14 Kai peltoizet kai pelloni piendaruized ylenä jäliközoiduttu.
and the fields and the sides of the fields have been neglected

15 Kui jo ei ole armahien askeluizeñi astujaizi.
and there are none of my dear steppers to walk

16 Eigö pienoizi pihamuahuizile pepettelemää.
and no small ones to putter in the yard.

17 Oppikkoa vain ygö armahad andelaized elelä uuzil elin (i) tilaizil.
Try dear giver to live in the new circumstances.

18 Ylen sulavis soguiziz suzien suzien da dien ker.
In harmony with strangers.

19 Oi kallis spoassaizeñi.
Oh my dear saint.

20 Anna suured (i) blauhostoveñiaized kaikil (i) rahvahaizil eliä yksisdummaizi.
Bless all people that they live in harmony.

21 Kui jo lien ollu ylen orboloin ozaized.
If only I had been left to the orphan's fate.

22 O katceldavannu.
Oh protector

23 Suojelle (n) Siñjisokolan siibyizil pienoizi pezäize (i) peitelessää.
Protect the small ones of Sinisokola, covered with wings in the nest.

24 O kalledit kantomut kui olen (i)
Oh dear ones who carried me. If only I had

25 orboin ozaizil jäänny yksil elintilaizil.
been left alone to the orphan's fate.

26 Oi kallehet kandajaizeñi.
Oh my dear bearer.

27 Älgää yllägiä yksinäizi eläjäizi.
Don't forsake me the lonely one.

28 Kui jo ollygö armahavia talaviaigaized annettu omil (i) eländaigaizil.
I have been given terrible winter time for my own life circumstances.

29 Mindä lien ollu valgeat tzaugevoatteivo varusteltu ennen kaikki aigaizi.
Why have the white clothes been prepared before their time?

30 Eigö lie voinu stiästellä vieluveräjizipiälici.
[The meaning of this line is obscure.]

31 On ajaa vied aigaized akkalaa lakkaized ollu.
There would have still been time before I would have had to become an old woman.

By framing her grief as a ritual performance of crying, Alina offers her individual body as a template for social meanings, rendering transparent the social, emotional, and bodily conditions of self. Specifically, emotional pain is somatized in her voice; not only does she cry her lament, but she utilizes techniques of textual and musical improvisation that reify vocal sonority itself. Jakobson (1960) has noted that such techniques are *autoreferential* in that they draw attention to the relationship between the form and content of the vocal utterance. Autoreferentiality characterizes the *poetic function* of language, which arises from the repositioning of "the principle of equivalence from the axis of selection into [*sic*] the axis of combination" (358), or in Saussurean terms, from the projection of the paradigmatic axis onto the syntagmatic axis. In other words, the overlay of paradigmatic and syntagmatic axes results in the sequential organization of similar linguistic elements that would in everyday speech be substituted for one another as members of a paradigmatic class.[3] Jakobson suggests that when similarity is placed in sequence, the distinction between selection and combination becomes blurred, leading to ambiguity and multiplicity of meaning. The poetic function is foregrounded in genres such as the *itkuvirsi,* where the principle of sequential equivalence is evidenced in alliterative texts, repetitive sighlike motives, and cycles of stylized weeping, which in turn produce a condensed and multilayered experience of communal mourning.

Alina improvises a text in the traditional formulaic and quasi-secret ritual language, ornamenting her text with vocables, alliteration, parallelism, and ritual names that refer to the deceased obliquely. In keeping with a name taboo for the dead, she calls to her mother with veiled expressions such as "my dear little golden flower sunshine, my dear little carrier, my dear little bearer," which in lament words is expressed as *kuldaine kukas paivaizeni, kallejen malittuizeñi majitciaizeñi, emozeni kallis kandajaizeni.* The text draws attention to its materiality and hence its embodied qualities by the alliteration of the "k" and "m" sounds, the internal rhyme of the diminutive ending *aizeni,* meaning "my little one who does or is *x*," and the parallelism of the three invocations to her mother. The autoreferentiality inherent in the alliterative names for the mother both metaphorically represents and metonymically invokes the intimate relationship between self and other, demonstrating Jakobson's assertion that the poetic function makes "anything sequent . . . a simile" (Jakobson 1960, 370).

Similarly, techniques of musical improvisation highlight the lament's material qualities, including the use of a descending, sighlike melody that is similar in form to "natural" crying; musical accents that further distort the already distorted text; and increasing microtonal and microrhythmic activity during the course of the lament as emotional tension grows. Paralinguistic features such as sobbing, sighing, moaning, swaying, covering the face, and trembling, likewise externalize emotional suffering, transforming the fragmented experience of individual pain into a socially coherent experience.

Figure 7.1 shows a transcription of the first few phrases of Alina's lament. Each sighlike phrase consists of a descending minor pentachordal contour with the duration of one breath, suffused throughout with stylized sobs. A specific skeletal melodic formula determines the overall shape of the melody: a terraced, descending minor pentachord with initial and cadential formulae. On the level of specific melodic movement within this general phrase structure, melodic contours and rhythms are text based, often going against speech accent. For example, in the spoken language, the first syllable of each word is accented. In the sung lament, syllables other than the first are accented musically by procedures such as melisma, prolonged duration, pitch, dynamics, or embellishments. On the smallest level of form, increasing microtonal and microrhythmic activity caused by intensified crying signals the lamenter's contact with the spirit world as she reaches a trancelike state and conveys messages between the worlds.

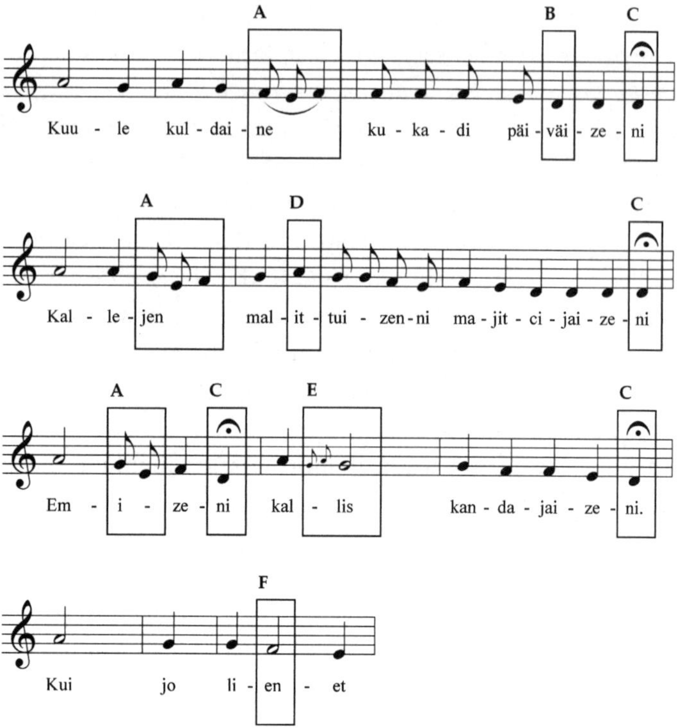
A
B
C
Kuu - le kul - dai - ne ku - ka - di päi - väi - ze - ni
A
D
C
Kal - le - jen mal - it - tui - zen-ni ma - jit - ci - jai - ze - ni
A
C
E
C
Em - i - ze - ni kal - lis kan - da - jai - ze - ni.
F
Kui jo li - en - et

Figure 7.1. A transcription of the first few phrases of Alina's lament.

Voice, Metaphysics, and Community

This brief analysis has been a mere sketch of the layers of meaning in a particular lament; a more detailed reading not only would require greater attention to the textual, musical, and paralinguistic features of the performance but also would need to place the analysis within the context of individual lives, the Karelian refugee experience, and the syncretism of Orthodox Christian and indigenous Karelian religious beliefs (see Tolbert 1987, 1990a, 1990b, 1994). Yet despite these limitations, it is clear that the lament gains its power from the embodied sonority of "crying with words," a power that can be attributed to the *iconic* and *indexical* processes (Peirce 1956 [1940]) that underlie heightened vocality. In contrast to conventional, arbitrary signs, such as words, icons and indices are interpreted as similar to or co-extensive with their objects, respectively, and thus have a necessary, or *motivated,* relationship with the material world. For example, the stylized weeping in the Karelian lament, with its sobbing, creaky voice, and sharp intake of breaths, is interpreted as similar to and therefore *iconic* to "crying with the eyes."[4] This stylized crying is co-present with culturally specific contexts of grief and mourning and is therefore an *index* of these situations. Furthermore, the stylizations of "crying with words" are iconic to stylizations in other cultural domains, such that "iconicity of style" indexes sociocultural identity and world coherence (Feld 1988; see also Feld 1984; Becker and Becker 1981; Turino 1999). Peircean *symbols,* on the other hand, have a conventional relationship to their objects and thus are free of the materiality of the sign/object relation that obtains with motivated signs. The relationship of words to their objects is the canonical example of conventional meaning; laments are symbolic to the extent that they are grounded in the conventions of local beliefs and practices (see Tolbert 2001b, 88; 2001a; 2002).

From an ethnomusicological perspective, conventional meaning is presupposed to underlie the cultural specificity of musical practices found throughout the world. However, the presence of stylized crying across a broad range of intercultural contexts indicates that the conventionalized iconicity of "crying with words" may have wider significance for an understanding of musical meaning as rooted in iconic and indexical processes. For example, genres of "sung-texted-weeping" (Feld 1982) or "ritual wailing" (Urban 1988) are found throughout the world, and in similar forms and contexts, suggesting that conventions of stylized, melodic weeping are based on bodily iconicity to panhuman experiences of "natural," albeit culturally inflected, crying. The lament is a potentially illuminating case study of the biocultural and socioemotional roots of musically mediated pain and transformation in that the interdependence of form, content, and emotional expression is particularly prominent in this genre (for an overview of the issues, see Feld 1990, 241–242; Feld and Fox 1994, 39–43).

The similarities among lament forms beg the question—are laments merely a special case of performative iconicity, or are they rather a highly transparent case of a more widespread phenomenon? A hint that the latter might be the case is suggested by the fact that it is almost too easy to say what a particular lament "means." For example, Alina

Repo's lament expresses the personal trauma of the refugee experience while mediating its collective dimensions through appeals to a group experience of sorrow and pain, a meaning that seems all the more obvious given its foundational iconicity to crying. However, from a Durkheimian perspective, performative elaborations of "icons of crying" (Urban 1988, 389–391) not only index cultural contexts of grief and mourning but also index the social transformations necessary to maintain society in the face of death, indicating that the transformative function of the lament, indeed of all ritual genres, is ultimately about the desire for sociality (Durkheim 1969 [1912]; Urban 1988, 393; 1996; Tolbert 2001a, 2001b, 2002).

Ethnomusicologists and anthropologists have long noted that ritualized performances of emotion such as the lament are core expressions of sociocultural identity and, as such, are invoked during rituals of transformation when the potential for emotional upheaval is particularly threatening to social stability. In the case of the Karelian lament, the *itkuvirsi* marks the deceased's transformation from a social being materially embedded in a community to an ancestor whose ongoing interactions with the community will from that point on need to be materially reenacted. This "work of sorrow" requires constant performance to sustain ongoing relationships and to reintegrate the group into a cohesive whole. Thus, "crying with words" not only represents an appropriate response to grief but, through this very appropriateness, also disseminates ideas about sociality throughout the community, thereby transforming the ephemeral nature of social relationships into enduring expressions of collective belief. From this perspective, the role of iconicity and indexicality as a means to guarantee sociality seems broadly applicable to any musical moment, implying that "crying with words" has significance beyond its reference to crying per se and has much to tell us about the socially grounded, emotionally motivated, and embodied nature of representation more generally.

More specifically, how does "crying with words" serve as a vehicle of cultural truth and thus guarantee sociality? As Tomlinson (1999, 4) notes, "[V]oice, employed in exceptional ways and in special, carefully demarcated circumstances, opens to perception invisible realms. Voice connects its bearers and hearers to ordinarily supersensible realities." Therefore, the autoreferentiality of "crying with words" draws attention not only to the tension between the form and content of the verbal message but to the concomitant metaphysical potential of vocality itself. The dialectic between the material form of stylized crying, that is, its form as a phenomenal object, and the noumenal idea it conveys, that is, the metaphysical realm of Tuonela, reveals the crying voice as that which simultaneously "makes the intelligible sensible" and "the sensible intelligible" (Urban 1996, 24). This continual dialectic between form and content suggests that cultural truths are in fact metaphysical truths. This is so because collective belief can only be instantiated in the *social* realm; the mediation between form and content takes place in the social arena and therefore mirrors the mediation between individual and collective experience more broadly.

The social mediation of form and content is highlighted in genres such as the *itkuvirsi*, which bring to the fore the dialectic between individual and collective experience, and hence between motivated and conventional signs. Individual experience of motivated signs can be substantiated by appeal to the material grounding of iconic and indexical reference, whereas conventional signs depend upon collective experience for their meanings. However, from a Peircean point of view, conventional symbols are built upon prior iconic and indexical reference, which suggests that the social bases of conventional meaning rest upon prior motivated meanings.[5]

To illustrate this idea with the Karelian lament, and following Urban's notion of *discourse circulation* (1996, xii–xiv, 241–257), ideas must be repeatable to gain currency; therefore, repeatable form in ritual genres announces itself as a potential vehicle of socially sharable, that is, conventional, meaning. However, form as a value unto itself focuses on the conventionality and potential arbitrariness of the sign, and content becomes potentially unmotivated. To recapture motivated meaning, the meanings of conventional signs must appeal to a sociality that is experienced as having a necessary connection to the material world. In the case of the Karelian lament, the lamenter uses phonetically altered ritual texts and stylized, melodic crying to produce formal patterns that advertise their status as replicable and hence sharable. However, as form becomes repeatable and sharable, content is guaranteed by socially mediated reference to motivated representational processes, in this case, to icons of crying and indices of grief. From this perspective, form is an embodiment of sociality; by "making the intelligible sensible" and the "sensible intelligible," "crying with words" produces both the meanings and objects of cultural truths. Thus, metaphysical truths are in essence social truths because they are negotiated through formal objects that become a focus for collective experience, allowing for "the construction of a noumenal understanding of the phenomenal world in terms of community" (Urban 1996, 251).

Intercorporeal Iconicity

To more fully understand how "crying with words" constructs "a noumenal understanding of the phenomenal world in terms of community" (Urban 1996, 251), it is necessary to broaden the discussion to encompass the phenomenological experience of heightened vocality more broadly (e.g., Barthes 1977; Burrows 1990; Tolbert 1992, 1994, 2001a, 2001b, 2002). Who is the being behind the lamenting voice, and what is she saying? As I have noted elsewhere,

> [W]e understand [vocality] in the most general sense as a vehicle for cultural truth because we hear [the voice] as the socially meaningful presence of another person. We understand [the lament] as an embodied voice, produced directly from a human throat or by instrumental proxy, yet retaining its identity as a "humanly organized sound" (Blacking 1973, 26). Even though we may perceive musical form, when hearing [the lamenting] voice we cannot help but hear more than pure structure. We grasp a social essence, one that is emotionally and corporeally informed. On some level, we glimpse the body behind the voice, a body whose voice refers to the imagined socio-emotional essence of its figurative producer (Barthes 1977). This voice is not merely an object, but a voice of an intentional being such as oneself, and one that therefore references states of arousal, attention, and emotion. Thus, an encounter with the voice is above all an intercorporeal encounter with a social presence, and we bring to it our social, corporeal, and enacting selves. (Tolbert 2001[b], 86–87)

This voice does not literally reference the subjectivity of its utterer but rather a figurative social essence whose voice is understood as an imagined product of figurative bodily movement. The primacy of bodily movement in the apprehension of voice is underscored by the fact that vocal production represents a physical interface between self and other, a literal site of internal gesture projected outward (Burrows 1990, 30). Perhaps most significantly, this vocal gesture is understood iconically in reference to one's own capacities for movement and thus indexes social meanings due to its status as an empirically verifiable *intercorporeal icon.* Elaborating on Merleau-Ponty's concept of the intercorporeal, the understanding of movement in terms of one's own capacity for movement has been theorized to account for intersubjectivity, in that it allows for movements of others to be interpreted as evidence of subjectivity and intention (Merleau-Ponty 1964; Sheets-Johnstone 1990, 112–133; 1994, 56–59; 1999; Wilkerson 1999). Thus "crying with words," through its intercorporeal iconicity to "crying with the eyes," indexes a "virtual person" (Watt and Ash 1998, 49) who possesses an intercorporeally intelligible "embodied subjectivity" (Grosz 1994, 22) and whose demonstrated contact with the deceased in *Tuonela* establishes an intercorporeally intelligible experience of the metaphysical realm.

Where might we find further support for the phenomenological experience of voice as a grounding of metaphysical truth? It is proposed here that the status of voice as intercorporeal icon, and hence its psychological validity as an expression of an embodied subjectivity, is mediated through the *body image.*[6] The body image is a map of how the body appears to ourselves, how we experience and understand ourselves as an embodied self. The body image was first described by physicians who worked with patients who had lost limbs in World War I and who suffered from painful sensations in these "phantom" limbs. The body image is thus not merely the perceptions and sensations of having a body that are congruent with the actual materiality of the body. It consists both of mappings of the body, that is, body schemas, and a psychological investment in a unified and coordinated body, one that is continually altered with experience. Most important for our purposes here, the body image remains attached to detachable parts of the body, which are perceived as intermediate objects, neither bodily or nonbodily. Schilder, a foundational researcher on the body image, elaborates as follows: "[O]bjects which were once connected with the body always retain something of the quality of the body-image in them . . . whatever originates in or emanates out of our body will still remain a part of the body-image. The *voice,* the breath, the odor, faeces, menstrual blood, urine, semen, are still parts of the body image even when separated in space from the body" (Schilder 1978 [1935], 213, cited in Grosz 1994, 81, emphasis added). It is significant that Schilder includes the voice as a detachable part of the body and hence an *emotionally* laden psychosomatic object. This implies that the voice has intrinsic psychological and social meanings due to its status as part of the body image and is therefore interpreted as iconic and indexical of a socially and emotionally grounded self.

Thus, the ability to understand voice as indicative of social essence arises from an understanding of voice as an effect of bodily movement as mediated through the body image and that is based on the more general ability to model movements and understand the movements of others as evidence of subjectivity and intention. Donald (1991, 1993, 1998, 1999) refers to this motor modeling ability as "mimesis" and theorizes that it represents the evolutionary emergence of uniquely human representational abilities. Perhaps the most persuasive evidence for the social basis of intercorporeal iconicity comes from studies in infant developmental psychology, which show that mimetic processes are crucial to the development of self. Newborn infants are able to imitate facial expressions and vocalizations (e.g., Meltzoff and Moore 1977), can distinguish themselves from others (e.g., Legerstee 1998), and have the ability to perform intermodal imitation, suggesting an innate body schema that underlies an innate, socially activated mimetic ability (Meltzoff and Gallagher 1996; Legerstee 1998; for an overview, see Trevarthen 1998, 1999b). Trevarthen proposes that vocality in particular is crucial to the mimetic processes underlying the development of self, positing an "innate communicative musicality" (1999a, 7) that comes into play during the infant's first social interactions (see also Dissanayake 2000). Thus, the voice has emotional significance in part because mimetic, socially motivated processes of self formation are indexed in any vocal utterance.

However, the intercorporeal and iconic underpinnings of self as expressed in the voice cannot be interpreted in a straightforward manner; indeed, the effectiveness of performative voices such as "crying with words" rests upon the fact that they exceed their putative referents. The iconic and indexical processes of self formation underlying vocality are in fact the basis for the symbolic, conventional use of the voice. Paradoxically, the conventional use of the voice depends on the reliability of voice quality as an index of bodily states; for example, restricted prosody can be an indicator of sadness or depression. This link between voice and emotional states is probably a residue from our primate heritage in that speech likely evolved from increasing voluntary control over previously involuntary emotion calls (e.g., Deacon 1997, 418–419; Donald 1991, 180–186). Thus, the voice articulates a dual potential; it is both an intentionally modeled vocal sound, yet it is also an unintentional index of an internal state. For example, the creaky voice and sobbing that are performatively represented in stylized crying, are dependable indicators of emotional states when "crying with the eyes." When "crying with words," the lamenter performatively asserts her "crying" as an authentic index of her grief, which links her intentionally modeled voice to the "natural" experience of crying and which can therefore be empirically verified through accommodation to individual experiences of crying. This tension between presentation and representation of emotion reveals the fact that for the voice to be interpreted as arbitrary sound, and therefore potentially unmoored from the social world, it must be anchored to the social world through "unfakable" bodily experience (Tolbert 2001b, 91; 2002). In the case of the Karelian lament, this "unfakable" bodily experience takes the form of an embodied and emotionally motivated presentation of self, one that can be substantiated through the intercorporeal iconicity of "crying with the eyes." In other words, "crying with words" indexes a figurative socioemotional essence as represented by the lamenter's body/self, leading those experiencing the ritual to believe that her voice indexes a person who has made spiritual contact with the other world and who, through the strength of her mourning, can mediate the mourning experience of all those present (Tolbert 1994).

Yet the lament's meanings do not end here. If first and foremost the voice indexes a social presence, "crying with words" makes those who hear it critically aware of the bodily conditions of representation and hence of the metaphysical grounding of culture and collective meaning in general. Thus, ritual performances such as "crying with words" not only reference the culturally appropriate response to grief but are a metacommentary on the iconic and indexical processes of self formation that allow for cultural meaning in the first place (see Tolbert 2001b, 91–92; 2002).

Whereas ritual practitioners in general use somatic techniques both to create cultural truth and to refer to the intersubjective processes of creating such truth, the embodiment of crying in the lamenting voice goes one step further in its assertion that cultural truth is guaranteed by an embodiment of *emotional* truth. When the Karelian lamenter "cries with words," those around her "cry with the eyes," both to make their communal grief palpable and to ground the chaotic, somatic expressions of grief in an intercorporeally convincing intelligibility. The fragility of society at moments of crisis requires the strongest confirmation of cultural truth; when the devastation of loss threatens the integrity of both the individual and the community, the public performance of grief counteracts this threat by revealing emotional experience as the guarantee of sociality itself. As the lamenter "cries with words," the members of the community reveal to one another, if only for a moment, the ephemeral, intersubjective, and materially embodied emotional truths that give meaning to their lives.

Notes

1. The title of this chapter references two remarkable works that explore the dynamics of metaphysics and expressive culture: Greg Urban's *Metaphysical Community: The Interplay of the Senses and the Intellect* (1996) and Gary Tomlinson's *Metaphysical Song: An Essay on Opera* (1999).
2. The case study of the Karelian lament presented in the first section of this chapter is adapted from my article "The Voice of Lament: Female Vocality and Performative Efficacy in the Finnish-Karelian *Itkuvirsi*" (Tolbert 1994) and reprinted with permission from Cambridge University Press. I am forever indebted to Alina Repo and the other Karelian lamenters who have taught me so much about their traditions. The first formal presentation of these ideas occurred at the Mind/Brain/Behavior conference on Pain and Its Transformations at Harvard University in May 2000. I am grateful to all the participants for their insightful comments and camaraderie. I would like to extend special thanks to the conference organizers, Sarah Coakley, Arthur Kleinman, and especially Kay Kaufman Shelemay, for their wonderful invitation to participate in cross-disciplinary dialogue on matters of music, mind, and brain.
3. See Culler (1976) for a discussion of Saussure's (1959) notions of the combinatorial and selective axes. Briefly put, Culler states that "syntagmatic

relations define combinatory possibilities . . . paradigmatic relations are the oppositions between elements that can replace one another" (1976, 60).

4. Urban (1988, 389–391) describes cross-culturally intelligible "icons of crying" found in ritual wailing in Amerindian Brazil, including sobbing, voiced inhalation, creaky voice, and falsetto vowels.
5. Peirce (1956 [1940], 102–103) describes signs as hierarchical in nature, such that indices are built upon prior iconic reference, and symbols upon prior indexical reference.
6. For general discussions of intercorporeality and the body image, see Grosz (1994, 62–85) and Weiss (1999).

References

Barthes, R. 1977. "The Grain of the Voice." In *Image, Music, Text.* New York: Farrar, Straus, and Giroux, 179–189.

Becker, J., and A. Becker. 1981. "A Musical Icon: Power and Meaning in Javanese Gamelan Music." In W. Stein, ed., *The Sign in Music and Literature.* Austin: University of Texas Press, 203–215.

Blacking, J. 1973. *How Musical Is Man?* Seattle: University of Washington Press.

Burrows, D. 1990. *Sound, Speech, and Music.* Amherst: University of Massachusetts Press.

Culler, J. 1976. *Ferdinand de Saussure.* Ithaca, N.Y.: Cornell University Press.

Deacon, T. 1997. *The Symbolic Species: The Co-Evolution of Language and the Brain.* New York: Norton.

Dissanayake, E. 2000. "Antecedents of the Temporal Arts in Early Mother-Infant Interactions." In N. Wallin, B. Merker, and S. Brown, eds., *The Origins of Music.* Cambridge, Mass.: MIT Press, 389–407.

Donald, M. 1991. *Origins of the Modern Mind.* Cambridge, Mass.: Harvard University Press.

———. 1993. "Précis of Origins of the Modern Mind: Three Stages in the Evolution of Culture and Cognition." *Behavioral and Brain Sciences* 16: 737–791.

———. 1998. "Mimesis and the Executive Suite: Missing Links in Language Evolution." In J. Hurford, M. Studdert-Kennedy, and C. Knight, eds., *Approaches to the Evolution of Language.* Cambridge: Cambridge University Press, 44–67.

———. 1999. "Preconditions for the Evolution of Protolanguages." In M. C. Corballis and S. E. G. Lea, eds., *The Descent of Mind: Psychological Perspectives on Hominid Evolution.* Oxford: Oxford University Press, 138–154.

Durkheim, E. 1969 [1912]. *The Elementary Forms of the Religious Life.* Trans. J. W. Swain. New York: Free Press.

Feld, S. 1982. *Sound and Sentiment: Birds, Weeping, Poetics, and Song in Kaluli Expression.* Philadelphia: University of Pennsylvania Press.

———. 1984. "Communication, Music, and Speech about Music." *Yearbook for Traditional Music* 16: 1–18.

———. 1988. "Aesthetics as Iconicity of Style, or 'Lift-up-over sounding': Getting into the Kaluli Groove." *Yearbook for Traditional Music* 13: 74–113.

———. 1990. "Wept Thoughts: The Voicing of Kaluli Memories." *Oral Tradition* 5(2–3): 241–266.

Feld, S., and A. Fox. 1994. "Music and Language." *Annual Review of Anthropology* 23: 25–53.

Grosz, E. 1994. *Volatile Bodies: Toward a Corporeal Feminism.* Bloomington: Indiana University Press.

Jakobson, R. 1960. "Closing Statement: Linguistics and Poetics." In T. A. Sebeok, ed., *Style in Language.* Cambridge, Mass.: MIT Press, 350–377.

Legerstee, M. 1998. "Mental and Bodily Awareness in Infancy: Consciousness of Self-Existence." *Journal of Consciousness Studies* 5(5–6): 627–644.

Meltzoff, A. N., and S. Gallagher. 1996. "The Earliest Sense of Self and Others: Merleau-Ponty and Recent Developmental Studies." *Philosophical Psychology* 9(2): 211–233.

Meltzoff, A. N., and M. H. Moore. 1977. "Imitation of Facial and Manual Gestures by Human Neonates." *Science* 198: 75–78.

Merleau-Ponty, M. 1964. *The Primacy of Perception.* Ed. J. Edie. Chicago: Northwestern University Press.

Peirce, C. S. 1956 [1940]. *The Philosophy of Peirce: Selected Writings.* Ed. J. Buchler. London: Routledge and Kegan Paul.

Saussure, F. de. 1959. *A Course in General Linguistics.* Ed. C. Bally and A. Sechehaye. Trans. W. Baskin. New York: Philosophical Library.

Schilder, P. 1978 [1935]. *The Image and Appearance of the Human Body: Studies in the Constructive Energies of the Psyche.* New York: International Universities Press.

Sheets-Johnstone, M. 1990. *The Roots of Thinking.* Philadelphia: Temple University Press.

———. 1994. *The Roots of Power: Animate Form and Gendered Bodies.* Chicago: Open Court.

———. 1999. *The Primacy of Movement.* Philadelphia: John Benjamin's.

Tolbert, E. 1987. "On Beyond Zebra: Some Theoretical Considerations of Emotion and Meaning in Music." *Pacific Review of Ethnomusicology* 4: 75–97.

———. 1990a. "Magico-Religious Power and Gender in the Karelian Lament." In M. Herndon and S. Ziegler, eds., *Music, Culture and Gender.* Berlin: Institute for Comparative Music Studies, 41–56.

———. 1990b. "Women Cry with Words: Symbolization of Affect in the Karelian Lament." *Yearbook for Traditional Music* 22: 80–105.

———. 1992. "Theories of Meaning and Music Cognition: An Ethnomusicological Approach." *The World of Music* 34(3): 7–21.

———. 1994. "The Voice of Lament: Female Vocality and Performative Efficacy in the Finnish-Karelian *Itkuvirsi.*" In L. Dunn and N. Jones, eds., *Embodied Voices: Representing Female Vocality in Western Culture.* Cambridge: Cambridge University Press, 179–194.

———. 2001a. "The Enigma of Music, the Voice of Reason: 'Music', 'Language,' and Becoming Human." *New Literary History* 32(3): 451–465.

———. 2001b. "Music and Meaning: An Evolutionary Story." *Psychology of Music* 29(1): 84–94.

———. 2002. "Untying the Music/Language Knot." In L. P. Austern, ed., *Music, Sensation and Sensuality.* New York: Routledge, 77–95.

Tomlinson, G. 1999. *Metaphysical Song: An Essay on Opera.* Princeton: Princeton University Press.

Trevarthen, C. 1998. "The Concept and Foundations of Infant Intersubjectivity." In S. Braten, ed., *Intersubjective Communication and Emotion in Early Ontogeny.* Cambridge: Cambridge University Press, 15–46.

———. 1999a. "Introduction." *Musica Scientiae* (Special issue 1999–2000): 7–11.

———. 1999b. "Musicality and the Intrinsic Motive Pulse: Evidence from Human Psychobiology and Infant Communication." *Musicae Scientiae* (Special issue 1999–2000): 155–215.

Turino, T. 1999. "Signs of Imagination, Identity, and Experience: A Peircian Semiotic Theory for Music." *Ethnomusicology* 43(2): 221–255.

Urban, G. 1988. "Discourse, Affect, and Social Order: Ritual Wailing in Amerindian Brazil." *American Anthropologist* 90: 385–400.

———. 1996. *Metaphysical Community: The Interplay of the Senses and the Intellect.* Austin: University of Texas Press.

Watt, R., and R. Ash. 1998. "A Psychological Investigation of Meaning in Music." *Musicae Scientiae* 2(1): 33–53.

Weiss, G. 1999. *Body Images: Embodiment as Intercorporeality.* New York: Routledge.

Wilkerson, W. 1999. "From Bodily Motions to Bodily Intentions: The Perception of Bodily Activity." *Philosophical Psychology* 12(1): 61–77.

Music, Trancing, and the Absence of Pain 8

Judith Becker

> Our normal waking consciousness, rational consciousness as we call it, is but one special type of consciousness, whilst all about it, parted from it by the filmiest of screens, there lie potential forms of consciousness entirely different. . . . No account of the universe in its totality can be final which leaves these other forms of consciousness quite disregarded. . . . They forbid a premature closing of our accounts with reality.
>
> *William James*

The focus of this chapter is a type of consciousness that lies outside "our normal waking consciousness," the phenomenon of religious trancing and the often accompanying absence of normal pain response.[1] Religious trancing, or religious ecstasy, is nearly always accompanied by music. The analgesic properties of music and trance are often dramatically enacted in rituals of religious trance. From the Sun Dance ritual of the Lakotas to the self-flagellation of Shi'a Muslims to the self-stabbing of the Balinese *bebuten* trances, trancing individuals perform feats of physical endurance that are unthinkable in ordinary body-mind states of consciousness. These are musical situations that may not be, in any direct way, about pain or suffering or healing but that may result in extraordinary stamina and a modulation of the sensation of pain.

Many kinds of music can, it seems, express sorrow, and most any kind of music can help a patient realign his own bodily rhythms and contribute to healing and the ensuing diminution of pain.[2] By contrast, music that accompanies religious trancing is not expressive of painful experiences nor symbolic of pain nor aimed at the reduction of pain. Rather, it is music whose primary function is to address, summon, or present an unseen world of gods, of deities, and of spirits. I suspect that the power of music to create an imaginary world, to invoke the presence of the denizens of heaven or hell, while entraining the minds and bodies of the trancers helps propel the trancers into a process of consciousness characterized by intense emotion, remote from their quotidian ways of interacting with their world. In this chapter I suggest that it is the alternate self of religious trance, the trance consciousness accompanied by intense emotion, that provides the analgesic, the means by which Balinese daggers do not penetrate the skin, and fatigue is for another day.

The Houghton Mind/Brain/Behavior Colloquium at Harvard University has as one of its aims the bridging of the chasm between humanistic and biological methods of research. Scholars who pursue cultural studies like anthropology and ethnomusicology have difficulty connecting their work with "hard sciences" like neurophysiology. We follow different heuristic procedures, look for different kinds of evidence, and have a different standard of evaluation and different formats for presenting research. We do not speak the same language; scientists have little motivation to learn to speak ours, and ethnomusicologists who are motivated to read the literature of neurophysiology face formidable challenges in locating the "cingulate cortices" or in deciphering "thalamocortical modulation."

Aside from the usual difficulties of communicating across disciplinary boundaries, a special problem arises in the study of the relationship between music and trancing. Rarely has trancing been addressed by neurophysiologists. There are good reasons why not. Trancing has been marginalized, distrusted by established religions, and classified as a pathology in the Western world since the eighteenth century (Decker 1986, 36; Inglis 1989, 116). Earlier, in the European medieval period, worse yet, trance was evidence of demonic possession (Caciola 1994). Trancing is surrounded by mystery and ofttimes suspected of being a bizarre form of chicanery.

Another reason for the lack of scientific study of trancing with music has to do with the difficulty of knowing where to start. We have had no way to imagine the neurophysiology of trance, nor a theory of consciousness that would provide a framework to begin to study the neurophysiology of trance. Trancers are spectacularly in motion from the onset until the completion of the trance, ruling out electrodes, PET scans, and MRIs. Neurobiologists study dreams (Hobson 1994), meditation, or pathological states of consciousness resulting from illnesses or injuries, situations where subjects can be examined and talked to (Squire 1987; Alkon 1992; LeDoux 1996). Trancers are on the move and not amenable to interviews. Trance consciousness remains opaque, unstudied, and suspect as the domain of religious fanatics and the mentally unstable. In my work, I hope to begin to demystify religious trancing and to argue for a reconfiguring of trance as a natural, nonpathological (but for us obscure) form of consciousness that often brings feelings of both joy and peace.

We know that any kind of music, even the piano, can act as a stimulator to trancing (Rouget 1985) and that loud sounds, often loud drumming, are among the most common types of musical accompaniment to trancing. Many firsthand accounts of experienced and skillful trancers testify to the catalytic role of music in the transition into trancing, in the sustaining of trancing, and in the transition back to normal consciousness (Friedson 1996, 6; Kapferer 1991, 264; Rouget 1985, 72). But the "why" of all this remains, from a secular, scholarly perspective, largely speculation.

It is my belief that recent theories of the biology and neurophysiology of consciousness (Maturana and Varela 1987; Dennett 1991; Edelman 1992; Damasio 1994, 1999) open up a way to begin to imagine trance consciousness and its musical accompaniment as a special kind of consciousness precipitated by strong emotions and characterized by a more or less complete replacement of the sense of "I-ness."

Specifically, the theory of consciousness developed by neuroscientist Antonio Damasio in his book *The Feeling of What Happens: Body and Emotion in the Making of Consciousness* (1999) provides a model upon which one can hypothesize about trance consciousness in a way that begins to integrate what we already know about trance phenomenology with neurophysiology. Rendering thinkable the properties of trancing, such as amnesia and insensitivity to pain, in terms of neural activity and chemical action seems a first step toward moving trance from a "marvel" (Hacking 1995, 143) to a position whereby it may become a serious focus for scholarly, scientific research.

Ethnographic data, based upon my own research, provide the basis for what follows.

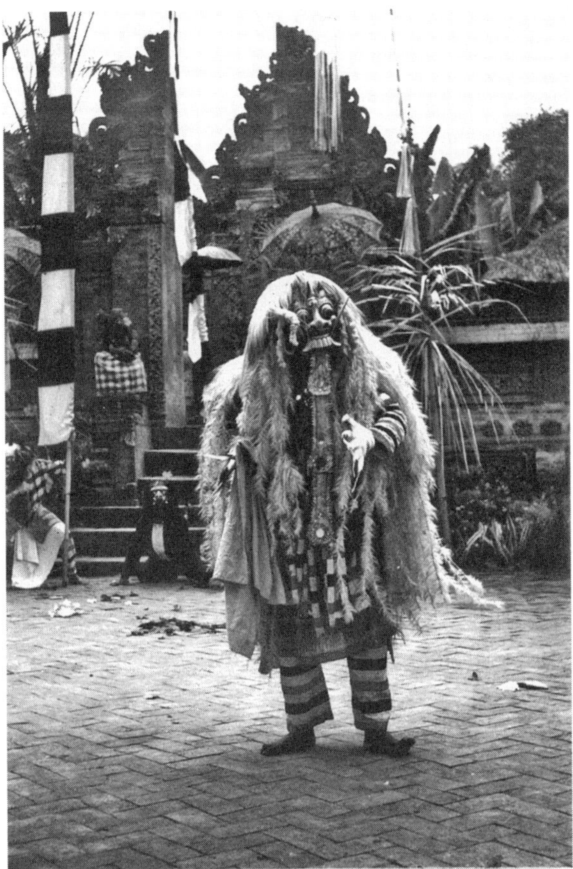

Figure 8.1. Rangda, Balinese witch.

Brief Description of the Rangda/Barong Ceremony

The Rangda/Barong ritual of Bali, Indonesia, is an event invoked to restore the balance between the world of people and the "other" world of the deities, spirits, and demons. If some misfortune befalls a village, such as crop failure, pestilence, or frequent cases of mental illness, the village will stage a ritual encounter opposing the great witch Rangda and her followers against the mythic beast Barong and his followers (see Figure 8.1).

The cast of performers in this ritual may include up to twenty other minor demons who may dance, cavort, or misbehave in amusing or threatening ways. A group of young men of the village volunteer to go into trance, to become the helpers of the beast Barong, and at the climax of the drama arm themselves with daggers and attack the witch Rangda.

Before the ceremony begins, all the participants are put into trance at the temple to the accompaniment of long lines of classical poetry sung slowly, in unison, by a chorus of women from the village. At the dénouement of the drama, which may take several hours, the witch Rangda puts a curse on the human followers of Barong, whereupon they turn their daggers against themselves, pressing the blades against their sternum or upper arm or sometimes on their cheek or just above the eyeball (see Figure 8.2).

Seldom do the trancers cut themselves. Gradually, as the force of their anger subsides, they fall to the ground in the classic "crisis" of trance (Rouget 1985, 38). They are then disarmed and removed to the temple where they are slowly brought out of trance. Throughout the public, theatrical part of the ceremony, the gamelan ensemble plays continuously (see Figure 8.3).

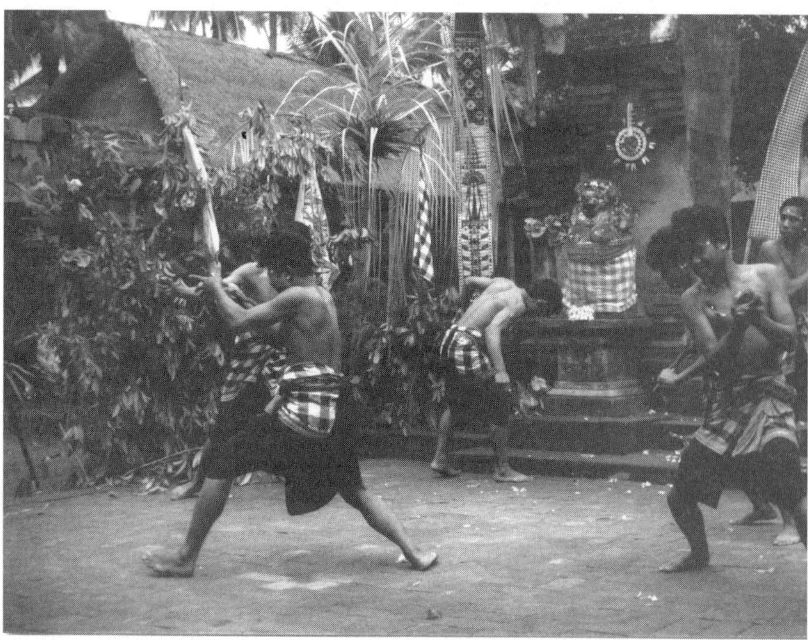

Figure 8.2. Bebuten trancers.

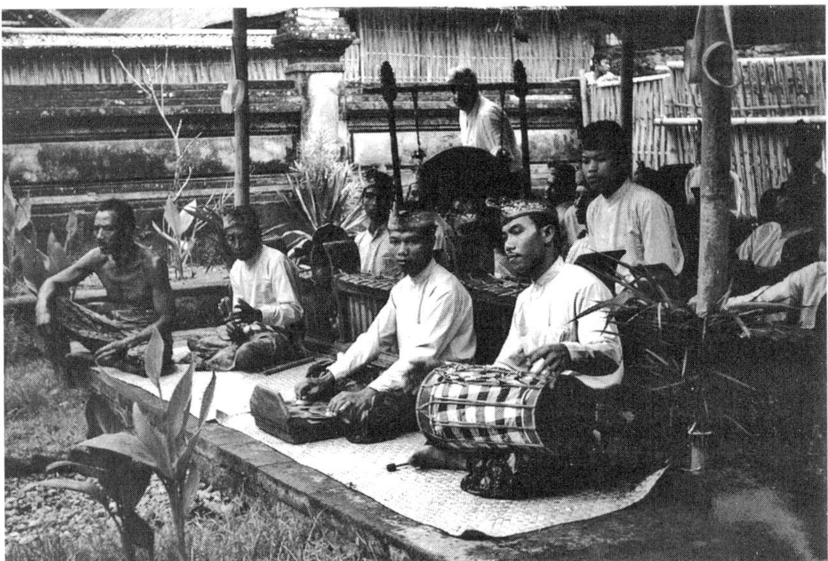

Figure 8.3. Balinese gamelan ensemble.

Different melodic motifs are associated with the numerous characters of the drama. At the point in the drama when the struggle between Rangda and the entranced human followers begins, the gamelan plays a short, loud, and furious ostinato pattern. It is important to note that the music does not *cause* the trance nor the self-stabbing. Members of the audience are also hearing the music but seldom go into trance. Sometimes a designated trancer will withdraw if his trance is shallow. And sometimes, contrary to expectations, an audience member may be overcome with rage and frustration and join the circle of trancers, be given a dagger by one of the attendants, and begin leaping about while stabbing himself.

The violent encounter between Rangda and Barong always ends in a standoff but somehow serves to restore cosmic balance. The young men come out of the trance feeling exhausted but relaxed, with faint memories of their spirit encounter.

The Emotions of Trance

> As for me, it is as if there were someone ordering me to stab. When it's like that, if I don't get hold of a kris [dagger], I should

> die, so strong is my anger. (Quoted from Rawa [Belo 1960, 128])

> When I come up to that tower, when the curtain opens like that, as soon as I step up to approach Rangda, I see a strong fire coming from her eyes. I just—"Oh! (slaps his hands together) I do this! I just jump! I feel myself just floating—because of the excitement, the aroma, the fragrances . . . whenever they pick up the music (sings "janga janga janga"), whenever you sing that song (sings a bit of gamelan "encounter" music) people just go crazy. I want to attack her! (I Wayan Dibia, interview, 1996)

Trancing always seems to be accompanied by strong emotions. In my research those emotions most commonly in evidence are joy (Pentecostals, Sufis), sadness (Sufis), or anger (Balinese *bebuten* trancers). The strong emotions of trancers link the music, insensitivity to pain and fatigue, and the perceptions of trancers that they have been in close contact with spirits, deities, demons, or a transcendent God. Emotion, music, and the numinous seem to be a unit, music reinforcing emotion, and both propelling the trancer into a sense of closeness with the holy, the unseen, the spiritual world.

In the Barong/Rangda ritual, the continuously playing gamelan creates the aura of a differing reality, a sound-mediated reality that renders plausible the appearance of deities and demons in the realm of humans. As one after another of the multitude of characters in the drama appear, the gamelan plays leitmotifs for each, both signaling their presence and making real their transition from the "other" world. The presence of these beings is in itself emotion producing. One is not likely to be indifferent to the denizens of the "other" world who so strongly affect one's everyday life. Without their signature tunes, without the aural envelop of the mythmaking music, their presence would not be nearly so affective. Music "sets the stage," fills the aural environment, and embraces all in its imaginary world.

In Bali, there are many categories of trance that relate to the nature of the possessing spiritual being. Some of these terms are: *kalinggihan,* possessed by an ancestor or a deity; *kasurupan,* to be chosen to be possessed, not necessarily in accordance with one's own will; *ngadep,* to have one's body borrowed; *kapangluh,* to be possessed by a refined spirit. Those who perform the roles of the attackers of Rangda are classified as *bebuten,* "possessed by *buta,*" a category of low spiritual beings, coarse of mind and body with only primitive emotions. Were the trancers to be possessed by a higher spiritual being, they would not exhibit anger as their dominant emotion and would move more slowly and smoothly. Because they are *bebuten,* they behave predictably like *buta.* They are filled with rage and a desire to attack the perceived generator of their anger, the great witch Rangda.

What Is Emotion?

In his famous and controversial theory of the emotions, William James claimed that the physiological component of arousal is primary and precedes the interpretation of the subsequent emotion (1950 [1890], 2: 442–485). The "feeling" of anger is the feeling that results from an increased heartbeat, an increase of blood to the face, an angry facial expression, an aggressive bodily stance, shallow breathing, and so on. Anger, the emotion, *is,* according to James, what one *feels* when enacting this display.[3] Following James, but with much more sophisticated knowledge of the neurophysiology of emotion and a more nuanced and inclusive theory of emotion, Damasio claims that the term "emotion" should be applied to the autonomic arousal of specific cortical and subcortical structures and that "feeling" that generally follows "emotion" should be applied to the complex cognitive, culturally inflected, and secondary interpretation of "emotion": "The term *feeling* should be reserved for the private, mental experience of an emotion, while the term *emotion* should be used to designate the collection of responses, many of which are publicly observable" (Damasio 1999, 42).

The generation of the initiating physiological emotion, in this theory, is not under conscious control. We normally understand that we do not will ourselves to feel anger or sadness or elation. Damasio cites the one exception he found, which he believes to be rare, of the pianist Maria Joao Pires, who claims to be able to either hold back or enhance her emotional involvement while listening to music or playing music.

Damasio was skeptical and submitted her to a test including skin conductance response and rate of heartbeat. One listening test was a "hold back emotion" listening; the other was an "emotional release" listening. She not only demonstrated her conscious control over bodily reactions believed to be autonomic, but she repeated the experiment and with the same results for a colleague who was sure someone had erred in the first experiment (Damasio 1999, 50).

I believe that control of the autonomic bodily responses of emotion and the ability to affect the intensity of those physiological responses constitute one definition of a trancer. One of the startling aspects of religious trancing worldwide is its stereotypicity. Trancers behave exactly the way in which they have learned to behave, and trance behavior is narrowly circumscribed by time and place. In my hometown, Pentecostal trancing can be witnessed each Sunday morning between 10:30 AM and noon, in a particular church, with all trancers following basically the same gestural script. Likewise, in the Rangda/Barong ceremony, the trancers who attack Rangda and then turn their knives against themselves do so on cue, so to speak. Very rarely do they enter trance before the proper narrative moment. Precisely at the point in the drama at which they begin trancing, their actions, gestures, and the duration of the trancing are predictable. Trance behavior is much more circumscribed, more stereotypical than everyday behavior. Trancers follow a script that determines the time of the onset of trance, the duration of trance, behavior during trance, and the style of withdrawal from trance.

How do they do it?

I believe they do it by control over the physiology of emotional arousal. To use the vernacular, they are able to turn on strong emotions at will. Trancers are not able to describe this process any more than pianist Maria Joao Pires could describe the opening and shutting of her floodgates of emotion. Like riding a bike, or learning via biofeedback, once you learn, you do not forget. You know that you know but cannot describe the knowing to another. The trancers at a Barong/Rangda ritual "permit" emotional arousal upon hearing music and finding themselves players in a religious drama. I suspect that strong emotional arousal helps precipitate the onset of a changed core and changed extended consciousness, a trancing consciousness characterized by its limitations, its focus, and its noetic quality.[4]

The Feeling of Emotion, Numinous Experience, and Musical Stimulation

A theory of consciousness and a theory of the emotion-stimulating properties of music may forward our understanding of the conjoining of music, religious trancing, and pain reduction. What follows is a plausible hypothesis to help stimulate dialogue and begin to bridge the scientific and humanistic approaches to extraordinary kinds of consciousness. The theory of consciousness presented here is modeled on that proposed by neurophysiologist Antonio Damasio (1994, 1999).

I suspect that many of the first-person descriptions of trance experience, such as the sense of timelessness, of living in the eternal present, and the sense of closeness to the divine are related to the strong emotions enhanced by music of the trance experience. Emotional arousal stimulates neurons in the hypothalamus, basal forebrain, and brain stem to release chemical substances into several other regions of the brain including the cortical areas associated with what are called the "higher" functions of the brain (see Figure 8.4).

At the neuronal level, the intensity of the feeling of emotion is partially a result of the action of the chemicals released in response to the inducer of emotion. Neurochemicals can be either inhibitory or excitatory. In addition, at each synapse the impulse can be either modulated, duplicated exactly, reduced, increased, or delayed. As input from the

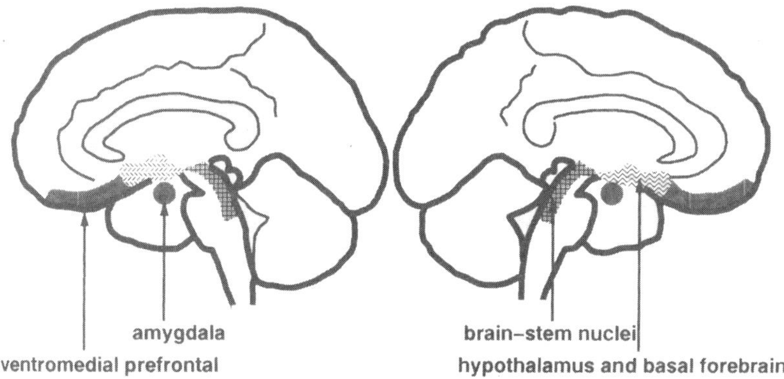

Figure 8.4. Principal emotion induction sites. Only one of these four sites is visible on the brain's surface (the ventromedial prefrontal region).

senses percolates to different parts of the brain and the nervous system, it gets processed at every stage. In Cytowic's words, "the neuron . . . is a storyteller that accentuates some features, completely ignores others, and is our fragile link to the physical world" (1989, 3). All perception is shaped, filtered, and processed.

> The result of these coordinated chemical and neural commands is a global change in the state of the organism. . . . But the brain itself is changed just as remarkably. The release of substances such as monoamines and peptides from regions of nuclei in the brain stem and basal forebrain alters the mode of processing of numerous other brain circuits, triggers certain specific behaviors (for example, bonding, playing, crying) and modifies the signaling of body states to the brain. In other words, both the brain and the body proper are largely and profoundly affected by the set of commands although the origin of those commands is circumscribed to a relatively small brain area which responds to a particular content of the mental process. (Damasio 1999, 67)

The chemicals released in the brain of the trancer who is imagining himself or herself in the company of beings from the spirit world, who is emotionally excited by the sounds of the gamelan may well include some of the natural opiates or endogenous opioid peptides (Fields 1987, 114–117). Peptides such as beta-endorphins are potent natural painkillers. Long-distance runners, some anorexics, and meditators have been found to have elevated beta-endorphin levels (Hooper and Teresi 1986, 80). I suspect that those in trance do also. The ability to withstand turning a dagger on oneself and the abatement of the pain of arthritis at a concert seem to be related phenomena. Balinese trancers not only do not feel pain when stabbing themselves, but they also rarely display any resultant physical trauma, such as open, bleeding wounds. Do the chemicals released by emotional arousal have the ability not only to impede the sensation of pain but to prevent the physical damage that would normally accompany the pain as well? Hearing the music enhances the emotion and the resultant stimulation of the production and release of certain hormones and monoamines, resulting in more intense feelings of rage. Along with rage, the trancers feel themselves to be in the presence of spirits from another realm, some of whom have temporarily taken over their bodies; for a while at least, the unseen world of powerful spirits is coterminous with their everyday Balinese world. They are enacting a cosmic narrative that is profoundly emotional, a drama that has changed the chemistry of their brains.

One result of this chemical bath can be the sensation of the slowing down of the mind processes as images are continually processed.

> The changes related to cognitive state are no less interesting. . . . The full range of alterations is not completely understood yet, but here are the most important I envision . . . a change in the mode of cognitive processing such that, for example, the rate of production of auditory or visual images can be changed (from slow to fast or vice versa) or the focus of images can be changed (from sharply focused to vaguely focused): changes in rate of production or focus are an integral part of emotions as disparate as those of sadness or elation. (Damasio 1999, 79–80)

The slower the processing of neural images becomes, the more removed one feels from the "time" of living bodies progressing from sunrise to sunset in a nonstop succession of activities and neural images. Slowing the mind is one aim of meditation and, I suspect, a by-product of trance consciousness as well.

Damasio's Theory of Consciousness and the Balinese Trancers

Damasio posits two levels of consciousness: core consciousness and extended consciousness, the equivalents of his core self and autobiographical self. We do not normally experience a distinction between these levels of self, but Damasio's clinical studies indicate that this distinction can be experimentally demonstrated. Condensing pages of vivid descriptions, Damasio summarizes his theory in Figure 8.5.

One of the aspects of Damasio's theory of consciousness that seems to make it relevant to the trancing experience is his belief that consciousness is the act of attributing to one's self whatever it is that one has just experienced through or in one's body. Until the experience is felt as *one's own,* there is sentience but not yet consciousness. Trancers have full consciousness but not the feeling that what they experience

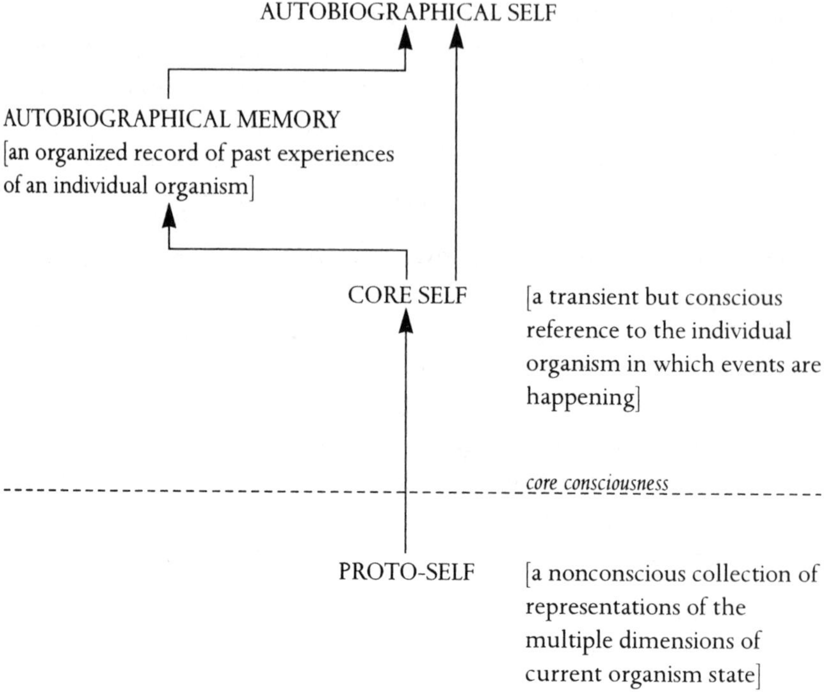

Figure 8.5. Kinds of self. The arrow between the nonconscious proto-self and the conscious core self represents the transformation that occurs as a result of the mechanism of core consciousness. The arrow toward autobiographical memory denotes the memorization of repeated instances of core-self experiences. The two arrows toward autobiographical self signify its dual dependency on both continuous pulses of core consciousness and continuous reactivations of autobiographical memories.

belongs to their autobiographical selves. The trancing experience belongs to the trance persona, not the autobiographical self of the Balinese peasant who trances.

Core Consciousness: The Core Self

For Damasio, core consciousness is an awareness of one's body in relation to the enveloping environment. Imagining oneself in the woods of northern Michigan, the information basic to core consciousness would include the following parameters: physical positioning (I am in the woods), emotional state (I am happy), thermal state (It is a bit chilly here), visceral state (I am starting to feel hungry), aural impressions

(Did I hear a bear?), and all other immediate bodily impressions (see Figure 8.6).[5]

This type of consciousness is clearly not simple but already complex. According to Damasio, core consciousness changes from moment to moment, from birth till death. "Core" relates not to what we might imagine as enduring, as primal, as stable, but rather to the kind of consciousness of the "here and now," the immediacy of one's bodily relationship to the enveloping environment at the present moment.

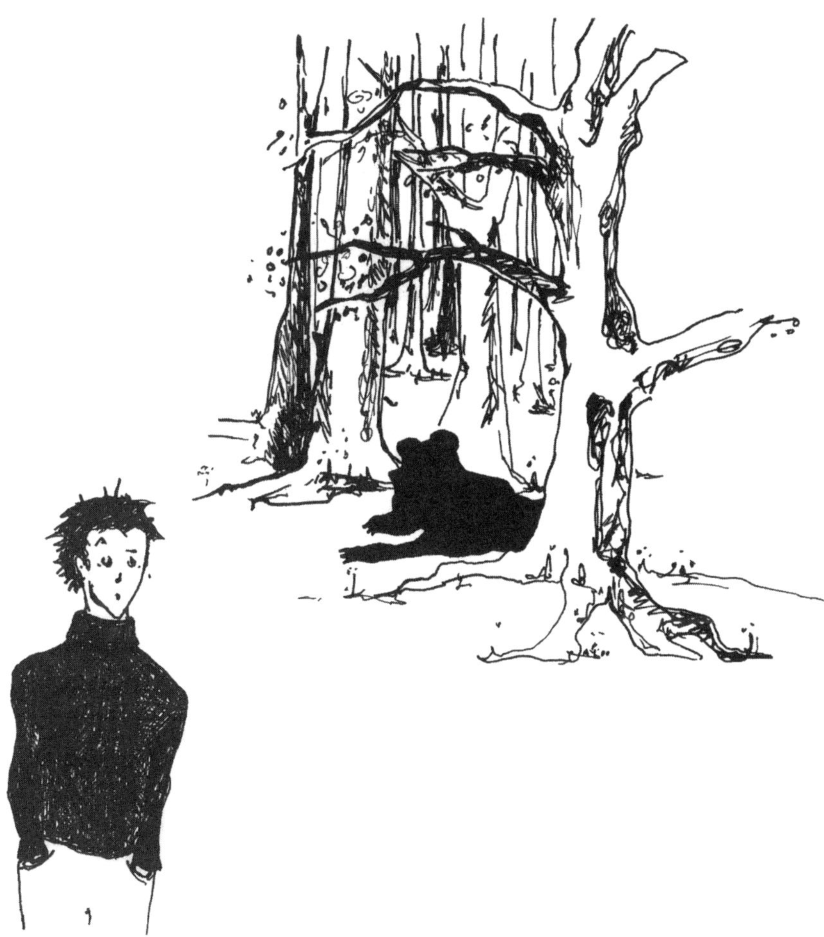

Figure 8.6. Person in woods with a bear behind a tree.

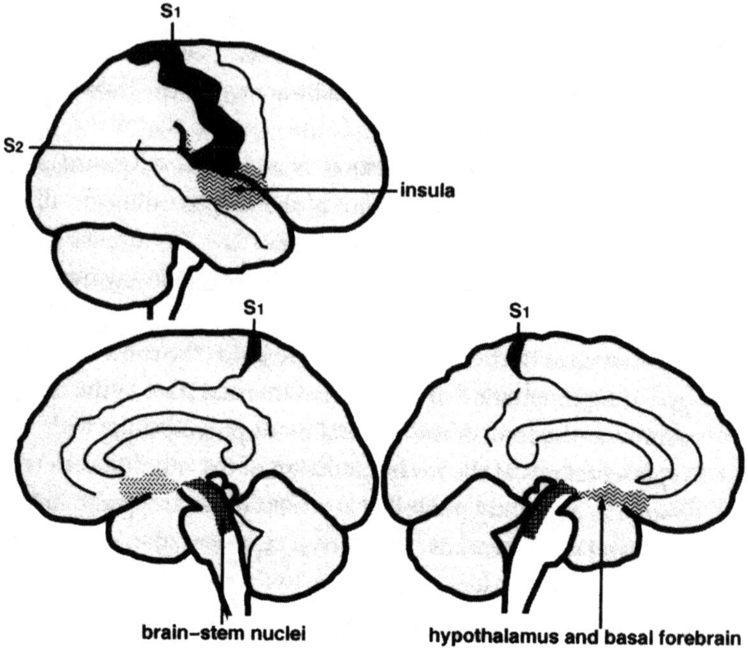

Figure 8.7. Location of some proto-self structures. Note that the region known as the insula is buried inside the sylvian fissure and is not visible on the cortical surface.

Preceding core consciousness, according to Damasio, there needs to occur a juxtaposition in the brain of two different first-order neural mappings. The first neural mapping is of the moment-by-moment internal physical state of the organism, called "body-map" or "proto-self." The body-map or proto-self is ceaselessly updated and results from neural patterns at several levels in the brain, including the brain stem nuclei, the basal forebrain, the hypothalamus, and parts of the somatosensory cortices. We are not conscious of the proto-self (see Figure 8.7).

> *The proto-self is a coherent collection of neural patterns which map, moment by moment, the state of the physical structure of the organism in its many dimensions.* This ceaselessly maintained first-order collection of neural patterns occurs not in one brain place but in many, at a multiplicity of levels, from the brain stem to the cerebral cortex, in structures that are interconnected by neural

> pathways. . . . The proto-self is not to be confused with the rich sense of self on which our current knowing is centered this very moment. *We are not conscious of the proto-self.* Language is not part of the structure of the proto-self. The proto-self has no powers of perception and holds no knowledge. (Damasio 1999, 154)

The second first-order neural mapping that precedes core consciousness is the mapping of images received from the senses or images internally generated, called "object-map." An "object" can be an entity projected from one of the senses, such as the sensation of seeing a bear or hearing a melody, or an entity generated internally such as a vision or a memory (see Figure 8.8).

An "image" is a neural pattern corresponding to an object conveying not only the look, sound, or feel of the object but also one's emotional response to it, its relationship to other objects, and one's own intentions regarding the object.

> By *object* I mean entities as diverse as a person, a place, a melody, a toothache, a state of bliss; by *image* I mean a mental pattern in any of the sensory modalities, e.g., a sound image, a tactile image, the image of a state of well-being. Such images convey aspects of the physical characteristics of the object and they may also convey the reaction of like or dislike one may have for an object, the

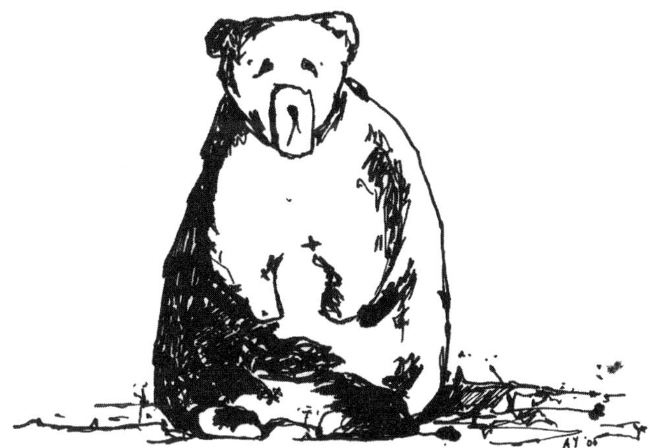

Figure 8.8. Object-map of bear projected by the visual cortext.

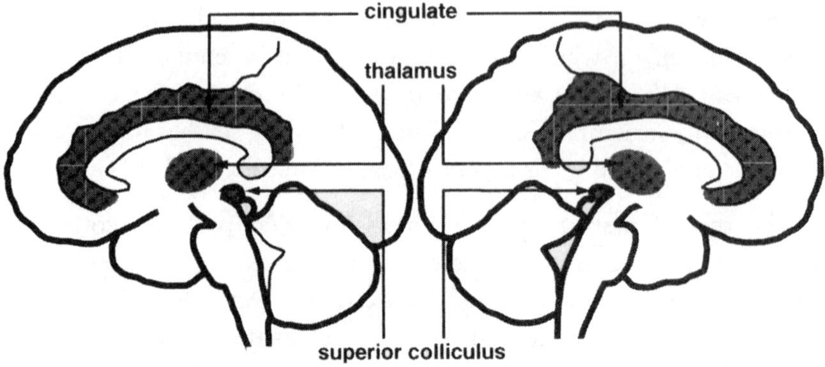

Figure 8.9. Location of main second-order structures.

> plans one may formulate for it, or the web of relationships of that object among other objects. (Damasio 1999, 9)

Core consciousness is the result of second-order mappings of the *relationship* between these two kinds of first-order mappings, that is, a mapping of the "object" (what is perceived or thought about) and the body-map or proto-self (see Figure 8.9).

The second-order mapping of the relationship between them results in a new body-map and a new core consciousness, now, a startled man in the woods of northern Michigan (see Figure 8.10).

Damasio also holds that an enhancement of the object-map, or the image of whatever is perceived or thought about, results from the second-order mapping of the relationship between body-map and object-map. The man sees not just a bear but a special sort of bear (see Figure 8.11).

> The neuroanatomy underlying the imaged account of the relationship and the enhancement of object image includes the cingulate cortices, the thalamus, and the superior colliculli. . . . The subsequent image enhancement is achieved via modulation from basal forebrain/brain-stem acetylcholine and monoamine nuclei as well as from thalamocortical modulation. (Damasio 1999, 193–194)

The sense of a *changed* body-map, a result of the relationship between the object-map and body-map, gives rise to the sense that these

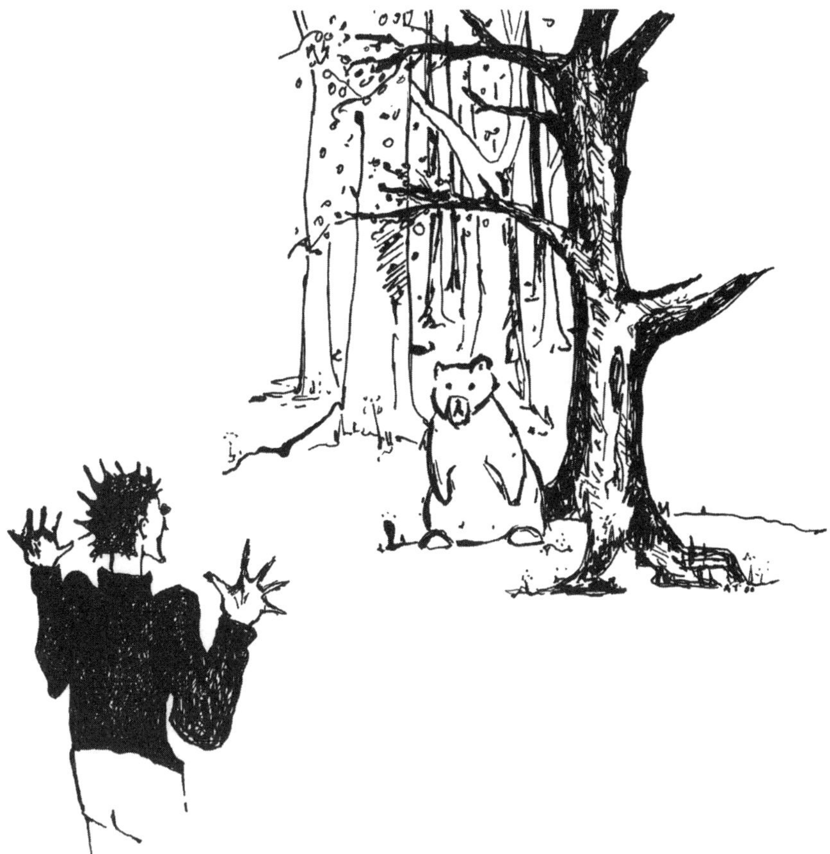

Figure 8.10. A startled man.

images belong to a *self*. Now, a terrified man has no doubt that the terror belongs to him (see Figure 8.12).

The core self, core consciousness, is the sense of *my* having these images and *my* knowing that they belong to *me*. This kind of here-and-now sense of a self, a knower of one's immediate situation, is Damasio's core consciousness.

Music and Core Consciousness: "Becoming the Music"

Trancers' core consciousness includes the fact that trancers are aware of the changing events around them, of themselves in relation to those

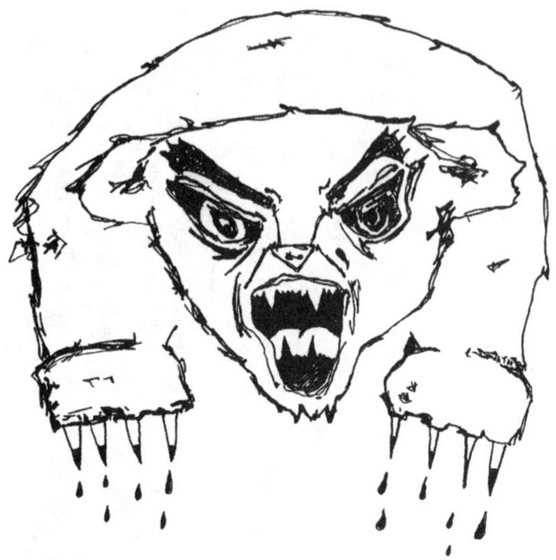

Figure 8.11. Enhanced image of bear.

events, and they respond appropriately moment by moment. For example, in one ritual I witnessed, the elaborate headdress of the man playing Rangda became loose. Even though in trance, Rangda momentarily stopped her infernal prancing about, stood still until an attendant had repaired the loose headdress, and then, after a moment's stillness, began the drama again in earnest.

In the Barong/Rangda ritual, the trancer also hears the Balinese gamelan play without pause. The drama is totally enveloped in the brilliant, vibrant, shimmering sounds of the gamelan. The rhythms of the gamelan and the intricate drum patterns are at every moment adjusted to the movements of whoever is at the center of attention at any dramatic moment. Drummers carefully watch the dancing, prancing characters and align melodies, tempos, and rhythms to every large and small gesture. Gamelan, drummers, and actors become one in a rhythmically coordinated domain.

The dramatic climax of the ritual, the hostile encounter between the trancers and Rangda, is accompanied by fast, loud, short temporal cycles played on the gamelan (see Figure 8.13).

In Balinese gamelan music, short, loud temporal cycles with no melodic elaboration indicate the presence of demons and fighting. No

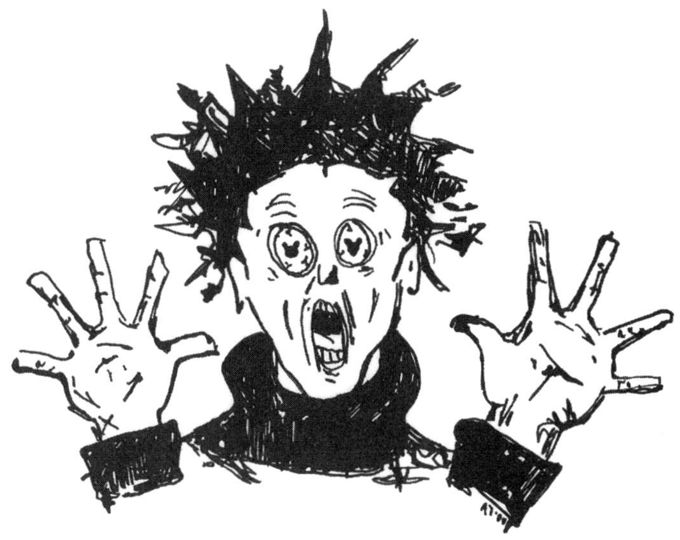

Figure 8.12. A terrified man.

Balinese music is more demonic, louder, or more minimalist than that which signals the encounter between the witch Rangda and the entranced men who attempt to thwart her power. The driving, incessant ostinatos of these themes are iconic of the emotions of fear and rage and the action of fighting. They undergird and sustain the manic frenzy of both the witch and her attackers. It is reasonable to assume that the gamelan music has a physiological impact on the men who participate and that groups of neurons in the brains and bodies of the trancers are firing synchronously with the gamelan rhythms. The clanging bronze keys of the metallophones, the booming gongs, and the pulsing rhythms of drums and cymbals, all synchronized, become one with the body and brain of the trancer.[6]

Gamelan music as object-map (sound) is juxtaposed with the body-map of the trancer. The second-order mapping of the relationship between the two results in a changed body-map and changed sense of core self. A "musicked" core consciousness must have a specific neurological pattern (see Figure 8.14).

Musicians from our culture often use an expression such as "I become the music" to describe their sense of self when playing music. Within the

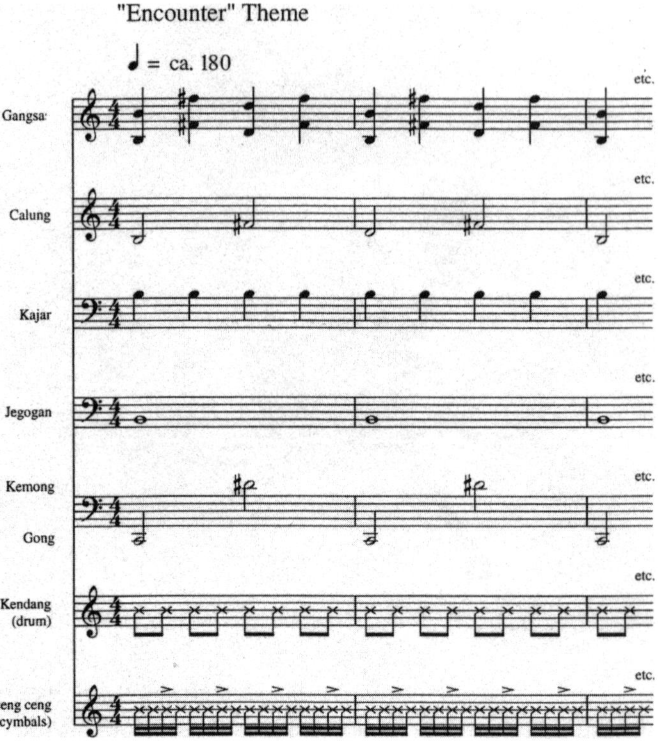

Figure 8.13. "Encounter" music.

frame of a "musicked" core consciousness, the phrase "I become the music" does not appear so metaphorical. As T. S. Eliot expressed it in *The Four Quartets:* "[Y]ou are the music while the music lasts." What are the ways in which the trancers' body-maps, their proto-selves, unknowing and unawares, respond to the insistent gamelan ostinatos? And how does this "musicked" proto-self change core consciousness?

Extended Consciousness: The Autobiographical Self

Damasio's core consciousness is complemented by extended consciousness that is linked to our personal history and our sense of who we are. For this reason his alternate term for extended consciousness is the term "autobiographical self." While core consciousness is constantly recreated moment by moment, we believe in a certain continuity or

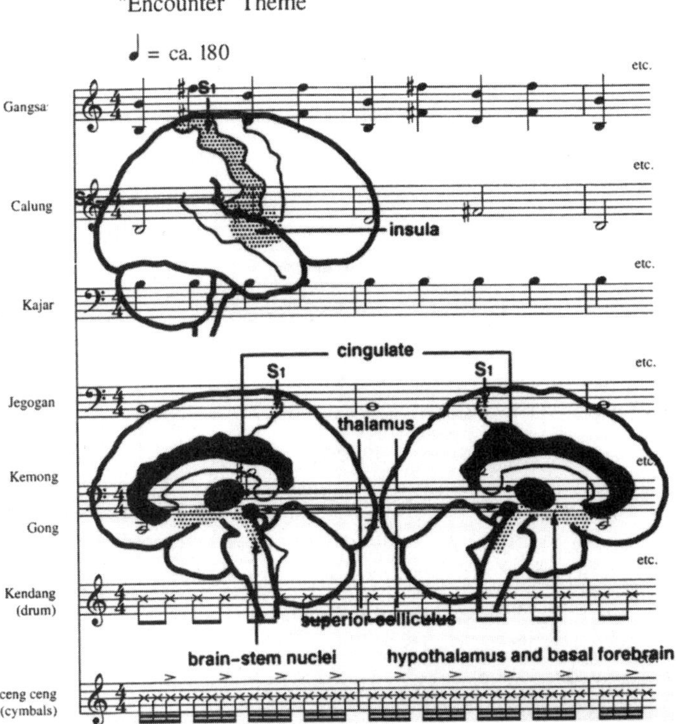

Figure 8.14. A "musicked" core consciousness.

"nontransient collection of unique facts and ways of being" in the establishment of the autobiographical self.

> Our traditional notion of self, however, is linked to the idea of identity and corresponds to a nontransient collection of unique facts and ways of being which characterize a person. My term for that entity is the *autobiographical self.* The autobiographical self depends on systematized memories of situations in which core consciousness was involved in the knowing of the most invariant characteristics of an organism's life—who you were born to, where, when, your likes and dislikes, the way you usually react to a problem or a conflict, your name, and so on. (Damasio 1999, 17)

Extended consciousness, according to Damasio, relates to the notion of identity and involves long-term memory, a sense of personal history, the narrative of one's own life. In humans, extended consciousness is a languaged consciousness encompassing not only a personal but a cultural history as well. Core consciousness becomes extended consciousness when multiple other maps, or neural patterns, are stimulated by the object-map, the body-map, and the second-order relationship map.

An image, an idea, a melody become richly overlaid with emotion, with knowledge about one's past experience with the image, and with values associated with the image.

Music and Extended Consciousness in Trancing: The Loss of the Autobiographical Self

WE ASKED: "And when they are stabbing their own breast, are they not even a little conscious of themselves?" To which Rena answered: "Not at all. I do not remember myself [*awak*] even a little bit; all I remember is the desire to stab my breast."

GM: "And if you have no kris [dagger], and, for instance, you try to get one from someone else, can't you remember who gave it to you?

RENA: At such a time I don't remember myself at all. For instance, if my headcloth should fall off and someone picked it up and did not return it to me, I would not be able to remember who it was who picked it up.

GM: What does it feel like when you have just been sprinkled with holy water?

RENA: When you've had holy water, then for the first time you feel like a person who has just awakened and got up from his bed. (Belo 1960, 105)

One of the salient features of possession trance is the apparent absence of, or inactivity of, or substitution for the autobiographical self. Trancers temporarily lose the sense of their private, autobiographical self in favor of the sense of the special self of trance possession.[7] Trancers' extended consciousness includes long-term memories of previous encounters with Rangda that become activated upon seeing Rangda again. They know what to feel and how to behave in relation to Rangda. This alternate trance self is necessarily impoverished in relation to their usual autobiographical self. The years of daily experiences, of interactions with persons and things, the laid-down memories of personal history have not occurred in relation to the extended self of trance possession. The entranced self is only experienced for a few minutes, or perhaps an hour or so, say, every few weeks. While the experience of the trance self lasts, the autobiographical self is forgotten.

The amnesia of trancers is in striking contrast to meditators who have crystal-clear memories of the processes and contents of their minds during meditation. Trance amnesia, I suspect, may be a result of the absence or inactivity of the autobiographical self during the trance period. The repertoire of pieces used in the Rangda/Barong ritual is largely specific to that ritual. All the memories, all the neural dispositions summoned by hearing the gamelan melodies, will refer to other instances of the same ritual. The possessed self is a self whose personal history and culture are largely circumscribed by the ritual event and the cosmology it invokes. The extended consciousness of the trancers, and thus their physical and cognitive behavior, is prescribed and stylized. They dance, they gesture, they react to others in the drama not as autobiographical selves but as the persona that the drama requires. Not until they are later brought out of trance within the inner sanctum of the temple is their full, rich, Balinese autobiographical self restored.

Could it be that the lifetime of associating the pains and fatigues of everyday life to the autobiographical self sets up the neural patterns whereby the pains and fatigues experienced while trancing are not associated with the trancing persona but with the absent autobiographical self? Could it be that the neural pattern dispositions for the autobiographical self are temporarily inactive, or not attended to by the trancers, and that the trancing body does not interpret its body-map as "fatigue" or "pain"? Could it be that the "I" who experiences the pain and fatigue is not, at the moment, paying attention?

> Knowing that you have pain requires something else that occurs after the neural patterns that correspond to the substrate of pain—the nociceptive signals—are displayed in the appropriate areas of the brain stem, thalamus, and cerebral cortex and generate an image of pain, a feeling of pain. But note that the "after" process to which I am referring is not beyond the brain, it is very much in the brain and, as far as I can fathom, is just as biophysical as the

> process that came before. Specifically, in the example above, it is a process that interrelates neural patterns of tissue damage with the neural patterns that stand for you, such that yet another neural pattern can arise—the neural pattern of you knowing, which is just another name for consciousness. If the latter interrelating process does not take place, you will never know that there was tissue damage in your organism—if there is no you and there is no knowing, there is no way for you to know, right? (Damasio 1999, 73)

Damasio's theory of the distinction between core consciousness and extended consciousness may be a way of thinking about the phenomenology of possession trance in terms of neurophysiological processes. A theory of consciousness, of the processes of consciousness, of the neural activity of producing consciousness needs to apply to extraordinary as well as to ordinary states of consciousness. Trancing may be an exceptional kind of consciousness, but its prevalence worldwide, its institutionalization within religious practices, and the fact that in locales where it is not deemed pathological its practitioners are ordinary people leading ordinary lives should lead us to reexamine our attitudes and our medicalized, pathological trance categories such as "multiple personality *disorder*" (Hacking 1995, 17) or "dissociative *disorder*" (Decker 1986, 48; Prince 1930, 288–294). Balinese *bebuten,* Sufi *hal,* and Pentecostal "slain in the Spirit" are not illnesses. They are socially sanctioned religious practices that bring comfort, solace, and an experience of the numinous to their practitioners. William James called trancing not only "natural" but also a "gift": "Mediumistic possession in all its grades seems to form a perfectly natural special type of alternate personality, and the susceptibility to it in some form is by no means an uncommon gift, in persons who have no other obvious nervous anomaly" (James 1950 [1890], 1: 393). Damasio's theory of the distinction between core consciousness and autobiographical consciousness allows one to imagine the neurophysiology of trance as the substitution of a different self during trancing, a trancing self who enacts a prescribed role within a stable, sacred narrative.

Music enhances the sense of a different imaginary world, provides a rhythmic template for the trancing body, increases emotional excitement, and facilitates the experience of a different self. The persona of the trancer may continue to ascribe his or her physical afflictions to the nontrancing persona and thus experiences a body-state that is often impervious to pain and fatigue. Concomitantly, the chemical bath stimulated by the emotions of the drama, the holiness of the event, and the accompanying music may be a powerful analgesic as well. In a phenomenon as complex as is trancing with music and not feeling pain nor fatigue, we need all the theoretical help we can muster. And currently some of the most compelling theories are coming from neurophysiology.

Notes

Epigraph: From James (1982 [1902]), 388.

1. I prefer the gerund "trancing" to the more common "trance state," as trancing is always a transitional, moving practice—a process that changes from moment to moment and that steadily moves toward its completion and fulfillment.
2. Research by musicologists on music and pain is nearly always framed around the issues of music as expressing painful experience, music as iconic of pain, or music as a symbolic representation of pain (Meyer 1956; Dahlhaus 1982; Kivy 1989). The literature on music as physical therapy does not address the ways of representing pain musically but speaks to the phenomenon of realizing greater freedom of physical movement while listening to music, which in itself may lead to the alleviation of pain. Oliver Sacks vividly describes the almost magical contribution of listening to Mendelssohn's Violin Concerto to his learning to walk again and to the ultimate rehabilitation of his smashed leg (Sacks 1984).
3. William James's theory of the emotions has been largely dismissed by contemporary psychologists and neurophysiologists. James never adequately allowed for the reverse process in the generation of emotion, that is, the idea that strong emotions can be initially generated by thought and then be reflected in the body. Ironically, Asian theatrical traditions, especially Kathakali from South India, have long trained actors to "feel" emotion by first embodying its physical characteristics. In the West, the Jamesian approach to emotion was also followed by the Polish director Jerzy Grotowski and his disciples (Grotowski 1968). A number of social scientists and psychologists have called for a reopening of a discussion of the Jamesian theory of emotion. See especially Solomon 1984; Ekman 1992, Ekman and Davidson 1993; Ekman, Levenson, and Friesen 1983; Zajonc 1984.
4. Trancers feel that they have been given access to a special kind of knowing, a special state of knowledge. William James posited that the two primary

qualities of mystic states are ineffability and their noetic quality (James 1982 [1902], 380).

5. William James also used the "bear" example (James 1950 [1890], 2: 450).
6. Studies of what is called "rhythmic entrainment" describe how the rhythms of body and brain become synchronized when groups of people listen to or dance to strongly rhythmic music. Rhythmic entrainment facilitates feelings of oneness, unity with other people, and unity with the holy and helps coordinate communal action (see Chapple 1970; Hall 1977; Condon 1986; Rider and Eagle 1986; Vaughn 1990; Wallin 1991; McNeill 1995).
7. What is more difficult to explain is the fact that experienced, skilled trancers oftentimes do remember their trances. Is this "lucid trancing" related to the phenomenon of "lucid dreaming" in which a self seems to occupy two different positions simultaneously? Is the "lucid trancer" simultaneously the trance persona *and* his/her autobiographical self?

References

Alkon, D. L. 1992. *Memory's Voice: Deciphering the Mind-Brain Code.* New York: HarperCollins.

Becker, J. 2004. *Deep Listeners: Music, Emotion, and Trancing.* Bloomington: Indiana University Press.

Belo, J. 1960. *Trance in Bali.* New York: Columbia University Press.

Caciola, N. 1994. "Discerning Spirits: Sanctity and Possession in the Later Middle Ages." Ph.D. dissertation, University of Michigan.

Chapple, E. D. 1970. *Culture and Biological Man: Explorations in Behavioral Anthropology.* New York: Holt, Rinehart and Winston.

Condon, W. S. 1986. "Communication: Rhythm and Structure." In J. Evans and M. Clynes, eds., *Rhythm in Psychological, Linguistic and Musical Processes.* Springfield, Ill.: C. C. Thomas, 55–77.

Cytowic, R. E. 1989. *Synesthesia: A Union of the Senses.* New York: Springer-Verlag.

Dahlhaus, C. 1982. *Esthetics of Music.* Trans. W. W. Austin. Cambridge: Cambridge University Press.

Damasio, A. R. 1994. *Descartes' Error: Emotion, Reason, and the Human Brain.* New York: Grosset/Putnam.

———. 1999. *The Feeling of What Happens: Body and Emotion in the Making of Consciousness.* New York: Harcourt Brace.

Decker, H. 1986. "The Lure of Nonmaterialism in Materialist Europe: Investigations of Dissociative Phenomena, 1880–1915." In J. M. Quen, ed., *Split Minds/Split Brains.* New York: New York University Press, 31–62.

Dennett, D. C. 1991. *Consciousness Explained.* London: Little, Brown.

Edelman, G. M. 1992. *Bright Air, Brilliant Fire: On the Matter of the Mind.* New York: Basic Books.

Ekman, P. 1992. "Facial Expressions of Emotion: New Findings, New Questions." *Psychological Science* 3: 34–38.

Ekman, P., and R. J. Davidson. 1993. "Voluntary Smiling Changes Regional Brain Activity." *Psychological Science* 4: 342–345.

Ekman, P., R. W. Levenson, and W. V. Friesen. 1983. "Autonomic Nervous System Activity Distinguishes among Emotions." *Science* 221: 1208–1210.

Fields, H. L. 1987. *Pain.* New York: McGraw-Hill.

Friedson, S. M. 1996. *Dancing Prophets: Musical Experience in Tumbuka Healing.* Chicago: University of Chicago Press.

Grotowski, J. 1968. *Towards a Poor Theatre.* New York: Simon and Schuster.

Hacking, I. 1995. *Rewriting the Soul: Multiple Personality and the Sciences of Memory.* Princeton: Princeton University Press.

Hall, E. 1977. *Beyond Culture.* Garden City, N.Y.: Anchor Books.

Hobson, J. A. 1994. *The Chemistry of Conscious States: How the Brain Changes Its Mind.* London: Little, Brown.

Hooper, J., and D. Teresi. 1986. *The 3-Pound Universe.* New York: Dell.

Inglis, B. 1989. *Trance: A Natural History of Altered States of Mind.* Toronto: Grafton Books.

James, W. 1950 [1890]. *The Principles of Psychology,* 2 vols. New York: Dover Publications.

———. 1982 [1902]. *The Varieties of Religious Experience.* New York: Penguin Books.

Kapferer, B. 1991. *A Celebration of Demons: Exorcism and the Aesthetics of Healing in Sri Lanka.* Washington, D.C.: Smithsonian Institution Press.

Kivy, P. 1989. *Sound Sentiment: An Essay on the Musical Emotions.* Philadelphia: Temple University Press.

LeDoux, J. 1996. *The Emotional Brain: The Mysterious Underpinnings of Emotional Life.* New York: Simon and Schuster.

Maturana, H., and F. Varela. 1987. *The Tree of Knowledge: The Biological Roots of Human Understanding.* Boston: New Science Library.

McNeill, W. H. 1995. *Keeping Together in Time: Dance and Drill in Human History.* Cambridge, Mass.: Harvard University Press.

Meyer, L. 1956. *Emotion and Meaning in Music.* Chicago: University of Chicago Press.

Prince, M. 1930. *The Dissociation of a Personality: A Biographical Study in Abnormal Psychology.* London: Longmans, Green and Co.

Rider, M. S., and C. T. Eagle, Jr. 1986. "Rhythmic Entrainment as a Mechanism for Learning in Music Therapy." In J. Evans and M. Clynes, eds., *Rhythm in Psychological, Linguistic and Musical Processes.* Springfield, Ill.: C. C. Thomas, 225–248.

Rouget, G. 1985. *Music and Trance: A Theory of the Relations between Music and Possession*. Trans. B. Biebuyck. Chicago: University of Chicago Press.

Sacks, O. 1984. *A Leg to Stand On*. New York: Summit Books.

Solomon, R. C. 1984. "The Jamesian Theory of Emotion in Anthropology." In R. Shweder and R. LeVine, eds., *Culture Theory: Essays on Mind, Self, and Emotion*. Cambridge: Cambridge University Press, 238–254.

Squire, L. R. 1987. *Memory and Brain*. Oxford: Oxford University Press.

Vaughn, K. 1990. "Exploring Emotion in Sub-Structural Aspects of Karelian Lament: Application of Time Series Analysis to Digitalized Melody." *Yearbook for Traditional Music* 22: 106–122.

Wallin, N. L. 1991. *Biomusicology: Neurophysiological, Neuropsychological, and Evolutionary Perspectives on the Origins and Purposes of Music*. Stuyvesant, N.Y.: Pendragon Press.

Zajonc, R. B. 1984. "On the Primacy of Affect." *American Psychologist* 39: 117–123.

Response:
Music as Ecstasy and Music as Trance

John C. M. Brust

The late British neurologist McDonald Critchley said, "Music can bring about a veritable perceptual spectrum, ranging from the simple reception of auditory sense data to impressions which in sensitive subjects are so evocative, overwhelming and transcendental as to defy description" (1977a, 217).

Critchley defines "ecstasy" as cosmic consciousness, the "mystical" change in self-awareness. In states of ecstasy there develops a curious state of merging whereby the subject becomes identified with external reality, which itself is endowed with a feeling of complete personal significance. He cites William James, who gave the following features to so-called mystical ecstasy: transience, passivity, ineffability, and noetic quality. Critchley cites a conductor of international renown, an acquaintance of his who during music would imagine himself released, as it were, from his own body and transported to the rafters of the theater. From that lofty vantage point he would visualize himself in miniature, confronting yet dominating his orchestra.

I think there is an obvious resemblance of Karelian lament to ecstasy, but the embodied status of representation makes it rather more concrete and literal than the more abstract nature of most music, which is able to produce ecstasy without text or iconic imagery.

Ecstasy resembles trance. I was interested that you never used the word "hypnosis," which is how I would characterize trance. Unlike ecstasy, trance produces amnesia and is more determined by suggestibility and expectation. Response to suggestions produces altered perception, memory, or action, including the loss of pain perception. During trance or hypnosis, stimuli are unconsciously registered and stored, rather like procedural memory, when you can learn how to do motor tasks even though you have a severe amnesic disorder. You won't remember having taken the lessons, but you'll unaccountably have learned how to serve a tennis ball. At a prearranged signal, memory returns for events during a trance. This kind of unconscious perception, memory, and action has nothing to do with Freudian notions of the unconscious. Indeed, during hypnosis, so-called recovered memories are largely inaccurate and determined by suggestibility.

I want quickly to describe four types of positive phenomena that neurologists encounter in music. They are positive, unlike amusia, the loss of musical ability, although some of them are pathological, and some are trivial or probably even normal. "Musicogenic epilepsy" refers to the ability of music to trigger a seizure. It tends to occur in musically talented people. It can occur with any type of music, depending on the person: classical, pop, salsa, or single pieces. There is a report of a portion of Rimsky-Korsakoff's *Snow Maiden* triggering seizures (Critchley 1977b, 344). There is a report of a patient whose seizures were triggered by the second movement of Beethoven's Fifth Symphony (Sutherling et al. 1980). It's probably related more to the sound pattern than the emotional structure of the music. There's a description of church bells in a particular pattern within an octave range that triggered seizures (Poskanzer, Brawn, and Miller 1962).

I was able to find a report of rock music producing a pain in the face, perhaps as a seizure phenomenon (Yanagada 1983). However, pain as a seizure manifestation, other than postictally, is most unusual.

Critchley also described musicophobia preceding a seizure. The patient heard *Waltz of the Flowers*, by Tchaikovsky, and after fifteen seconds "[h]er face took on a restless and pained expression and respirations became labored, the eyelids began to open and shut. She appeared distressed, her fingers clutching the bed clothes, her lips performing rapid smacking movements, then a vacant stare and she went into a grand mal seizure" (Critchley 1937, 13).

It's been suggested that Joan of Arc's visions might have been musicogenic seizures. At her trial, she described: "I heard the voices three times, once in the morning, once at vespers, and again, when the *Ave Maria* rang in the evening" (Foote-Smith and Boyne 1991).

The second type is musical partial seizure. These are seizures that consist of hallucinated music. Again, it can be almost any type of music, and it varies with the person. I saw one patient, an older man, whose seizures took the form of hearing Glen Gray and the Casa Loma Orchestra playing "Sweet and Low." He had never been particularly fond of the Casa Loma Orchestra, but when I pointed out to him what was coming out of the radio these days, he decided he could live with it. In one of his summary papers in the 1960s (Penfield and Perot 1963), Wilder Penfield described musical partial seizures with a male chorus and orchestra performing "White Christmas," a radio jingle, organ music without words, an orchestra playing in a musical hall that was simultaneously visually hallucinated, and so forth.

The third type is release hallucination and tends to occur in older people who are losing their hearing. They start hallucinating music. A woman heard Irish jigs and Christmas carols; as her hearing got worse, it degenerated into rock and roll and then finally frank tinnitus. Some patients have been able to dial a tune with it, which is interesting. When they start hearing the music, if they think hard enough about it, they can pick something more to their liking, as if they were changing stations.

Finally, synesthesia refers to one stimulus producing an inappropriate sensory response. In this case, sound produces visual hallucinations, generally just colors or maybe simple geometric shapes but not LSD-like panoramas. Sometimes a particular tone will produce a particular color—for example, G sharp is red, D is green. There was a very well studied teenage boy who had the same hallucination every time, yet he did not have absolute pitch (Rizzo and Eslinger 1989).

The mechanism of these four phenomena is simply not understood. So it's not really surprising that something as complicated as music being able to induce trance or ecstasy is not very well understood, either.

Steven Pinker puzzled about this in his book *How the Mind Works* (1997). He refers to music as auditory cheesecake. He thinks that it's an accident that just happens to be there. As he puts it, perhaps it is a resonance in the brain between neurons firing in synchrony with a sound wave and a natural oscillation of the emotion circuits. Perhaps it is some kind of spandrel or a crawl space or short circuit or coupling that came along as an accident of the way auditory emotional language and motor circuits are packed together in the brain.

So as we say in our field, more work needs to be done in this area. It is surprising how little research money is devoted to these topics.

References

Critchley, M. 1937. "Musicogenic Epilepsy." *Brain* 60: 13.

———. 1977a. "Ecstatic and Synaesthetic Experiences during Musical Perception." In *Music and the Brain: Studies in the Neurology of Music,* by M. Critchley and R. Menson. Springfield, Ill.: C. C. Thomas.

———. 1977b. "Musicogenic Epilepsy (1) The Beginnings." In *Music and the Brain: Studies in the Neurology of Music,* by M. Critchley and R. Menson. Springfield, Ill.: C. C. Thomas.

Foote-Smith, E., and L. Boyne. 1991. "Joan of Arc." *Epilepsia* 32: 810–815.

Penfield, W., and P. Perot. 1963. "The Brain's Record of Auditory and Visual Experience." *Brain* 86: 595.

Pinker, S. 1997. *How the Mind Works.* New York: W. W. Norton.

Poskanzer, C., E. Brawn, and H. Miller. 1962. "Musicogenic Epilepsy Caused by Only a Discrete Frequency Band of Church Bells." *Brain* 85: 77.

Rizzo, M., and P. J. Eslinger. 1989. "Colored Hearing Synesthesia: An Investigation of Neural Factors." *Neurology* 39: 781.

Sutherling, W. W., L. M. Hershman, J. Q. Miller, and S. I. Lee. 1980. "Seizures Induced by Playing Music." *Neurology* 30: 1001.

Yanagada, H. 1983. "Facial Pain Induced by Music." *Anesthesiology* 58: 388.

Response:
Thinking about Music and Pain

Kay Kaufman Shelemay

In responding to the excellent essays of Elizabeth Tolbert and Judith Becker, it is important to note that Tolbert and Becker address musical processes that stand in somewhat different relationships to pain. Let me map out three important ways in which music relates to pain, only two of which are touched on in Tolbert and Becker's essays. I would then like to contribute a short discussion about the specialists who transform pain through their musical expertise and practices.

As we have learned from Tolbert's nuanced discussion of the Karelian lament, Karelian women express the pain of loss through a musical-expressive form incorporating pitched melody, wailing, and weeping. The Karelian lament constitutes at once a representation and experience of pain. In this case, pain has been experienced prior to its "vocalization" in a lament, the performance of which sets into motion a cathartic process through which pain can be expressed and acknowledged in socially sanctioned ways. The lament, as discussed by Tolbert, transforms pain into musical expression, moving the coded sound from the body of the singer into the realm of community sensibility. Lament in this instance can be said to provide (to use Arthur Kleinman's original term) a "language" through which acute pain can be vocalized; the pain discharged through this musical channel existed prior to its vocalization. In the case of the Karelian lament, the individual suffering gives voice to the pain.

In contrast, Becker takes a close look at music and trance, investigating the Balinese Barong-Rangda ceremony during which the trancers participate in a musical process that (if successful) will serve to block the pain that might otherwise be experienced during the course of the ritual to be performed subsequently. In this case, music provides an analgesic in advance of what would otherwise be a painful stimulus: in the Barong-Rangda ritual, dancers stab themselves with short daggers *(kris)*. Becker draws on the theory of consciousness proposed by Antonio Damasio to provide a hypothesis through which one might more fully imagine "trance consciousness." While one of Becker's goals is to move consideration of trance from the category of cultural "marvel" to a framework accessible to scientific research, she implicitly raises a number of other issues in her essay. In contrast to Tolbert's lamenting Karelian women, who sing to rid themselves of pain they have already experienced and internalized, Becker's male trancers move into an altered state to avoid pain and do not themselves perform or generate the musical sound that is transformative. Rather, they move toward trance in response to the "long lines of classical poetry sung slowly, in unison, by a chorus of women" and then maintain this state while accompanied by the gamelan during their frenzied dances. In the Balinese Rangda ceremony, music's analgesic properties are initiated by an external source.

Neither Becker nor Tolbert discusses the disturbing potential of music to cause pain. Music's ability to trigger pain can be achieved through intermittent, excessive decibel levels of pitched or unpitched sounds. Such processes may be viewed as the domain of torture; indeed, one can recall the "harassment campaign of light and noise" used intermittently by U.S. government forces during the siege of David Koresh and the Branch Davidian community at Waco (Riley et al. 1993). Inflicting pain through musical sound operates in a different relationship to cultural values and expectations than does music of lament or trance. In the latter contexts, the expressive and palliative potentials of music in relation to pain are strongly shaped by existing cultural expectations. In contrast, the use of music to *cause* pain might be characterized as "acultural"—the pain arises from its sheer magnitude. It is absent or defeats any expectations and inflicts what Elaine Scarry (1985) has termed "a splintering of consciousness."

In each of these three cases, the musical specialist stands in a different relationship to pain. Only in the instance of the lament does the individual experiencing the pain herself perform, giving voice to the pain state.[1] While many cultures appear to generate trance states with varying degrees of analgesic properties, the performance of the music in most cases seems to be separated from the trancer, who more often than not dances or performs some sort of expressive motion (Rouget 1980). Indeed, to initiate and maintain a trance state most often requires a third party or parties who provide the sonic component. Similarly, the possibility of inflicting pain through musical sound can only be achieved by a third person acting on the body and consciousness of another. Thus any "scientific study" of the manner in which pain is transformed through music requires somewhat different approaches in terms of the channels through which sound is initiated and those through which it is perceived. We have heard some discussion of growing capabilities to track pain through scanning procedures, thereby ascertaining the processes through which pain activates multiple cortical regions. An experimental model tracking the palliative effect of music would appear possible only when charting the impact of music from an external source as it was received, whether seeking to palliate or cause pain. Rather than debating only the pathways pain travels, we might shift to a lateral focus, tracking and following musical pathways. Whether we need to distinguish neurologically between music that mitigates pain and music that causes pain remains to be determined.

The relationship between music and pain clearly varies according to its setting—some traditions privilege music as an expression or representation of pain; others tend to emphasize music's palliative powers. (I'm frankly not sure what cultures would claim practices of causing pain through music!) However, common aspects of the relationship of music and pain are suggested by Becker's and Tolbert's essays, and I'd like to follow up with these now, looking briefly at the intersection of music, ritual, and belief with pain therapies and the centrality of musicians to the practice of healing in these contexts.

Both essays (and many others in this volume) make clear the direct or indirect relationship of the music/pain axis to ritual complexes and further highlight the powerful role that religious practitioners play in palliating pain. I note Tolbert's cautious linkage of laments to indigenous Karelian religious practices as well as to Eastern Orthodox Christianity. Becker's case study of Balinese trance is subsumed within the Barong-Rangda ritual, an occasional observance intended to reestablish social and spiritual balance. These are only two instances of the transformation of pain located at an intersection of music, ritual, and belief. Music is a particularly common channel through which the experience of and response to pain is managed and mediated.

If we are to make connections between neuroscientific and humanistic inquiry, I suggest that we need to delve more deeply into the ways in which musicians are implicated in and give shape to the musical processes associated with ameliorating pain. To date, there have been only a few in-depth studies of music's role in rituals of healing and renewal, including Roseman's (1990) exploration of Temiar healing in Malaysia and Friedson's (1996) work on Tumbuka healing in Malawi. The production of the musical components in these contexts is not the outcome of casual musical processes but stems from esoteric therapies learned and transmitted with great care. One barrier to the study of music and healing is that these practices and their inner workings have been masked from researchers and are often highly secret domains within their own societies. Let me provide two brief additional examples of the ways in which musicians link modalities of cultural healing.

Among several forms of musical healing I've encountered in the Ethiopian highlands, perhaps the most prominent and pervasive is the close involvement of Ethiopian church musicians *(dabtara)* with healing practices. In addition to performing the musical liturgy during Christian rituals in the church, the *dabtaras* are famous for producing amulets in the form of scrolls *(asmat),* which contain magical texts and incantations thought to drive away spirits that cause disease. *Dabtaras* also "perform" these same incantations as oral therapies over the sick, transforming the magical formulae encoded in the scrolls into the realm of musical and ritual practice. The particular blend of oral and written therapies partakes of a dualism that pervades many other aspects of Ethiopian expressive culture. One traditional Ethiopian proverb about pain localizes appropriate therapies: "For a headache, shout on it! For a stomach ache, eat on it!" (Levine 1965, 227).

A veil of secrecy surrounds these healing practices on the fringe of Orthodox Christianity, and Ethiopian *dabtaras* do not openly discuss their work as healers; indeed, I studied with leading church musicians who never mentioned healing while providing detailed oral histories about their lives and careers.[2] Within Ethiopian church circles, the *dabtara*'s role in healing is subject to something approaching a formal taboo, as noted in this brief passage in the one published personal history by a *dabtara:* "We have not included the divination text [Awde-Negast] here, which deals with astrology, in the above mentioned categories of holy books. This is because it has been banned by the Ethiopian Orthodox Church as being outside its approved disciplines. . . . This is the main reason for its exclusion from the list of holy books and wholesome learning" (Imbakom 1970, 2).

Yet despite widespread reticence to acknowledge the power of *dabtaras* in the domain of healing outside official church duties, traditional church iconography explicitly celebrates the transformative power of sacred chant and the protection it offers against pain. Here we can view one of the two most widely reproduced representations of Saint Yared (see Figure R8.1), the church musician commemorated annually for formulating the corpus of Ethiopian Christian liturgical music under divine inspiration in the sixth century. The painting portrays the musician as so transported by his own singing and dancing that he does not feel the spear of Emperor Gabra Masqal that has accidentally pierced his foot. If Yared's performance suggests that Ethiopian Christian chant itself provides an analgesic against pain, the look of surprise on the emperor's face marks his own startled recognition of music's power. Here we find the transformative power of musical performance linked not just to a ritual context but also to the life and person of one powerful individual. In a very real sense, each *dabtara* is Saint Yared's heir and derives from him both the power of sanctioned chant and the unofficial power to heal.

I found similar associations of musicians and musical healing much closer to home when I studied a paraliturgical hymn repertory *(pizmonim)* among Jews of Syrian descent in the United States. It was obvious early on that one of the most beloved hymns from late-nineteenth-century Aleppo, "Refa Siri" (Heal Me), was a prayer for the healing of pain, as noted in its first verse:

> Heal my pain, oh faithful Lord,
> Because you are the master healer.
> Fortify the weakness of my mind
> And give strength to my soul

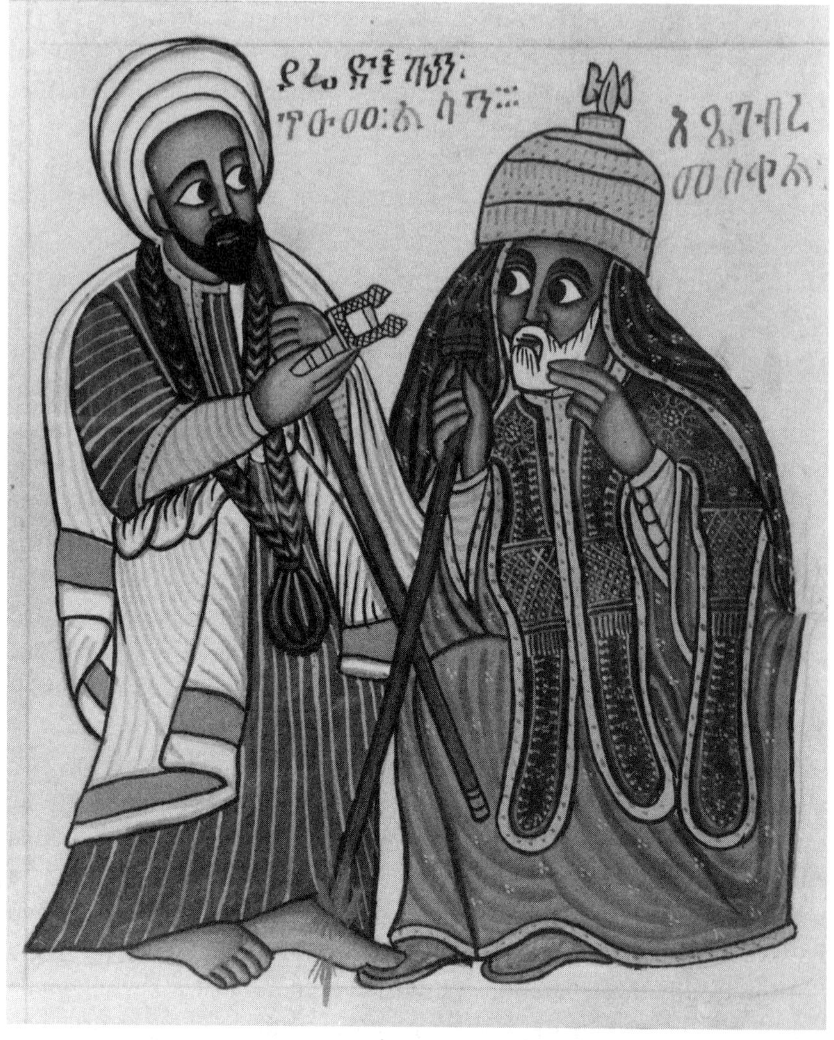

Figure R8.1. This traditional Ethiopian painting shows Saint Yared performing liturgical chant and dance in front of Emperor Gabra Masqal.

This *pizmon,* composed in the late nineteenth century, is still sung today throughout the Syrian Jewish diaspora when an individual who has recovered from an illness or surgery is called forward in the synagogue. Oral traditions about this song commemorate its specific association with a painful incident in Aleppo during which the song's composer, Rabbi Raphael Taboush, lost his eyesight; Raphael's name, spelled *refa'el* in the song's Hebrew acrostic (not reproduced here), literally means "heal me, Lord." Ethnographic interviewing and observation revealed other hymns composed by Taboush that are also connected in their textual content and associated oral traditions with healing practices. Beyond providing links to the healing powers of song, one must acknowledge the instrumental role of a particular musician who first composed, performed, and rendered these songs efficacious. The musician as healer—in the Syrian Jewish tradition, specifically Taboush as healer—is integral to an understanding of the palliative powers of music in all its aspects (Shelemay 1998).

This is not to ascribe the genesis of healing practices to a single individual. For instance, in Syrian practice, we know of healing traditions that predate the musical therapies of Taboush. The historian Abraham Marcus (1989, cited in Shelemay 1998, 222–223) has found remarkable descriptions from eighteenth- and nineteenth-century Aleppo of healing practices among that city's Jews: in addition to employing physicians, Syrian Jews called in rabbis to pray at the bedside of the sick in order to help combat the work of holy spirits and also hired Muslim holy men to apply their powers of intercession and exorcism. While healing and charming are technically forbidden to Jews by biblical injunction (Deut. 18:11), traditional healing practices, including the use of amulets, were evidently widespread among Jews in Aleppo. But as certain individuals were instrumental in perpetuating musical remedies for pain and illness, one finds that musical efficacy continues to be dependent in the Syrian tradition on personal associations. For instance, *pizmonim* are still used to palliate physical dysfunction and psychic pain in present-day Brooklyn, sometimes within the context of regular religious rituals. One of the most widespread oral traditions among Brooklyn Syrians requires that the individual to be healed must be named in the song. As an example they tell of a man in the community named Abraham who was trying unsuccessfully to conceive a child. During this period, when he attended Sabbath morning synagogue rituals, the participants would sing a *pizmon* containing the phrase "the seed of Abraham," seeking to ensure, through the power of song with its references to the patriarch who conceived a child at an advanced age, that the Brooklyn man's efforts would be successful.

These brief examples from my own research across far-flung domains of Christian and Jewish practice, reinforce Tolbert's and Becker's insights into the power of music to transform pain in strikingly different religious, geographical, and cultural contexts. This is a telling commentary on the potential of music to express specific cultural values while standing in common cause to palliate pain.

All of these examples also raise provocative questions regarding the gendering of musical processes through which pain is transformed. We have seen that Balinese males are guided into trance by female voices, then supported in their altered states by music performed by the all-male gamelan. In contrast, Tolbert's lamenters are exclusively women. There are clear gender divides in Ethiopian healing as well; *dabtaras* who mitigate pain and illness are always male, whereas use of trance in traditional Ethiopian *zar* cult healing is the provenance of women. It appears that men more often control forms of musical prophylaxis, while women are more closely associated with, and instrumental in, situations in which pain is already established and must be exorcised. In summary, the power of music to mediate or palliate pain is clearly shaped, depending on cultural and social factors, by both men and women; healers within a given society may also model themselves after specific individuals who through their own experiences are considered to have invested music with healing powers.

Music may be more important than we have conventionally suspected in the management of pain. Given music's multiple roles in transforming pain, it may be appropriate to offer here a final ethnomusicological response to a comment in Clifford Wolff's essay that pain is a biological necessity and that human beings need pain in order to survive. It might be worthwhile to consider that music may also be a biological necessity, one that enables human beings to survive at those very moments when they cannot avoid pain.

Notes

1. In some traditions, the lament is performed not by the individual in psychic pain but by professional lamenters. A salient example is the highland Ethiopian lament, where a professional female leader is often supported by a choir; both the ensemble and its laments are known as *musho,* highlighting the union of singer and song (Powne 1968, 77–78).

2. A dissertation written by Allen Young provides rare data on these healing practices in the Ethiopian highlands (Young 1970).

References

Berliner, P. 1978. *The Soul of Mbira: Music and Traditions of the Shona People of Zimbabwe.* Chicago: University of Chicago Press.

Damasio, A. R. 1999. *The Feeling of What Happens: Body and Emotion in the Making of Consciousness.* New York: Harcourt Brace.

Friedson, S. M. 1996. *Dancing Prophets.* Chicago: University of Chicago Press.

Imbakom Kalewold, A. 1970. *Traditional Ethiopian Church Education.* Trans. M. Lemma. New York: Teachers College Press.

Levine, D. 1965. *Wax and Gold: Tradition and Innovation in Ethiopian Culture.* Chicago: University of Chicago Press.

Levy, I. 1969. *Antologia de liturgia judeo-espanola,* vol. 4, no. 225. Jerusalem: Marian Book Mfg.

Marcus, A. 1989. *The Middle East on the Eve of Modernity: Aleppo in the Eighteenth Century.* New York: Columbia University Press.

Powne, M. 1968. *Ethiopian Music.* Oxford: Oxford University Press.

Riley, M., et al. 1993. "Tragedy in Waco." *Time Magazine,* May 3.

Roseman, M. 1990. *Healing Sounds from the Malaysian Rainforest.* Berkeley: University of California Press.

Rouget, G. 1980. *La musique et la transe.* Paris: Gallimard.

Scarry, E. 1985. *The Body in Pain: The Making and Unmaking of the World.* Oxford: Oxford University Press.

Shelemay, K. K. 1992. "The Musician and Transmission of Religious Tradition: The Multiple Roles of the Ethiopian Dabtara." *Journal of Religion in Africa* 22(3): 242–260.

———. 1998. *Let Jasmine Rain Down: Song and Remembrance among Syrian Jews.* Chicago: University of Chicago Press.

Young, A. 1970. "Medical Beliefs and Practices of Begemder Amhara." Ph.D. dissertation, University of Pennsylvania.

Discussion:

The Presentation and Representation of Emotion in Music

NICHOLAS WOLTERSTORFF: I want to ask Elizabeth Tolbert a question about the music itself. What I found absolutely striking about all three Karelian laments is that at the end of each phrase the singer wept. It was most marked in the first case, but it was close to weeping in all three cases. It seemed to me that a great deal of the power of these laments depended on this weeping. If one imagined that absent, they would still be powerful, but it would not be the same sort of power.

It seems that there is a mixture of things going on. There is musical and literary representation of pain, but there is also something awfully close to the real thing or a near mimic of the actual thing. That goes beyond iconicity.

ELIZABETH TOLBERT: That's actually what I was trying to say, that you have a presentation of emotion, a representation of emotion, and an experience that is constituting a social world in which to place your emotions. The fundamental iconicity of crying makes it seem as though this only happens in the lament, but it happens in every kind of music. In the lament you are overfocused on the iconicity of crying and underfocused on the idea that you can't understand music as an individual utterance. Music is always a social utterance in that it requires a group of people who understand it and a person performing it who provides a phenomenal object that you can invest with meaning.

WOLTERSTORFF: Is the singer so intensely involved that she is actually overcome by grief?

TOLBERT: Yes, but I don't think it's the same *as* grief. It's somewhat similar to a trance state in that even though she is using aspects of the autobiographical self to focus everybody's attention, and to focus her performance, in a certain way she is offering her personal pain as a sacrifice so that everyone else can mourn. And she can lose her autobiographical self. So, yes, she gets more and more worked up and usually ends just sobbing uncontrollably. But it's a different way of being overcome than someone crying on their own. I have seen these people get into an incredible state, and then the next second they are out of it. It's not that it's not real; it's more like a trance state. If you understand emotion as being merely personal, then you would ask if it is real or not. But if you understand it as transformative or social or mediating between individual and social emotion, then it's "real" in a different way.

Discussion:
Neurobiological Views of Music, Emotion, and the Body

SARAH COAKLEY: I would like to ask Howard Fields and Clifford Woolf to say something at this point. A whole area of discussion that was left undeveloped after the presentation of your own papers was the question of how you both perceive sufficient flexibility in the brain's response to pain. Despite the fact that you both reject the gate theory in its classic form, you seem able in principle to accommodate cultural variables in your approach to pain, and these are of course particularly evident in this musical material. I think we'd all like to hear more from you about that.

HOWARD FIELDS: In science we look for mechanisms and explanations as opposed to descriptions. In this triangle of music and emotion and the body, a question that comes up in my mind is the difference between what's genetic and what's learned. It seems as though there is a genetic, instinctive component that ties music to emotion. I think of things like work songs and lullabies and laments. I wondered whether there was a structural similarity between the lullaby and the lament, because the lament seemed to involve a bodily component such as rocking movements. Likewise, march music and rap music seem to trigger violence or a defensive anger. It seems as though there is a music for almost every emotion. My question is whether this is something that came about instinctively or is learned, in which case there would be two different ways of approaching the neurobiology.

The other thing that came to mind was the movie *A Clockwork Orange,* by Stanley Kubrick, where the evil protagonist loves to commit acts of violence to Beethoven. In the process of curing the protagonist, he is given a drug that nauseates him and makes him vomit while the music is played for him and videos of violent acts are shown. By the time the treatment is finished, he becomes paralyzed and nauseated when he hears the music. That is a case where the meaning of the music takes on an opposite polarity by association.

How could music come to be connected to emotion and then back to the body? William James (1884), in the James-Lang theory of emotion, theorized that the nervous system plays out a physical embodiment of emotion through the sympathetic nervous system, the motor system, and perhaps facial expression. He suggested that you actually feel your body changing under the afferent drive from the brain, and that plays back into your somatosensory system to give you the emotion. I don't think anybody believes that anymore, but it's an idea that has relevance to what we're talking about.

Antonio Damasio (1994) has put forward the idea of a "somatic marker": that you interpret emotions by virtue of association, by calling up a representation of the way your body felt in a similar situation in the past. It involves a representation of the body instead of the real body.

There was a great functional imaging study that was done at Massachusetts General Hospital by Rauch et al. (1995). They got people who were either spider-phobic or snake-phobic. They dangled an empty box in front of them and then dangled the snake or spider. They imaged the subject under both conditions and subtracted them to get the pattern of activity that was associated with the phobia. Of course the limbic system was activated, but what was more interesting to me was a strong activation of the somatosensory pathway. The fear was activating through a central pathway, the somatosensory system, implying an activation of a "virtual body."

If we conceptualize emotion as a reactivation of a virtual body, a representation of a body, perhaps music has ties directly to the somatic representation. Of course this is testable, which means it has a real possibility of being proven wrong.

COAKLEY: Do we come away from this session assuming, as John Brust seemed to suggest, that the processes by which trance works, especially musically, are really not yet understood?

LAURENCE KIRMAYER: I'd like to speak to that because I know there is as yet no literature in this area. I was at Oxford recently at a conference on neurosciences and brain imaging of hysteria. The current literature in this area finds no simple physiological correlates of trance. The people who study hypnosis and trance think of it as a very complex cognitive performance that is socially shaped, that follows a script, and that involves all kinds of internal strategies to partition information and avoid looking at or revising certain things.

Yet there are specific cognitive processes that are going on. There is now at least one set of neuroimaging studies looking at people with hysterical paralysis (Halligan et al. 2000). This is not the same thing as pain, but there are analogies in that people with spontaneous hysterical paralyses or with hypnotic re-creation of that have specific activation of frontal fields. There is no somatosensory cortex involvement that distinguishes them from people with intentional movements, but there is a frontal lobe process that points to the limbic system and to issues of attention and affect. As with many of these studies, it's at such a crude level that a million different processes could be implicated. Some kind of psychological analysis is needed to specify what those processes are, so that we can draw some meaning from the localization.

CLIFFORD WOOLF: One of the major contributions that Patrick Wall made (1988), apart from integrating the psychology with Ron Melzack's work on the gate control theory, was the notion that the nervous system is a dynamic process, and it changes. People obviously recognize that it changes during development and maybe also in the face of disease states. But Wall played a major role in integrating the notion that the modifiability of the nervous system is integral to the way it functions.

Michael Merzenich, a colleague of Howard Fields's, has studied music in this context (Kilgard and Merzenich 1998; see also Zhang, Bao, and Merzenich 2001). There is no question that music will change our brains. If you measure the distribution of the way tones interact in the cortical areas, you find a neuroanatomical architectural scaffold that is changeable. It can enlarge, and it can be modified. That's true of the somatosensory cortex and all other parts of the brain. So we need to see this in a dynamic context.

TU WEIMING: Maybe we should introduce a different cultural perspective here. A long time ago, Jaeger (1959) described the Greek mode as very visual and the Judaic mode as very aural. Many of the terms we now use in the West are influenced by the Greek mode: "insight," "vision," and such notions. Chinese culture is now being studied to determine whether the aural or the visual is privileged. For example, the Chinese character for "sage" uses the radicals for "ear" and "mouth," emphasizing aural perception. There is a very early assumption that aural perception is closer to the heart, that it moves more deeply than sight. With sight, you have to cast your vision out and try to grab something. Our discussions here have privileged the aural, but we should also think about the importance of sight linked to the experience of pain, for example, in looking at the crucifixion. It's a totally different issue, but it's fascinating that even in very broad, generalized cultural terms, you have different motifs and different orientations. I'm not sure whether or not they can be scientifically studied.

JEAN JACKSON: Kay Kaufman Shelemay said that the issue of pain being used to punish is something that perhaps occurs only in fiction, but I have an actual example. There was a judge in California who in a certain sense let the punishment fit the crime. Bitter complaints had been made against people who were brought in for playing enormously loud rap music. Their punishment was being put into a room and forced to listen, without covering their ears, to Gene Autry or Wayne Newton or somebody that they found excruciatingly painful. They reported pain, and they were allowed to come to a point of empathy with the folks to whom they had given pain.

JOHN BRUST: There is a Gary Larson cartoon in that regard. The caption is "Charlie Parker in hell," and he's in a cell, listening to fusion.

JACKSON: There are lots of fictional examples of music being used to punish, for example, with Gilbert and Sullivan!

COAKLEY: Shouldn't we consider whether rap could not also be a cathartic trance? We've been sneering here about rap, but is it not also performing some cultural function that could be transformative?

KIRMAYER: That is certainly possible. On a more personal note, my brother is a musician who plays very intense avant-garde jazz, like the late phase of John Coltrane. Some of my relatives who dutifully go to concerts to show their appreciation say they cannot stand it, that it's physical pain. I have a friend who says it gives him a heart attack. There is an issue of training one's ear or understanding a vocabulary so that it ceases to be a noise or an assault.

ELIZABETH TOLBERT: There is an assumption underlying all of this that music is supposed to have a powerful effect. I think this is connected, at least in Western culture, with the split between language and music. Music is supposed to be unmediated, going directly to the heart; language is supposed to be mediated and reasoned. This relates to the split between reason and emotion, mind and body.

We need to understand that, even in language, things like the tone of voice are communicating something that is not just linguistic. Language isn't just language as it's idealized. Music is not just music as it's idealized. Music is not a direct way of understanding. We're always enculturated beings, and there's no way we can isolate culture. There's no way we can say this is biological, and this is not biological. Biological is already cultural, and culture is already biological. Somehow we have to try and get away from ideas that lead us to choose whether associations between certain musics and certain emotions are innate or learned. They are innately learned because this is how we learn to understand anything. They have a form and they have a meaning, and you learn that in the context of everyday experience.

FIELDS: But it's *conceivable* that there could be "unlearned," genetic aspects to the effect of music on the body.

TOLBERT: I think that could be the effect of *sound,* perhaps, and not just music per se.

FIELDS: All right. Let's say a sound that's not necessarily music makes you feel good. The question is: How is it that a sound makes you feel good? Is it because your auditory system is linked to your reward pathway, so that it's something akin to the way you would feel if you took amphetamines or cocaine? Or does it happen through the process of association? A song, for example, is associated with warmth and being fed because you heard it when your mother comforted you when you were hungry. And now, when you lose someone you love, you sing that song to yourself as a way of re-creating that soothing feeling. That would be learned.

These are completely different things in a neurobiological sense. If you get pleasure from something, it's either a primary reward that you don't have to learn, like food when you're hungry or drink when you're thirsty, or it's through association with some other thing that is primarily rewarding.

RICHARD WOLF: But how could you possibly distinguish them methodologically? Even in the case of having hunger satisfied, if a vegetarian is given a piece of meat, or if you're given food that is absolutely repulsive but will fill you up, it will be a very ambiguous situation. The question is how you can distinguish *neurologically*. I understand that there are certain pathways that can be studied, for example, opiates excite certain responses, but the subjective experience of feeling good does not seem to be something you can really get at.

FIELDS: I'm not so sure. Barry Everitt at Cambridge has done a very interesting study (Cardinal et al. 2002). He looked first at the primary rewarding effects of drugs such as cocaine; then when cocaine was administered to an animal, a tone was played. After several pairings of tone and cocaine, the animal would press a lever to hear that tone. As with the suffering and the sensory aspects of pain, it turns out that the primarily rewarding and the learned rewarding mechanisms involve different parts of the brain. So you could say that if different brain regions are involved in learned and primary rewards, at least in theory there's a way to get at it through experiment.

WOLF: But that's proposing that a mouse doesn't bring any kind of baggage to the experiment, which is probably true. But you can never assume that with a human.

References

Cardinal, R. N., J. A. Parkinson, J. Hall, and B. J. Everitt. 2002. "Emotion and Motivation: The Role of the Amygdala, Ventral Striatum, and Prefrontal Cortex." *Neurosci. Biobehav. Rev.* 26(3): 321–352.

Damasio, A. R. 1994. *Descartes' Error: Emotion, Reason, and the Human Brain.* New York: G. P. Putnam's Sons.

Halligan, P. W., B. S. Athwal, D. A. Oakley, and R. S. J. Frackowiak. 2000. "Imaging Hypnotic Paralysis: Implications for Conversion Hysteria." *Lancet* 355: 986–987.

Jaeger, W. W. 1959. "The Greek Ideas of Immortality." *Harvard Theological Review* 52(3): 135–147.

James, W. 1884. "What Is an Emotion?" *Mind* 9: 188–205.

Kilgard, M. P, and M. M. Merzenich. 1998. "Plasticity of Temporal Information Processing in the Primary Auditory Cortex." *Nat. Neurosci.* 1(8): 727–731.

Rauch, S. L., C. R. Savage, N. M. Alpert, E. C. Miguel, L. Baer, H. C. Breiter, A. J. Fischman, P. A. Manzo, C. Moretti, and M. A. Jenike. 1995. "A Positron Emission Tomographic Study of Simple Phobic Symptom Provocation." *Arch. Gen. Psychiatry* 52(1): 20–28.

Wall, P. D. 1988. "Recruitment of Ineffective Synapses after Injury." *Adv. Neurol.* 47: 387–400.

Zhang, L. I., S. Bao, and M. M. Merzenich. 2001. "Persistent and Specific Influences of Early Acoustic Environments on Primary Auditory Cortex." *Nat. Neurosci.* 4(11): 1123–1130.

Discussion:
Ritual and Expectation

HOWARD FIELDS: I think this conference has been exceptionally successful so far in trying to understand how ritual and music can change the experience of pain. As I watched the videotapes used with the musical presentations, it occurred to me that a ritual is a group exercise that is out of the ordinary, a kind of costumed docudrama. There's a problem, and people hope it is going to be solved. I think what is going on is that their *expectation* is being changed (see Prince and Fields 1997 for an earlier, and more extended, discussion of "expectation" in the medical management of pain). "Expectation," which is an acceptable word in science, is equivalent to "belief" among nonscientists. It has two parts to it: hope and faith. Hope, we might say, is the thing you desire, and faith is the likelihood or the probability that your desire will be achieved.

Ritual and music don't really change hope that much, but they do influence faith. I think music is an incredibly important aspect of ritual, which is much less powerful without music. The key is that words and music are different in a fundamental way. Here's my proposal: music has a special way of mitigating doubt or improving faith because it's nonpropositional. Since it's nonpropositional, it can't be false. Even if it is harshly dissonant, you can't falsify music. It's there, so it is in some way shielded from doubt. Doubt is always linguistic in its expression. Music can be bad, but it can't be untrue.

Going back to pain and transformation, I'm suggesting ritual and music change pain by changing expectations. The music may work in part by a kind of a procedural learning that mitigates doubt, which can so easily be expressed in words. When we look at expectation, then we're back to something that can be studied with the tools of neuroscience. Likewise, if we think of faith as a kind of probability, the likelihood of occurrence, then we can go back to neurobiology.

One big problem is that about 99 percent of pain research has focused on the spinal cord, but 99 percent of the pain experience is in the brain, where culture, society, and expectation come into play. The intersubjective factors that are external to the person, out there in the world, and which largely determine the operation of the nervous system, are really what the brain is all about. What's going on in the "body" (that is, as understood here in contradistinction from the brain) plays a very small role in what happens in the brain.

This is where expectation comes in. This is where music and ritual can alter the actual message that's sent to wherever the "magical" event is that results in our subjective feeling of pain. At the moment we're not making any progress on that, that I can discern. That's where neuroscience ends, at least for now.

Reference

Prince, D. D., and H. L. Fields. 1997. "The Contribution of Desire and Expectation to Placebo Analgesia: Implications for New Research Strategies." In A. Harrington, ed., *The Placebo Effect: An Interdisciplinary Exploration.* Cambridge, Mass.: Harvard University Press, 117–137.

Pain, Ritual, and the Somatomoral

Beyond the Individual

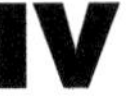

Pain and Humanity in the Confucian Learning of the Heart-and-Mind

9

Tu Weiming

Cheng Hao (1032–1085), a principal Neo-Confucian thinker, made an intriguing observation about humanity. He noted that the most fitting term for understanding the Confucian idea of humanity is *buren,* a common expression in Chinese medical books explaining the paralysis of the arms and legs, which literally means the absence of humanity. In this view, the sensation of pain is an essential feature of being human; an inability to feel pain is considered a major deficiency not only in terms of health but also in respect to morality. It is human to feel pain, while the inability to do so is detrimental to our humanity. This positive attitude toward pain is predicated on the belief that embodiment and sensitivity are two essential features of humanity:

> A book on medicine describes paralysis of the four limbs as absence of *ren* (humanity). This is an excellent description. The man of *ren* regards Heaven and Earth and all things as one body. To him there is nothing that is not himself. Since he has recognized all things as himself, can there be any limit to his humanity? If things are not parts of the self, naturally they have nothing to do with it. As in the paralysis of the four limbs, the vital force no longer penetrates them, and therefore they are no longer parts of the self. (*Er-Cheng yishu* 2A:2a–b)

The key word *ren,* consisting of a "human" radical and a sign normally interpreted as "two," often translated as "humanity," is variously rendered as benevolence, goodness, human-heartedness, perfect virtue, love, or altruism. Late Berkeley Sinologist Peter Boodberg (1953) suggested that "co-humanity" is the most appropriate translation, for humanity is always a relational concept. Cheng Hao's interpretation, in the tradition of Mencius, stressed the human capacity for communication and sympathy. A full appreciation of his deceptively simple paragraph requires a cosmological account of embodiment and the idea of humanity as all-embracing sensitivity.

Embodying Heaven, Earth, and the Myriad Things

The cosmological insight underlying the human capacity for embodiment is succinctly captured in Zhou Dunyi's (1017–1073) "An Explanation of the Diagram of the Great Ultimate." While Zhou's assumptive reasoning for the advent of the human is complicated by his creative adaptation of culturally specific ideas such as *yin-yang* and the Five Agents, the outline of his explanation is readily comprehensible. He first offers a familiar account of the evolutionary process whereby Heaven, Earth, and the myriad things came into being. Through movement and tranquility, the Great Ultimate (which is also referred to as the Ultimate of Non-being because it cannot be defined as a thing) generates the two primordial forces of *yin* and *yang*. The transformation of *yang* and its union with *yin* give rise to the Five Agents (water, fire, wood, metal, and earth). With elegant simplicity, Zhou concludes his narrative of the cosmic story by stressing union, integration, interaction, and transformation: "When the reality of the Ultimate of Non-being and the essence of *yin*, *yang*, and the Five Agents come into mysterious union, integration ensues. *Qian* (Heaven) constitutes the male element, and *Kun* (Earth) constitutes the female element. The interaction of these two vital energies engenders and transforms the myriad things. The myriad things produce and reproduce, resulting in an unending transformation" (*Zhouzi quanshu*, in Chan 1963, 463). Zhou articulated a strong belief in the continuity and communicability of all modalities of being. From an evolutionary perspective, since everything is made of the vital energy *(qi)*, there is consanguinity among all things: stones, plants, animals, and humans.

Wing-tsit Chan notes that *qi* means both matter and energy, a distinction not made in Chinese philosophy. Although he prefers to translate *qi* as "material force," rather than either "matter" or "ether," he acknowledges that *qi,* in the classical sense, denotes the psychophysiological power associated with breath and blood. It is, therefore, permissible to render it as "vital force" or "vital power" (Chan 1963, 784). While *qi* is the "matter-energy" that underlies all things, it is not simply the building block of reality. The reductionist language of monads and particles fails to convey the moving power and hidden dynamism that *qi* signifies. *Qi* is never static; it is becoming as well as being; it is existence in process. The cosmos, made of *qi,* is the "great transformation" *(dahua).* Since it encompasses all modalities of being in the process, everything (air, water, stone, plant, animal, or human) is imbued with *qi* as a vital and dynamic component of the cosmic process. Human beings ought to be aware that they are an integral part of this "great transformation" (Tu 1992, 91–92).

Zhang Zai (1020–1077), in the same spirit, straightforwardly articulated his faith in the human capacity to be organically connected in the universe:

> Heaven is my father and Earth is my mother, and even such a small creature as I finds an intimate place in their midst.
>
> Therefore that which fills the universe I regard as my body and that which directs the universe I consider my nature.
>
> All people are my brothers and sisters, and all things are my companions. (*Zhang zi quanshu* 1:1a)

Zhang's idea of embodiment makes it explicit that forming one body with the universe is not an abstract ideal but a lived reality. While only the sage's virtues can be compared with the creative forces of Heaven and nature, each human being can find a proper niche in the cosmos. Human sensitivity is such that our capacity for caring is limitless; it can embrace a blade of grass or a distant star.

Zhou's and Zhang's worldviews provide an inclusive humanist vision. We humans are not only anthropological but also cosmological beings. Made of the same stuff as all other beings in the cosmos, we feel at home in the midst of it and have developed a capacity to admire the beauty of nature and to form a spiritual communion with mountains, rivers, trees, and stones. Maintaining a sustainable harmonious relationship with the world around us is our moral obligation. Furthermore, our sense of intimacy and connectedness compels us to actively participate in the cosmic process.

The uniqueness of being human lies in the stuff that the human body and mind-heart is made of—the highest quality of the vital energy of the Five Agents. The principle or pattern *(li)* that makes us what we are is often referred to as the Heavenly Principle *(tianli)*. Human intelligence, rationality, moral sense, and above all, sensitivity are the result of the Heavenly Principle. Cheng Hao proudly announced that although he received much of his learning from his teachers, he had to personally acquire an experiential understanding of how the Heavenly Principle works. Whether or not the Heavenly Principle takes an active role in crystallizing the most refined and delicate vital energy to create the human form, it is still the ultimate reason underlying the order of things that makes us unique and yet intimately connected with Heaven, Earth, and myriad things. Xunzi in the third century BCE emphasized the importance of rightness (a sense of duty): "Fire and water possess energy but are without life. Grass and trees have life but no consciousness. Birds and beasts have consciousness but no sense of duty. Man possesses energy, life, consciousness, and, in addition, a sense of duty. Therefore he is the noblest being on earth" (Watson 1963, 45). Although Xunzi underscored a sense of duty as distinctively human, he fully acknowledged that energy is a constitutive element in all modalities of being and thus is indispensable to human existence. Zhou, following the tradition of the *Book of Change,* singled out human spirituality in terms of the cardinal virtues, such as humanity and rightness, as the ultimate reason that enables the sages (the most authentic expressions of humanity) to form a unity with Heaven.

While we humans, like fire, water, grass, trees, birds, and beasts, are products of the vital energy in the "great transformation," we are, strictly speaking, not creatures but co-creators of the cosmic process. Although the belief that Heaven engenders and the human completes may have predated the Confucian tradition (see Chang 1983, 33–55), the Confucian idea that human beings ought to form a partnership with Heaven is predicated on an ethic of responsibility. The Confucian statement in the *Analects* that human beings can make the Way great, but the Way cannot make human beings great (*Analects* 15:28) may lead to the false impression that humans act as creative agents on their own. The injunction is, rather, that we humans are obligated, by a sense of awe and reverence, to make ourselves worthy of what the Heavenly Principle empowers us to do as partners. The *Doctrine of the Mean* (XXII) states that through self-realization human beings actively participate in the transforming and nourishing process of Heaven and Earth and thus form a trinity with Heaven and Earth (see Tu 1989, 77–79). Accordingly, we can rise above our earthly existence by cultivating the virtues inherent in our nature. Indeed, "[t]he character of the sage is 'identical with that of Heaven and Earth; his brilliancy is identical with the sun and moon; his order is identical with that of the four seasons; and his good and evil fortunes are identical with those of the spiritual beings.' The profound person cultivates these moral qualities and enjoys good fortune, whereas the belittled person violates them and suffers evil fortune" (Chan 1963, 463–464).[1] For Cheng Hao, the virtue that most profoundly empowers us to realize our own nature and therefore form one body with Heaven, Earth, and the myriad things is humanity *(ren)* as sensitivity.

In the perspective of embodiment, our biological evolution shows that we are organically connected with all modalities of being in the cosmos. A sense of continuity links the myriad things to our existence. We owe our existence to Heaven and Earth. The same vital energy that makes stones, plants, and animals also makes us. We are created out of the evolving cosmos, not as islands but as streams flowing with and into each other as an integral part of the cosmic transformation. Virtually all things between Heaven and Earth are relevant to us. Our sensitivity enables us to "embody" an ever-expanding universe not only in the symbolic sense but also in the physical experience of connection and communication. The animal kingdom, the biosphere, and the inorganic universe as well as all members of the human community are related to us in a communion of subjects, rather than as a collection of objects (see Berry 1990; Berry and Swimme 1994).

This idea of the human as the most sentient and sensitive being in the universe extends the horizon of the meaning of pain beyond the evolutionary perspective. The concept of pain as heightened self-awareness performing the useful function of warning is well recognized. However, this interpretation only scratches the surface of its significance.

A distinction between pain and suffering must be made in this connection. While the former can be explained in evolutionary terms, the latter requires a more complex explanatory model. If suffering, associated more with chronic pain than with acute pain, is conceived as an inevitable experience in the human need for embodiment, the biochemical and neurophysiological sources of pain are necessarily intertwined with psychological, social, cultural, and cosmological concerns. The psychological tension generated by our inability to communicate, participate, and integrate in a communal setting is a case in point. This is not to say that somatic pain, like anger, disappointment, or despair, is actually caused by nonphysical reasons. Rather, in our attempt to analyze the etiology of pain in terms of a holistic vision, we cannot ignore the obvious fact: the universal human sensitivity toward embodiment raises doubts about treating pain as simply the experience of an isolated individual.

The matter is complicated by the realization that the absence of pain causes the greatest concern. The Confucians believe that we humans experience pain more fully, if not more acutely, than other animals because we are the most sentient and sensitive. Indeed, our emotional vulnerability, psychological responsiveness, and intellectual sensibility are all closely connected with our sensitivity. Since human beings are easily touched, affected, moved, and provoked by the world around them, pain is a natural result of the human condition. Yet the inability to experience pain signifies that some part of the body is no longer an integral aspect of the energy flow, as if it has been "cut off" from the cosmic process. If humanity is understood as sensitivity, this insensitivity can be interpreted as a form of inhumanity. If we lose the sensations of pain and itch, as a Chinese proverb notes, we are no longer human.

Humanity as Sensitivity

The locus classicus for defining humanity as sensitivity is the *Book of Mencius*. In characterizing the uniqueness of being human, Mencius acknowledged that the difference between humans and animals is extremely small. Yet this little difference that distinguishes humans from other animals is truly consequential, for it can make the human great. The traits that we humans share with fellow members of the animal kingdom constitute what Mencius referred to as the "small body," such as the instinctual demands for sex and food. Only that which makes us unique is called the "great body." The great body is none other than "a heart sensitive to the suffering of others" (*Mencius* IIA:6).

In the famous story about seeing a young child about to fall into the well, Mencius insisted that we would certainly be moved to compassion on such an occasion. This ability to commiserate with the child indicates that our ability to feel our own pain enables us to empathize with the suffering of others. "From this," Mencius concluded, "whoever is devoid of the heart of compassion is not human." However, a heart sensitive to the suffering of others is only the germ of humanity. If we are able to develop it, "it will be like a fire starting up or a spring coming through." "When it is fully developed, we can take under our protection the whole realm within the Four Seas, but if we fail to develop it, we will not be able even to serve our parents" (*Mencius* IIA:6).

A salient feature of the great body is its fluid unpredictability. It is both a minimum condition and a maximum realization of humanity. We cannot imagine anyone without it. We must constantly develop our great body, our human sensitivity, recognizing that no matter how we try to expand and enlarge it, there is always room for improvement. The method of self-cultivation lies in the extension of that which we naturally possess: "For every man there are things he cannot bear. To extend this to what he can bear is humanity." We cannot bear the suffering of those we love. If we can extend that sensitivity toward those about whom we feel indifferent, our humanity will be greatly enlarged. Thus, Mencius noted, "if a man can extend to the full his aversion to harming others, then there will be an overabundance of humanity" (*Mencius* VIIB:31).

A heart sensitive to the suffering of others is the great body because the potential of its growth is limitless. It was the reason that humane government in the past was established: "No man is devoid of a heart sensitive to the suffering of others. Such a sensitive heart was possessed by the former Kings and this manifested itself in compassionate government. With such a sensitive heart behind compassionate government, it was as easy to rule the Empire as rolling it on your palm"

(*Mencius* IIA:6). On the other hand, if we allow our "small body," instinctual demands, to overwhelm us, we will not be able to serve our parents well. With sympathy, humane governance is realizable, but without it, family disintegration is unavoidable. The critical idea is "extension." The quality of our humanity depends on how it is being extended. "A humane man extends his love from those he loves to those he does not love. A ruthless man extends his ruthlessness from those he does not love to those he loves" (*Mencius* VIIB:1). The choice is ours: "Benevolence [humanity] is the heart of man, and rightness his road. Sad it is indeed when a man gives up the right road instead of following it and allows his heart to stray without enough sense to go after it. When his chickens and dogs stray, he has sense enough to go after them, but not when his heart is strayed. The sole concern of learning is to go after this strayed heart. That is all" (*Mencius* VIA:11).

A sense of priority is vitally important. If we do not vigorously cultivate our great body so that our sensitivity is enhanced, selfish desires and negative environmental influences will mislead us: "The organs of hearing and sight are unable to think and can be misled by external things. When one thing acts on another, all it does is to attract it. The organ of the heart can think. But it will find the answer only if it does think; otherwise, it will not find the answer. This is what Heaven has given me. If one makes one's stand on what is of greater importance in the first instance, what is of smaller importance cannot displace it. In this way, one cannot but be a great man" (*Mencius* VIA:15). The ability of the heart to think is not merely a cognitive reflection on the proper course of action to take but an act of the will to enhance the power of the great body to transform our private ego into a fitting expression of the self. In other words, through both the cognitive and affective dimensions of the heart, we learn to expand our feeling of commiseration so that it can flow from a tiny stream into a mighty river. To cultivate our sensitivity to the suffering of others, we must keep reminding ourselves that our heart is always present and constantly alert. Without self-cultivation, there is no guarantee that we will be able automatically to preserve the sensitivity of the heart.

Sympathy, as the most prominent feature of the heart, is closely linked to pain and suffering. The Chinese character *xin,* rendered here as "heart," involves both the cognitive and affective dimensions of consciousness. It signifies both intellectual awareness and moral awakening. Therefore, it is often translated as "heart-and-mind." While pain and suffering are not means of redemption and sanctification in the Confucian tradition, they are purifying experiences relevant to our sense of aliveness and our recognition of the existence of others. Surely, the Christian idea of martyrdom that embraces pain as an integral part of trial and sacrifice is absent here, but the notion that the agonizing experience of pain can make one whole is not at all incompatible with the Mencian view of human greatness: "That is why Heaven, when it is about to place a great burden on a man, always first tests his resolution, exhausts his frame and makes him suffer starvation and hardships, frustrates his efforts so as to shake him from his mental lassitude, toughen his nature and make good his deficiencies" (*Mencius* VIB:15).

The great burden that Heaven is supposed to have placed on the cultural heroes is the same burden that all human beings must shoulder. Strictly speaking, the burden is not an externally imposed command but is instead an internally motivated sense of duty. The committed Confucian scholars "must be strong and resolute, for their burden is heavy and the road is long" (*Analects* 8:7). Since life lived with a sense of duty to realize one's humanity is the burden, and only with death does the road come to an end, the burden is heavy and the road is long.

By stating that sympathy is the defining characteristic of true humanity, Mencius privileges feeling as the basis for knowing, willing, and judging. If the full distinctiveness of being human is sensitivity, then intelligence, rationality, and moral sense are no longer seen merely as cognitive functions of the mind but as affective activities of the heart as well. Actually, the separation of the mind and heart as two discrete faculties is itself problematical. It is difficult to imagine that our ability to know, to reason, or to will is not organically intertwined with our feelings. Learning to be human, in this sense, is learning to be sensitive to an ever-expanding network of relationships. Our ability to feel the suffering of others and our inability to endure the suffering of those close to us empower us to embody our family, community, nation, and the world in our sensitivity. We first learn as children that we are not isolated individuals but centers of relationships through sympathetic bonding with our parents. Filial love can thus be conceived as the cultural code that is built into the biological reality of human relatedness. Egoism as a form of insensitivity must be overcome so that the small body can be extended from the isolated individual to the family. However, if we cannot extend our sympathy beyond our parents and family, even though we may have transcended egoism, we will still suffer from nepotism. The scope of our sensitivity and our humanity will still be extremely limited. By implication, we must also transcend parochialism, ethnocentrism, and chauvinistic nationalism, to allow our sensitivity fully to embody the human community as a whole.

Nevertheless, as Zhou Dunyi and Zhang Zai's "anthropocosmic" vision clearly indicates, the full meaning of being human, as dictated by the Heavenly Principle, extends beyond anthropocentrism. Since human sensitivity knows no limit, we must move beyond the human community to extend our sympathy to nature and the cosmos as a whole. Therefore, embodying Heaven, Earth, and the myriad things in our sensitivity is the full expression of humanity. Since our sensitivity enables us to embody all things, and since our true nature helps us to establish a reciprocal relationship with all people, the proper way of enhancing our humanity is readily available to us: "All the ten thousand things are there in me. There is no greater joy than to find, on self-examination, that I am true to myself. Try your best to treat others as you would wish to be treated yourself, and you will find this is the shortest cut to humanity" (*Mencius* VIIA:4). Notwithstanding the ontological assertion of forming one body with all things and the soteriological promise of complete self-knowledge, full humanity can only be realized through vigorous spiritual and ethical discipline. The task is to refine and expand the natural feeling of sympathy so that a heart sensitive to the suffering of others continues to grow.

Mencius once remarked that he was good at cultivating his "flood-like *qi*" *(haoranzhiqi),* which is translated by Wing-tsit Chan as "strong, moving power." When queried about what he really meant, he responded: "It is difficult to explain. This is the *qi* which is, in the highest degree, vast and unyielding. Nourish it with integrity and place no obstacle in its path and it will fill the space between Heaven and Earth. It is a *qi* which unites rightness and the Way. Deprive it of these and it will collapse. It is born of accumulated rightness and cannot be appropriated by anyone through a sporadic show of rightness" (*Mencius* IIA:2). The accumulated rightness that gives birth to the "flood-like *qi*" is a sustained and balanced effort to cultivate our sympathetic heart so that it can flow into a mighty current, uniting Heaven and Earth. The heart that can feel pain and is sensitive to the suffering of others has the potential of embodying all things in its sensitivity.

Certainly, this does not mean that physically handicapped people, including those who actually suffer from paralysis of the four limbs, have lost their ability to form one body with the universe. Although the heart that is sensitive to the suffering of others may take its own pain as a point of reference, it is also the stress, the tension, the discomfort, the uneasiness, or the sense of alienation that can prompt a sympathetic response in the heart. The cultivation of the heart refers to the general state of being, rather than to a specific condition of the physical body. In fact, the experience of excruciating pain may actually inhibit us from any desire for communication. Neither the absence of a sensation of pain nor the experience of immobilizing pain necessarily affects the sensitivity of the heart. Yet there are at least two ways that our natural capacity for embodiment and sensitivity can be diminished: inertia and limitation.

Inertia occurs when selfish desires and environmental influences significantly undermine the capacity of the heart to expand. As the heart becomes desensitized by the interaction of things, it may lose its alertness to the extent that it becomes, like the paralysis of the four limbs, nonresponsive to the suffering of others. The loss of sympathy in the heart because of inertia is a major deficiency in one's well-being. Understandably, Mencius insisted, "A great man is one who retains the heart of a new-born babe" (*Mencius* IVB:12).

Limitation, especially self-imposed, refers to all the limited and limiting physical and mental blocks that have prevented the heart from further growing: egoism, nepotism, parochialism, ethnocentrism, chauvinist nationalism, and anthropocentrism. While it is both necessary and desirable to realize ourselves through the nourishing environment of family, community, society, nation, and the world, if we confine ourselves only to one of them, our humanity will be curtailed. Nepotism may appear more expansive than egoism and anthropocentrism more expansive than ethnocentrism; yet they still hamper the full growth of the sympathetic heart. If the inability to bear the suffering of others is confined to family members, fellow countrymen, or human beings, the heart's full potential for embodiment and sensitivity is still far from being realized.

Wang Yangming (1472–1529), in his "Inquiry on the Great Learning," offers a comprehensive vision on this:

> Therefore when he [the small man or an ordinary person] sees a child about to fall into the well, he cannot help a feeling of alarm and commiseration. This shows that his humanity forms one body with the child. It may be objected that the child belongs to the same species. Again, when he observes the pitiful cries and frightened appearance of birds and animals about to be slaughtered, he cannot help feeling an "inability to bear" their suffering. This shows that his humanity forms one body with birds and animals. It may be objected that birds and animals are sentient beings as he is. But when he sees plants broken and destroyed, he cannot help a feeling of pity. This shows that his humanity forms one body with plants. It may be said that plants are living things as he is. Yet, even when he sees tiles and stones shattered and crushed, he cannot help a feeling of regret. This shows that his humanity forms one body with tiles and stones. This means that even the mind of the small man necessarily has the humanity that forms one body with all. (Chan 1963, 659–660)

Thus, the personal experience of pain is being transformed into a virtue of sympathy that frees us from the predicament of being an isolated individual. As we realize that the self, as a center of relationships, can become connected, through a concerned consciousness, with all modalities of being in the universe, our anxiety of being alone is overcome. Our ability to feel intimately related to an expanding world, far from a figment of the mind, is solidly grounded in our nature. Surely, the heart sensitive to the suffering of others is highly differentiated in terms of its varied responses—alarm and commiseration, "inability to bear," pity, and regret—but its sympathetic capacity is rooted in the personal experience of pain. On the other hand, what Mencius feared as the loss of the original heart is also a real danger in the human condition. Actually, only when our hearts and minds are not "aroused by desires and obscured by selfishness" can we form one body with Heaven, Earth, and myriad things. Wang Yangming further explained:

> When it [the mind] is aroused by desires and obscured by selfishness, compelled by greed for gain and fear of harm, and stirred by anger, he [the small man] will destroy things, kill members of his own species, and will do everything. In extreme cases he will even slaughter his own brothers, and the humanity that forms one body will disappear completely. Hence, if it is not obscured by selfish desires, even the mind of the small man has the humanity that forms one body with all as does the mind of the great man. As soon as it is obscured by selfish desires, even the mind of the great man will be divided and narrow like that of the small man. (Chan 1963, 660)

Nevertheless, the possibility of recovering our true nature is always there. The original substance of the heart-and-mind is never totally lost. Even though "the humanity that forms one body" disappears completely, the authentic possibility of "a feeling of alarm and commiseration" is still present. In the last analysis, it is the human body, rather than speculative thought, that enables us to embody all things in our sensitivity.

The Body as the Locus of Sympathy

In "A Confucian Perspective on Embodiment," I argue that since the heart-and-mind *(xin)* is not a Cartesian *res cogitans* because it experiences the visceral sensations of pain, it is organically integrated with the flesh of the body, involving "breath and blood." Accordingly, embodiment is more than an imaginary act; it is an experiential understanding,—indeed, a real sense of interconnectedness. The body, so conceived, is not a static structure to be observed, dissected, and analyzed as an object but should be seen as more akin to energy fields. It is like a moving stream rather than an island. The body made of *qi* is an open system, encountering, enduring, engendering, and transforming (Tu 1992, 88–89).

Our bodies are the human forms of the vital energy, an integral part of the cosmic process engendered by the Great Ultimate. More appropriately perhaps, "our bodies are the gifts entrusted to us by our parents and by Heaven." This may have inspired Wang Gen to say: "If we came into being through evolution or transformative birth *(huasheng)*, then Heaven and Earth are parents to us; if we came into being because of creation or formalistic birth *(xingsheng)*, then our parents are Heaven and Earth to us."[2] In either case, the distinctiveness of being human lies in continuity with, rather than rupture from, Heaven, Earth, and the myriad things.

The body so conceived is an attainment. We do not own our bodies. We become our bodies; as we learn to sit, stand, walk, run, and talk, we are empowered to express ourselves through our bodies. Although ontologically we are our bodies, in an existential sense, we must learn to become our bodies. The Confucian idea of the living body as the primary datum and an irreducible reality is diametrically opposed to the Cartesian view that the body, contrasted with the thinking mind, is not essential for self-identity. For the Confucians, the body is the proper home for the heart-and-mind. Furthermore, the heart-and-mind manifests itself through the lived body and expresses its true nature by the experiences and feelings of the body. This is the reason that Mencius asserted that only the sage could bring the bodily form to fruition: "Our body and complexion are given to us by Heaven. Only a sage can give his body complete fulfillment" (*Mencius* VIIA:38).

Surely our bodies are biological realities, but as gifts from our parents and Heaven, they are endowed with a particularly delicate and subtle vital energy that predisposes them to be sensitive and responsive to all things with which they come in contact. Both in principle and in practice, nothing lies outside the scope of human concerns. Our bodies are experientially in communication with all modalities of being. We are always involved in an interchange with an ever-expanding network of relationships. Even though the interchange can be empirically demonstrated in biochemical terms, our human sensitivity enables us to feel the presence of Heaven, Earth, and the myriad things not as others but as an inner reality of our own existence.

Confucians believe that the human capacity of limitless sympathy is not culturally learned, aesthetically imagined, or even intellectually willed. Wang Yangming made it explicit "that the great man can regard

Heaven, Earth, and the myriad things as one body is not because he deliberately wants to do so." Rather, it is "because it is natural to the humane nature of his mind that he do so" (Chan 1963, 659). In Mencian terminology, a heart sensitive to the suffering of others is a defining characteristic of our innate nature, that with which we are born. All human beings are endowed with the same heart, although not everyone, in fact, fully develops the sympathetic capacity (the great body) to become thoroughly compassionate, as does a sage. Thus, Wang Yangming maintained that "[f]orming one body with Heaven, Earth, and the myriad things is not only true of the great man. Even the mind of the small man is no different. Only he himself makes it small" (Chan 1963, 659). That sympathy, in varying degrees of intensity, can be extended not only to humans but also to birds, animals, grass, trees, tiles, and stones is not based on sagely attainment but rather on native intelligence and innate ability. This is why Mencius insisted that the sages are those who have first realized the commonality in all our hearts (*Mencius* VIA:7). We may add that in so doing they serve as a source of inspiration for us.

The all-inclusiveness of human sensitivity is, therefore, rooted in our ordinary senses such as seeing, hearing, smelling, tasting, and touching. The body, the psychophysiological stuff, is the confluence of energy fields and the convergence of dynamic processes. Neither the image of the body as a conglomerate of discrete organs nor the image of the body as a combination of static structures captures how the body interacts with the world. The Confucian conception of the body as a modality of *qi* may be visualized as a flowing stream constantly responding to the vicissitudes of the changing environment. Yet the uniqueness of being human is the endowment of the heart-and-mind as an integral part of the body. The body with the heart-and-mind as the center is never reducible to a reified corporeality. The exclusive dichotomy of mind and body, or spirit and matter, is alien to this way of thinking.

By conceptualizing the body as energy fields, health is measured by the overall pattern of their interaction. Each energy field is defined, not by its physical properties, but by its specific role in the processing, storage, and distribution of vital energy and thus in the maintenance of life (see Porkert 1974). Since the poor condition and functioning of one particular field affect the performance of all others, corrective means will have to be applied simultaneously to several seemingly unconnected areas. Treating a headache by solely focusing on the head, or foot pain by dealing exclusively with the foot, is often ridiculed in Chinese medicine as a superficial, partial, and temporary relief for conditions that may have deep roots elsewhere. The absence of observable symptoms of ailment, disease, discomfort, or pain does not necessarily mean health. If the primary purpose of medicine is healing rather than curing, health care, for the maintenance of life, must promote the enhancement of vitality not only as a preventive measure but also for its own sake. Medical intervention is directed at the intersection of the energy fields in order to restore the organic pattern of their natural flow. Isolated treatment, without a holistic grasp of the well-being of the total person, is at best one-sided. The diagnostic methods—inspection, auscultation, pulse palpation, and interrogation—are intended for gathering all relevant information as a basis for interpreting the overall condition of the patient.

Since the vitality of the body depends on the smooth functioning of numerous interconnected energy fields, medical wisdom entails personal knowledge of how energy, which is distributed throughout the body from the inmost organs to the surface of the skin, actually works. The discovery of the pathways by which energy travels, commonly known as the meridians, is a major discovery of traditional Chinese medicine. So are the famous acupuncture points, the several hundred "foramina" *(xue)* located near the periphery of the body that can serve as indicators of how various patterns of energy flow. Although these foramina are detectable by electronic devices, they are not physically fixed points attached to subcutaneous structures.

The amazing phenomenon of auriculo-acupuncture strongly suggests that the Chinese theory of correspondence, despite its seemingly impressionistic approach, can be further explored as a way of understanding the complex dynamism of the body. Treating stomach pain by inserting a needle in the area of the ear where the crus of helix vanishes shows that the digestive system is somehow linked to a certain region of the ear (Ziyin and Zelin 1994, 200). By inference, organs such as the heart, liver, spleen, lung, kidney, and others all have their representative domains reflected on the ear. Whether or not the ear is "essentially a framework of cartilage wrapped with skin," traditional Chinese medicine envisions the auricle as an inverted fetus lying there with the head down and the feet up (198, 200). With extensive research and empirical studies, scholars in China have identified ninety-nine acupuncture points along the surface and inner side of the ear (201). It seems that the concentration of auricular points as signs of the health of the body is unique. It is still a mystery why this is so.

It should be noted that, in the Confucian tradition, the audio perception is often singled out as particularly significant for the cultivation of sympathy. The art of listening is crucial for self-knowledge. Sound is considered more powerful than sight, smell, taste, and touch in penetrating into the innermost landscape of our heart-and-mind. The virtue of the ear is receptivity. Our ability to feel a sympathetic resonance with the world around us through sound is worth cultivating because it helps us to be in tune with our fellow human beings and with nature. Confucius remarked that his ear became *shun* (compliant, obedient, or attuned) at the age of sixty (*Analects* 2.4); this connotes a profound care, a desire to listen nonjudgmentally and receptively to all the sounds in the spirit of impartiality. A recommended translation of the Chinese word *sheng* (sage), consisting of the ear and the mouth radicals, is "audient" (Boltz 1982). The virtue of the great listener, as the image of the Buddha symbolizes, is sympathy and compassion.

Doctors treat pain by acupuncture to "restore proper phasing of the energy flow." Proper balance is necessary for the maintenance of health. Traditional Chinese medicine, taking advantage of the etymological proximity of "pain" *(tong)* and "release" *(tong,* which can also mean "flow," "penetration," "connection," and "open"), offers an explanation of how acupuncture works. Pain occurs when and where there is a blockage in the energy flow. The needle stimulates the affected area and releases the blocked energy. As a result, pain is relieved (Tu 1987, 148).

If the body, as the microcosm of the cosmos, can only function well when its dynamism and vitality are enhanced by communication and interchange, the heart-and-mind embedded in the body signifies that sensitivity is a defining characteristic of humanity. Sympathy is biologically grounded, but it is through the conscientious transformation of our instinctual demands that we allow the virtue of sensitivity to the suffering of others to define who we are. In the Confucian learning of the heart-and-mind, the building of a cultural code on biological reality is a twofold process: to recognize the minimum condition for human existence and to strive toward maximum human flourishing:

> The way the mouth is disposed towards tastes, the eye towards colors, the ear towards sounds, the nose towards smells, and the four limbs towards ease is human nature, yet therein also lies the Decree. That is why the gentleman does not describe it as nature. The way benevolence [humanity] pertains to the relation between father and son, duty to the relation between prince and subject, the rites to the relation between guest and host, wisdom to the good and wise man, the sage to the way of Heaven, is the Decree, but therein also lies human nature. That is why the gentleman does not describe it as Decree. (*Mencius* VIIIB:24)

The sensory perceptions of the body are our nature, but their full satisfaction also depends upon external conditions beyond our control; the virtues, such as humanity, cannot be realized without favorable external conditions, but they are also rooted in our nature. Confucians choose to accept the legitimacy of instinctual demands but to consider the fulfillment of virtues as a moral imperative. However, Mencius insisted that all human beings possess the heart of compassion as the germ of humanity. Is sensitivity of the heart to the suffering of others naturally endowed? Mencius maintained that sympathy is not welded to us from the outside but has always been within us. He acknowledged that "seek and you will get it; let go and you will lose it" (*Mencius* VIIA:3). Without self-cultivation, the heart cannot grow and may even be lost. This is why the difference between the great body and the small body is critical: "There are cases where one man is twice, five times or countless times better than another man, but this is only because there are people who fail to make the best of their native endowment" (*Mencius* VIA:6). The "flood-like *qi*" that fills up the space between Heaven and Earth symbolizes the fullest development of the great body, which has its beginning in the innate human sensitivity to the suffering of others. The same moral reasoning is applied to sages who compassionately embody all things and to the belittled men who fail to show any concern toward their closest kin. Those of us in between, while we worry about the danger of insensitivity, can always try to extend and expand our sympathy.

We may want to revisit Cheng Hao's definition of humanity. For Cheng Hao, "to the man of humanity, there is nothing that is not himself" means that regarding Heaven and Earth and all things as one body, the self, as an all-embracing sensitivity, embodies them experientially and holistically. The rhetorical question, "[S]ince he has recognized all things as himself, can there be any limit to his humanity?" suggests that, through a heart sensitive to the suffering of others, he is personally involved in the affairs of the cosmos, world, nation, community, and family to the extent that nothing is outside his orbit of concern. Any artificial imposition of a limit to his sensitivity and sympathy will adversely affect the inclusive nature of his humanity: "If things are not parts of the self, naturally they have nothing to do with it." The paralysis of the four limbs within the body as the microcosm is then analogized to show that, inspired by an ethic of responsibility, human beings as filial children of the universe must participate in the "transforming and nourishing process of Heaven and Earth" (see Chan 1963, 108). The body's vital energy should penetrate the macrocosm of the "great transformation" so that the "flood-like *qi*" can suffuse the space between Heaven and Earth. Only then can the painful experiences of alarm, unbearableness, pity, and regret be transformed into feelings of tranquility, equilibrium, impartiality, and joy.

Yuasa Yasuo, the contemporary Japanese thinker, concludes his original study titled *The Body, Self-Cultivation, and Ki-Energy* with a thoughtful note: "The view of human being[s] espoused by this philosophy ['a kind of practical anthropology developed by traditional philosophy and science in East Asia'] maintains that the human being is not a *homo faber* who conquers nature, but is an ecological, receptive being made alive by the invisible power working from beyond nature, for the human being is originally a being born out of nature" (Yuasa 1993, 188). As ecological, receptive beings born out of nature, the proper way for us to deal with pain and suffering as a species is to transform our anxiety, stress, and tension into creative energy and then to use the creative energy to enhance personal integration, to build a fiduciary community (Tu 1989, 39–66), and to establish a sustainable and harmonious relationship with nature (Tu 2001).

Notes

1. I translate *junzi* as "profound person" rather than "superior man."
2. Read Wang Gen's "Yu Nandu zhuyou" [Letter to Friends of the Southern Capital], in *Wang Xinzhai xiansheng quanji* [The Complete Works of Wang Gen, 1507 edition], in the Rare Books collection of the Harvard-Yenching Library, in Cambridge, Mass., 4.16b.

References

Analects. 1979. Trans. D. C. Lau. London: Penguin Classics.

Berry, T. 1990. *The Dream of the Earth*. San Francisco: Sierra Club Books.

Berry, T., and B. Swimme. 1994. *The Universe Story: From the Primordial Flaring Forth to the Ecozoic Era—A Celebration of the Unfolding of the Cosmos*. San Francisco: HarperSanFrancisco.

Boltz, W. 1982. "The Religious and Philosophical Significance of the Hsiang-erh Lao Tzu in the Light of the Ma-wang Tui Silk Manuscripts." *Bulletin of the School of Oriental and African Studies* 45(1): 95–117.

Boodberg, P. 1953. "The Semasiology of Some Preliminary Confucian Concepts." *Philosophy East and West* 2(4): 317–332.

Chan, W.-t., trans. and comp. 1963. *A Source Book in Chinese Philosophy*. Princeton: Princeton University Press.

Chang, K. C. 1983. *Art, Myth, and Ritual: The Path to Political Authority in Ancient China*. Cambridge, Mass.: Harvard University Press.

Er-Cheng yishu [Surviving Works of the Two Chengs]. 1963. In *A Source Book in Chinese Philosophy*, trans. and comp. W.-t. Chan. Princeton: Princeton University Press.

Leder, D., ed. 1992. *The Body in Medical Thought and Practice*. Dordrecht: Kluwer Academic Publishers.

Mencius. 1970. Trans. D. C. Lau. London: Penguin Classics.

Porkert, M. 1974. *The Theoretical Foundations of Chinese Medicine*. Cambridge, Mass.: MIT Press.

Tu, W. 1987. "A Chinese Perspective on Pain." *Acta Neurochirurgica* Suppl. 38: 148.

———. 1989. *Centrality and Commonality: An Essay on Confucian Religiousness*. Albany: State University of New York Press.

———. 1992. "A Confucian Perspective on Embodiment." In *The Mind in Medical Thought and Practice*, ed. D. Leder. Dordrecht: Kluwer Academic Publishers.

———. 2001. "The Ecological Turn in New Confucian Humanism: Implications for China and the World." *Daedalus* 130(4): 243–264.

Watson, B., trans. 1963. *Hsün Tzu* [*Xunzi*]. New York: Columbia University Press.

Yuasa, Y. 1993. *The Body, Self-Cultivation, and Ki-Energy.* Trans. S. Nagatomo and M. S. Hull. Albany: State University of New York Press.

Zhang zi quanshu [The Complete Works of Master Zhang]. 1963. In *A Source Book in Chinese Philosophy,* trans. and comp. W.-t. Chan. Princeton: Princeton University Press.

Zhouzi quanshu [Complete Works of Master Zhou]. 1963. In *A Source Book in Chinese Philosophy,* trans. and comp. W.-t. Chan. Princeton: Princeton University Press.

Ziyin, S., and C. Zelin. 1994. *The Basis of Traditional Chinese Medicine.* Boston: Shambala Publications.

Response:

Reflections from Psychiatry on Emergent Mind and Empathy

Laurence J. Kirmayer

I confess to an absolute surfeit of ideas and connections between things at this point in our discussion. At some moment this diagram will become sentient because there are so many connections.

In Tu Weiming's presentation there are a number of very broad, philosophical issues that I want to comment on from the point of view of psychiatry and the kind of attempt that goes on in clinical settings to integrate many different levels. Most of us adhere to what we could call emergent materialism. We accept that the human being is hierarchically structured, that emergent phenomena unquestionably exist by virtue of organization, that a neural network does things that an individual cell doesn't do, and so on.

One of the interesting philosophical questions, which links the biological view and the wider view of social cultural factors, however, is where mind itself emerges and whether it might emerge not simply at the level of brain but at the level of community and of interactions between people.[1] There are some phenomena we share with other animals that might occur just at the level of brain; but there certainly are other phenomena that emerge at the level of the linguistic community, and self-consciousness may well be one of them. The network that we then have to describe and understand involves other people, not just one person. There are things about our brain that make it especially good at such networks for evolutionary reasons.

I also wanted to say something very briefly about reductionism on another level. There are two kinds of reductionism that are important here. One is an ontological reductionism: Is it really only the building blocks that exist, and everything else is just an elaboration of those? The other is methodological reductionism.

I think one can reject ontological reductionism, because new things really do come into the world as a result of things becoming more elaborately arranged. Yet we can still accept methodological reductionism as one way to understand what's going on. We need to look for simple ways to take hold of the world, to make sense of what's going on. In talking about what the mediating structures will be, we must share a commitment to take one concept and see how far we can go with it, which is a certain kind of reductionism.

One last point on comparisons between Chinese medicine and Western medicine is quite important and will take us back to the social. In my understanding, in Chinese medicine the underlying assumptions about what the world is made of lead to an epistemology in which there is often no strong difference between a person's subjective report of his or her symptoms and the underlying problem. The account is an index, if you will, of the underlying problem. In contrast, for several hundred years, Western allopathic medicine has held the notion that verbal reports are deeply suspect in various ways, and we must see something in the body, or something lighting up in the brain, to know what's *really* going on.

One of the big appeals of Chinese medicine is not that it's holistic in any sense but that it does track people's experience. In Western medicine people are told, "You can't possibly have this pain, because there is nothing there"; or, "We fixed this pain, it's gone now." A terrible violence is done to people's experience because of the deep conviction that what is "real" must show up on our tests. This is a backdrop but quite pertinent to how people actually experience pain. The cultural models have profound influence both on interpersonal interaction, how a healer responds, and also on how a person conceptualizes his or her own pain.

I saw an exciting link to psychiatry in Tu's presentation around the issues of sympathy, empathy, and resonance. This has been a major concern in psychiatry, at least until recently. Nowadays, we're so biologized that we seemingly don't have to empathize with people as long as we can measure their antidepressant levels. In fact, all symptom reports in psychiatry are now taken as indices of an underlying disorder, not as narrative accounts of suffering.

But there is an older tradition in psychiatry that had a lot to do with human encounter, and some of us hope to return to that. It was preoccupied with understanding how to listen to another person, how to respond, and what the impediments to that are. I agree that we are so constructed that we feel other people's pain, and it's part of what lends us to the presence of another. But it's also palpably true that most of us spend a lot of time rather successfully fending off other people's pain, both individually and collectively.

Note

1. Arthur Kleinman calls this dimension of pain the "somatomoral" aspect—and hence the title of this part of the book. *Eds.*

Painful Memories

Ritual and the Transformation of Community Trauma

10

Jennifer Cole

We often think of pain as irreducibly private and physical, a process that occurs within individual bodies and has little to do with the social world. But as several scholars have pointed out, the experience of pain and suffering is also fundamentally social. In part, the social nature of pain results from the myriad ways in which the "social world and the body-self interfuse" (Kleinman and Kleinman 1999, 143; see also Erikson 1976; Kleinman 1999) so that the conditions of social existence manifest themselves in the lived body-self. But because pain is social, because of the variable ways in which it can be interpreted, it is also political. Studies in medical anthropology, in particular, emphasize the highly ideological nature of diagnosis and healing. In some cases, the interpretation and treatment of pain can have a depoliticizing effect, particularly when the suffering caused by wider social and economic processes is interpreted as an individual phenomenon. Women in poor Brazilian favelas, for example, embody the strain of living at the bottom of a stratified political and economic system through the idiom of *nervos,* a physical ailment that causes shaking, weakness, and headaches (Scheper-Hughes 1992). These women blame their own bodies for their weakness and for their inability to nurse their babies. They medicate themselves, and they do not turn an accusing eye on the Brazilian state. By contrast, many accounts of small-scale societies emphasize the way in which the sick individual body is interpreted as a sign of sickness in the wider social body; healing entails realignment of the social order. One thinks, for example, of Victor Turner's (1967)

Ihembi and the way in which his treatment involved the renegotiation of his lineage relations. And in some cases, the roots of pain and the way people respond to it may challenge the existing distribution of power. Take, for example, the ways in which the Mothers of the Plaza in Argentina, whose children had "disappeared," drew on their pain and grief to contest the politics of the Argentine state (see Suárez-Orozco 1992).

Unlike studies in medical anthropology, discussions of specific healing rituals have tended to sidestep questions of power in order to focus on the mechanisms of ritual efficacy. Perhaps one of the most famous attempts to understand how ritual healing works is that provided by Claude Lévi-Strauss. In his essay titled "The Effectiveness of Symbols" (1963), Lévi-Strauss analyzes a Cuna pregnancy chant sung by a shaman at a difficult birth. According to Lévi-Strauss's analysis, the shamanistic recitation narrates the patient's experience, thereby connecting physiological reactions to mythic categories. As Csordas and Kleinman (1996) observe, "the principal of efficacy in this interpretation is the inherent power of a correspondence or homology between symbolic acts and objects, metaphors, or cosmological structure and the thought, emotions, or behavior of those treated." It is the song's ability to create a narrative that links multiple levels of reality together that makes it effective.

By contrast, Tambiah (1977) and Schieffelin (1985) each use very different ethnographic data to argue that the way symbols "make sense of" and transform situations alone can not account for the processes through which healing might come about. Instead, they argue that we need to look closely at the ways in which the *experience* of ritual may work to "create the cosmology as an experiential reality for the participants" (Tambiah 1977, 98). In his study of a Thai healing cult, Tambiah (1977) shows how it is through the performance itself, and through the buildup of an illocutionary force created out of the repetition of ritual words, that the practice of meditation actually achieves its effect. Schieffelin elaborates on this performative approach in his analysis of Kaluli spirit séances. He argues that the real force of transformation comes about not so much from symbolic permutations as through the nondiscursive, rhetorical levels of performance and through the ways in which the spirit medium, in interaction with the audience, co-creates a new reality that recontextualizes a painful situation.

This chapter draws together assumptions about the profoundly ideological nature of healing with a focus on mechanisms of ritual efficacy through a discussion of a dramatic example of how people on the east coast of Madagascar used cattle sacrifice to heal their community after a war.[1] I argue that particularly in cases of social violence and healing the ability of ritual to assuage pain lies in its ability to draw pain into the process of producing—which is always, also, as many scholars have argued, a process of reconstructing—people's memories. To be sure, renarrativization and performance, the lynchpins of previous analyses of ritual efficacy, play a part in this process. But by focusing more specifically on *memory* as a mechanism that links individual bodies with wider social narratives, and *commits* people to a particular narrative by rooting it within their subjective sense of themselves, we have a powerful way to think about how ritual efficacy might be achieved. As we shall see, the process works through the production of affect—which following Massumi (1996) I see as the realm of visceral, bodily intensity and excitation—and its subsequent narration. However, precisely because the work of healing requires the harnessing of unstable, bodily affect, healing is only ever precariously, and temporarily, achieved.

The Rebellion

In March 1947, the same year that the British partition of India caused massive riots on the subcontinent, the peoples inhabiting the east coast of Madagascar rose in rebellion against the French colonial regime that had dominated their lives since colonial conquest in 1895. Malagasies armed with spears and the occasional gun attacked French administrative centers, military garrisons, police stations, French concessions, and Malagasy sympathizers with the colonial regime. Over the next two months, the revolt spread to cover most of the east coast of the island as bands of rebels moved from village to village, sometimes forcibly inducting men into the rebel army as they went.

Officials declared the rebellion over in December 1948, when they had defeated the last of the rebels. A full twenty months of fighting had passed. Author of one of the first history books to examine the rebellion seriously, Jacques Tronchon (1986) estimated that during the long campaign of 1947–1948, 550 French died, while 100,000 Malagasy were executed, tortured, starved, or driven into the forest. Even according to official French government accounts, 89,000 Malagasy died, about 2 percent of the entire population of 4 million; over 11,000 were killed as a result of military action (Allen 1995, 47; Tronchon 1986, 70–74).

Caught between the brutality of the French and that of the rebel army, Betsimisaraka—the name of the people who inhabit this region—suffered throughout the events. Civilians witnessed horrible atrocities as rebels killed people who had collaborated with the French regime. In many places rebels systematically mutilated their victims, and bodies were found riddled with spear wounds, cut into pieces, their genitals torn off. Others were carved into pieces and fed to dogs, or the dogs too were killed, tied to human bodies, and thrown in the water.[2] The French way of killing was equally brutal but more efficient. Senegalese and Moroccan soldiers attacked and burned villages suspected of harboring rebels, or they tracked the rebels through the forest, at times firing at anyone wearing a raffia shirt.[3] French planes flew low over villages, spraying them with machine-gun fire or dropping bombs and grenades that Betsimisaraka peasants often mistook for tobacco holders. Once people had fled into the forest, hunger, a less spectacular killer that eventually took more lives, exacerbated the initial violence. The rebel reports reveal a veritable obsession with food: my impression is that more people worked for them gathering food supplies than actually fought in battles, an observation that would correspond to the high rate of death by starvation documented by Tronchon (1986).[4]

But it was not only outsiders that inflicted pain and suffering the year that the rebellion occurred: local people also inflicted pain on each other. Based on evidence provided by survivors with whom I spoke, this pain was not for the most part the physical pain of torture. Rather, it was the kind of pain that results from watching your world fall apart, the pain that results from the breakdown of the social order. There was, for example, the pain suffered by one woman as she watched from the cover of the woods as a band of Creole settlers burnt her town. There was the sheer terror described by another woman who heard machine-gun fire while harvesting rice and was so terrified that she took her children and ran for days deeper and deeper into the woods. Others witnessed as their daughters were raped by French soldiers or taken as "wives" by rebel chiefs. And everywhere people betrayed each other—for example, by telling a rebel chief that a neighbor was really a French sympathizer and thus a traitor to the nationalist cause. Violence was ubiquitous.

In 1992, I went to do fieldwork in the region of Madagascar that had been most heavily hit by the violence I just described. At the time, there had been renewed anthropological interest in trying to understand nonliterate peoples' modes of historical consciousness. I chose Madagascar, and particularly the east coast, because the people there seemed to offer a unique combination of highly developed memorializing practices (the one thing most anthropologists know about Madagascar is that the people rejoice in the exhumation and reburial of their dead) with a turbulent history. Here, I hypothesized, was the perfect place to watch how people remember the painful and violent past. But what most struck me during the initial months of my fieldwork was the absence of any reference to the rebellion, as well as any sign of lingering pain. At the time, I thought that the rebellion was no longer a matter of importance. After all, we tend to assume that time heals, tissues regrow, and memory fades. With the passing of the years perhaps people had managed to put the events behind them and move on. Somewhat forlornly, I turned my attention to cattle sacrifice, which was people's primary healing ritual and with which they seemed deeply involved.

Several months into my stay, however, I found myself confronted by a curious phenomenon. At the time, Madagascar was in the midst of a political transition from a state socialist government to a more "democratic" regime subject to the demands of the International Monetary Fund and the World Bank. The transition entailed the holding of new elections. As propagandists from various political parties came through the town to woo votes, memories of the rebellion suddenly and spontaneously resurfaced with tremendous emotional force. Older people who had lived through the events began to talk about the failed rebellion incessantly. They talked openly about how they had fled into the forest, so terrified by the bombs and machine-gun fire that they couldn't even stop to bring food. They talked with rage about how they had felt tricked into joining the political party that had organized the rebellion, and they talked in more elliptical, guarded ways about the violence they had done to one another. And they talked about these events in such a way that witnessing them I felt that these were people who were not calmly reminiscing; they still seemed to feel pain. Surrounded by such an outpouring of pain and grief and the resurgence of what were clearly distressing, painful memories, I began to wonder how it was that I had thought they had moved beyond the events of the rebellion in the first place. Clearly my initial impression that they were not irrevocably traumatized by the events of 1947 needed revision.

What we have here is a story of the infliction of pain, its apparent erasure, and its sudden reappearance. But how does ritual fit in? People's fascination with cattle sacrifice gave me some clues; the archives point us in the same direction. Here I turn to what people did immediately following the rebellion.

After the War: Ritual Healing

Immediately after the rebellion, most civilians were still hiding, terrified, in the forest; the military sent planes loaded with leaflets telling people to come out of the forest because the fighting had stopped. In addition, the military used those Malagasy who had turned to the French for protection to work as guides, leading troops into the forest to relocate civilians who had gone into hiding. Faced with certain death by starvation in the forest, some people also returned to the town by choice. Typically they came crawling out of the bush, waving a white flag of surrender. After having checked in at military camps where a census was taken, survivors were then sent home to their villages, most of which had been burned to the ground either by irate settlers or by the occupying colonial army.

In the village where I would work, a military camp had been set up at one end of town, while the local inhabitants crammed together into the church, the only building left standing. By day, they were told to stick close to the village where French soldiers could protect them from marauding rebel bands. In the first few weeks after they "came up," most villagers worked on rebuilding their houses. As time wore on and the last rebels had made their submissions, people were gradually able to resume farming and to try and restore order to their lives.

From what I have been able to piece together from archival accounts and people's oral narratives, the period following the rebellion was characterized by an efflorescence of ritual activity. These rituals were organized by both the French colonial government and by the Betsimisaraka themselves. Comparing the problem of postrebellion Betsimisaraka society to France following the liberation, administrators in the area argued that they needed a way to reassert the authority that the rebellion had so seriously compromised. Their solution was to organize public tribunals in which respected Betsimisaraka elders and community members were made to judge and mete out punishment to people who had actively participated in the rebellion, in a process parallel to the contemporary Truth and Reconciliation Committee Hearings in South Africa. The punishment was called a "skin cleansing" *(sasahoditra),* and it involved anywhere from ten to twenty days of public labor, rebuilding the very school or maternity wards that they had destroyed in what one administrator referred to as a "frenzy of madness."[5] According to the local district chief, the "skin cleansing" was remarkably successful. "This practice of airing dirty laundry *en famille* has been an astonishing success," he observed. "The judges have judged with a zeal that compromises them definitively in our favor. The guilty have accepted their punishment with relief for the fear of the police which haunted them, as did the absence of punishment for a crime they considered to be sacrilege for they had raised their hand against their elders."[6]

But these official, colonially imposed kinds of rituals were matched by more intimate rituals that the Betsimisaraka themselves chose to perform. As one administrator described the local scene in 1949:

> The old customs have regained favor, people are attending more and more to their elders, there is a return to paganism that is almost disconcerting. This includes a wave of circumcisions around the month of September, the meticulous cleansing around the tombs which appears to be spreading in imitation of Europeans, and the numerous cattle sacrifices which appears to have exceeded

> 800 in this year alone.[7] Perhaps this return to traditional values is normal after a period of crisis like the rebellion, for we have ourselves experienced it in France after the armistice.[8]

Here, a little bit of local context is necessary. Like many Malagasy groups, the Betsimisaraka perceive ancestors as the root of all power, efficacy, and growth (see Cole 2001). People believe that their ancestors can bless and heal them, as well as cause them suffering and pain. During the rebellion, people called on their ancestors to help them in the struggle for independence; they also called on them simply in order to survive. Though considering their losses it would not have been surprising if Betsimisaraka had given up on the idea of ancestral power, the sheer fact of their survival despite defeat appears to have had the opposite effect.

Thus, many of those people who had made vows to ancestors during their flight and returned alive to the village felt obligated to fulfill their vow, called a *voady,* and repay the ancestral gift of life with a gift of their own. Sometimes the fulfillment of the vow meant the sacrifice of a bull, the most serious, powerful way to renew and negotiate their relations to ancestors. At other times, people made smaller vows that they could fulfill more simply. One woman I knew, for example, described how her father had returned periodically from their hiding place in the forest to gather rice that was still growing in their fields by the abandoned town. "He made a vow that when he really returned he would sleep for three nights at the foot of his ancestral prayer-post, next to where his ancestors house had stood." And he did.

While some rituals were performed at an intimate, family level, a number of sacrifices were also aimed at the level of the wider community. For the most part, these rituals appear to have been purifying rituals through which the community was cleansed and reconstituted after the violence of the war. As one old woman said, "[W]e killed a cow to cleanse the burned town. And we invoked the ancestors and said that if a Malagasy, master of the ancestors here, led Europeans to burn the town, then here was the cow that would judge him [before God]. But if the European's force which makes him a European [*mahavazaha an'azy*] made him burn the town, well, then, there was nothing we could do." Or as another older woman described what had happened: "We fled to the west, digging a huge hole in the ground where we hid all of our possessions, but they were all stolen by those who came up [out of the forest] first." [Jennifer: Did you sacrifice any cows when you came out?] "We killed two cows, to cleanse ourselves. . . . Malagasy had killed Malagasy, but they didn't mean to. So we washed that before God, and gave it to him to judge. There were those who did evil, but they didn't mean to for the government was too strong."

Based on what historical records tell us about those long twenty months during 1947–1948 as well as people's painful memories of the events, it seems safe to say that people in the region where I worked suffered deeply during the rebellion. We also know that they performed rituals in an effort to mark an end to the pain and social anarchy brought about by their experience of war. Given my experience of life in Ambodiharina, where people had indeed regained a sense of "everydayness," and where no survivor I spoke with described symptoms anything akin to posttraumatic stress disorder, these rituals appear to have assuaged social, and perhaps physical, pain. Again we return to the question: how? To explore this question further, I turn to Betsimisaraka beliefs and practices concerning cattle sacrifice.

Memory and Amnesia, Sickness and Health: Ancestors and Cattle Sacrifice in Betsimisaraka Social Practice

It has been suggested that interest in memory can be "considered screens on which a culture projects its anxieties about repetition, change, representation, authenticity and identity" (Roth 1989, 51). In nineteenth-century France, for example, people conceived of illness and suffering in relation to memory, and people were said to suffer from "too much memory" or certain kinds of forgetting, maladies that were always also discussions about what the relationship between past and present should be. These observations are relevant to the Betsimisaraka, whose cultural practice also reveals striking concern with the relationship between past and future; their conceptions of temporality are intimately intertwined with ideas about health and well-being. For Betsimisaraka, however, this focus on memory is embedded in an idiom of ancestors, which also links it fundamentally with power. Betsimisaraka hold that to live with ancestral blessing is to be healthy, prosperous, and happy. To live without it means one's life is fraught with pain, sickness, and death. That these ideas about ancestors are intimately tied to notions of memory is evident when we consider that Betsimisaraka ideology maintains that contemporary people should live as the ancestors live. Most people interpret this by saying that people should honor ancestral memory by living in the same places that their ancestors lived, farm their fields, honor their taboos, and maintain their tombs. This kind of memorializing behavior is said to maintain ancestral *hasina,* a word that means sacred efficacy and that people believe is a quality that imbues their lives and fortunes with prosperity and good health. In return for this kind of memorializing behavior, which pervades many aspects of rural Betsimisaraka daily life, ancestors are meant to bless their descendants and make them prosper. Power, memory, and ancestors are inextricably intertwined (see Cole 2001).

Ideally, people are supposed to live as their ancestors lived. In practice, however, the social order is, of course, constantly changing as people come to find old taboos inconvenient, decide to move their houses to new towns where they are more likely to be able to earn a living, or stop farming their ancestors' fields to pursue other interests. The problem as Betsimisaraka see it is that if people start to neglect or forget their ancestors, they are soon reminded because the ancestors come and make their recalcitrant descendant sick.

All this is not to say that Betsimisaraka do not recognize somatic causes of suffering—like many people, they have a pragmatic approach that recognizes that pain and suffering stem from both bodily and spiritual conditions, and they try to mix their interpretations and remedies appropriately. But people do maintain that Western medicine must be accompanied by the right actions in relationship to ancestors in order to actually work. Thus every illness requires that people treat the illness on both a material and a metaphysical level. This is where sacrifice comes into play, for Betsimisaraka believe that since it is ancestral wrath that makes them sick, if you can make good on your relationship to ancestors, you will be cured. What usually happens is that an ill person seeks out a diviner, who then reads divination beads and assesses the problem. If a sacrifice is required, the person is given "medicine against blame"—herbs that are believed to ward off ancestral anger and retribution until the person has amassed enough money for the sacrifice to be completed. At the same time, the sick person takes honey or rum (two substances believed to facilitate contact with ancestors), places it in the northeastern corner of the ancestral great house, and calls the ancestors, saying, "If you make me better, then I will sacrifice a bull to you in thanks." Betsimisaraka say that due to the "magical power of words" (see Tambiah 1985), the ancestors hear the vow and come and make the supplicant better. In return, the supplicant has to amass enough money to fulfill the vow and sacrifice a bull.

In most cases, the ritual sequence of a sacrifice is fairly simple. The chosen animal's legs are tied together, and the animal is thrown to the ground, its head facing east toward the ancestral prayer post. The young men who have wrestled the bull to the ground also usually take white clay, signifying ancestral blessing, and ritually wash the bull with water poured from a bamboo tube. At this point a ritual speech is delivered to the assembled community that states the reasons why the sacrifice is taking place. The respondent—a man who has been chosen by the villagers to assume this role—then verbally responds, acknowledging the reasons that the sacrifice is performed. So crucial is this response speech that people actually say that without it—and without the attendance of the villagers as witnesses—it is as if the sacrifice had never taken place. After the respondent has finished, the man in charge of communicating with the ancestors for that particular family steps up and seizes the bull by the tail (for direct access to the ancestors!). He lets out a piercing yell to get their attention and repeats the reasons that the bull is being sacrificed, but this time so that the ancestors will hear. His explanation done, he calls out a long list of ancestors' names. When the invocation is finished, young men come forward to kill the animal, which is usually done by holding the animal's head down with a pestle, while young men hack with a knife at the animal's throat. Though there are a few minor ceremonial details to finish off, the most important part of the ritual has now been performed (Cole 2001).

Before turning to look more closely at the sacrificial speech that forms the heart of the ritual, there are a number of points that I wish to make. Such sacrifices often take place *after* the person is already cured. Moreover, because Betsimisaraka conceive the material investments in the ceremony as belonging to an extended family, many family members will also use the sacrifice as their own opportunity to negotiate their relationships to ancestors. What begins as an attempt to heal an individual of pain and suffering ends up, by the time the culminating ritual is actually performed, as a much wider attempt to re-narrate a series of painful events in order to create what at least some participants hope will be a post-illness reality. The essence of the ritual is about re-creating the powerful, experiential reality of certain normative propositions through a process of scaffolding an individual's memories.

It was this kind of cattle sacrifice ritual that people performed when they returned from their flight in 1947, and it is this effort to create a post-illness reality that I want to explore here. Because the events of the rebellion happened forty-five years before my fieldwork, my argument is an inferential one. In particular, I suggest that by looking carefully at how sacrifice worked as a healing technique for assuaging physical and social pain in 1992–1994, some of which was, as we shall see, due to disruptions wrought during the colonial period that preceded the rebellion, we are in a better position to understand how collective and individual healing took place after the rebellion. The specific events occasioning the rituals I observed during 1992–1994 are not about the rebellion. However, the process of reweaving the social fabric, and engaging painful affect in the process of reconstituting people's memories, is a clear common thread linking these examples together.

As in any other sacrifice, Zakatiana, a man in his late forties, began his ceremony with a ritual greeting, in which he welcomed his guests to the event. His words were answered by the "respondent," a man who represented the other families gathered at the event. At this point, Zakatiana launched into the following narrative: "I promised to throw a sacrifice, but I didn't, and so I fell ill. A strong man had to carry me all the way to Marotsiriri [the Catholic dispensary], and I was not cured, and they carried me to Mahanoro [a town slightly farther away], and I was not cured; and they sent me all the way to Vatomandry [a town still farther away with a large hospital], but for six months I did not stand. My family carried me. 'Aha,' I said to my wife, 'I am ill.' And as my wife said, 'I will not leave my husband until he is dead.' [He recounts the conversation:] 'You won't leave me?' 'No, unless you are dead, I shall never leave you.' " At this point, Zakatiana emphasized the main reason for the ritual: "I was sick, now I am well. The ancestors have blessed me. Together we eat the bull."

Perhaps one of the most striking aspects of the sacrificial speech is the way it oscillates between what appear to be the two primary reasons for the ritual: first, that Zakatiana and his father and brothers have fathered many sons, and second, that Zakatiana was sick and has now recovered. What many people know is that it is precisely because Zakatiana produced many sons and did not immediately thank his ancestors that he fell sick in the first place. However, it is the triumphal line "I was sick, now I am cured. The ancestors have blessed me; together we eat the bull" that holds the ultimate key to understanding what is happening. For Zakatiana, like the other participants at the ritual, the ritual reaffirms one of the master narratives on which their understandings of their lives are premised: that ancestors bless their descendants and make them prosper and that, in turn, descendants recognize their ancestors with gifts of sacrifice.

Although Zakatiana's ritual was primarily about thanking the ancestors and demanding their blessing, it also incidentally reworked people's memories of the colonial past.[9] In particular, Zakatiana's ritual was also a house cleansing, a kind of ritual that transforms the meanings associated with tin-roofed houses. Thus, after having announced the primary reason for the sacrifice, Zakatiana continued his narrative with another story about Kasy, his paternal cousin who had gone to the city: "Along with that, we know that Kasy went out to seek for wealth. And at that time he decided to build a tin-roofed house in his ancestral land. And he built a tin-roofed house in his wife's town, and for that reason I announce to you that the reason we sacrifice the bull is to enter that house." Although space does not permit a detailed analysis here, houses have tremendous symbolic importance among Betsimisaraka as among many Malagasy peoples (see Bloch 1998; Cole 2001; Huntington 1988; Feeley-Harnik 1980; Thomas 1998). During the colonial period, Creole settlers and French colonial officials both inhabited tin-roofed houses, and these became important symbols of colonial domination, associated with the Chef de Canton and the Creole settlers who exacted taxes and impressed Betsimisaraka into work gangs. But Betsimisaraka also began to copy this style of house building, which was seen as a sign of prestige. Since Betsimisaraka believe that social identity is tied to place, people believed in symbolic terms that if you lived in a tin-roofed house, you in some sense became like a settler. It was during the colonial period that the belief emerged that if you lived in a tin-roofed house, you would suffer and die if you did not perform a ritual sacrifice. In effect, what the sacrifice does is to take the power and wealth that people accumulate through their associations with what are considered *vazaha*—foreign—ways of doing things and force them to recommit to the ancestral order. At the same time, and this is the point I want to emphasize here, the ritual takes what was once a symbol—and hence a potential site of memory—of the colonial order and recasts it as a sign, and memory, of ancestral power.

Finally, Zakatiana's ceremony, like most sacrifices, also asserted fundamental claims about people's relationships in the present. For example, referring to another member of his family, Zakatiana explained, "So too we know that Dez and Marie fought. Marie said, 'What is mine does not make you living (i.e., support you) nor does what is yours support me.' But now, Dez has bought that land and so we return those words that Marie spoke. May all that Dez plants prosper and make him living." In this case, the mention of the fight is a reference to a struggle over land, where a brother and sister fought, and the sister cursed the brother by saying, "What is mine doesn't make you living." Because Betsimisaraka believe in the magical power of words to effect change in the world, the brother was forced symbolically to remove these words over the body of the bull. The intended effect of the ritual is to erase, or remove, social tension and reinstate an ideal model of harmonious social relations. As the speech emphasizes, Dez had bought that land, and so, "May all that he does [on that land] make him prosper."

There are many variations on the themes I have addressed here and many different ways in which Betsimisaraka use cattle sacrifice to heal themselves, for as they are fond of saying, "Anything, anything can be washed on a bull." However, taken together, the various elements of the speech combine to produce the following master narrative: that Betsimisaraka live in a world of mutually nurturing ancestors and descendants, that they live in a world where the narrative of colonial power can be "washed" and reconfigured as a narrative of ancestral power, and that they live in a world that is free of social tension. Returning to the assumptions about the ideological nature of healing with which I began, we can see the profound links that Betsimisaraka make between healing individual bodies and the re-creation of the social order. Moreover, we can also see that particular efforts at re-creation are often also strategic efforts on the part of individuals to impose certain kinds of meanings. In Zakatiana's circumcision, for example, the discussion of Dez and Marie's fight was also an attempt to assert Dez's legitimate control over Marie's land, just as Kasy's house washing might also be read as the effort of a city dweller to soothe the envy of his rural kin. In the case of the rituals held after the rebellion, we can only guess at some of the social dynamics that took place, but it nevertheless seems likely that similar strategic considerations were also at stake.

Affect and Narrative: The Ritual Construction of Memory

Clifford Geertz once remarked that the Balinese cockfight represents the world to the Balinese as "they most deeply do not want it" (1973, 446). What seems to go on in sacrifice is just the opposite, as the people who sponsor a particular sacrifice use the ritual to create an ideal version of what they *wish* the world was like. This vision is most evident in the sacrificial speech that dominates the ritual event. The question remains, however, as to how this ritual relates both to the painful events of the rebellion and to the absence of pain and its reappearance that I witnessed during my fieldwork.

Let me return to Brian Massumi's (1996) conception of affect and its relation to symbolic processes that I mentioned earlier. According to Massumi, the domain of affect is located in a field of perception that is prior to language and images—it is the realm of visceral experience that strikes the senses, the body, and the brain. In other words, affect—pure intensity—exists prior to its representation in a meaningful system of signification but provides the raw material for various kinds of narrativization. In thinking through the question of how Betsimisaraka cattle sacrifice works to assuage pain, Massumi's model is useful, for Betsimisaraka sacrifice works as a healing ritual precisely through the narrative capturing of affect and the way it draws on people's pain in the process of making memories. Many neurobiologists have pointed out the close association between pain and memory: those drugs that alleviate pain also erase memory (Sandkuhler 2000). Likewise, social theorists from Durkheim (1995 [1912]) to Nietzsche (1923 [1887]) have pointed out that memory requires pain. In Betsimisaraka sacrifice, a contrary, if complementary, process plays out as Betsimisaraka use pain—in Massumi's terms, a form of affect—in the process of making less painful memories.

In some ways, given the prominence of the sacrificial speech, Betsimisaraka sacrifice shares a Lévi-Straussian focus on re-narration. After all, archival documents, which include Betsimisaraka testimony, suggest that Betsimisaraka were active participants in the events. If my informants are to be believed, however, the rituals held after the rebellion constructed a narrative that emphasized that "it was all the government's fault" and "they didn't really need to hurt one another," and these are the narratives that continue to circulate locally to this day. I believe that this interpretation is a result of the rituals that people performed at the time, though it is impossible to know whether people did not also project their concerns back onto their remembered version of the ritual. However, the focus on a narrative externalization in people's remembered version of the ritual in 1992 jibes with accounts by colonial officials in 1948, many of whom believed that Betsimisaraka tended to sidestep the question of their own guilt by externalizing responsibility and blaming the Merina.[10]

But it is hardly the narrative alone that accounts for how cattle sacrifice scaffolds people's memories, for it tells us little about why people feel committed to the memory at hand. It does not tell us how it is that people appropriate a particular narrative and use it to construct the memories through which they think about who they are, how it becomes something that they can "see" and envision in their mind's eye. In Massumi's terms, this process can only occur if the ritual succeeds in harnessing affect, by bringing affect together with a semantic network of meanings in the context of the rite. To start, individual affect is always, already there in the pain and suffering of the individual who sponsors the ritual. It is there as well in the anticipation of the many other attendees who—because of people's profound belief in the power of ancestral blessing—hope that they will somehow benefit from their participation in the rite. But affect is also collectively produced in many of the performative dimensions of the ritual emphasized by Schieffelin (1985) and Tambiah (1977). This production of affect that draws people into the construction of the ritual is built up in several ways. First, Betsimisaraka say that sacrifice only works if the wider community acts as a witness to the event. This need to witness is performatively incorporated into the ritual itself, when each of the guests comes and contributes a small amount of money to the proceedings. Though the money contributed is minimal, people always claim that it is the community's participation that makes the ritual effective. But the work of creating a performative reality and generating affect is visible in other ways as well, primarily in the call and response during which the crowd passionately asserts that the narrative presented by the speech-maker is true (recall: "your words are clear!" "Your words are true!"). The collective production of affect—and here it resembles nothing more than Durkheim's collective "effervescence"—is also visible in people's behavior as they cheer, fight, and scream over the body of the sacrificial bull.

Taken together, the different levels of affect, both the pain of the sponsor and the affect produced collectively during the rite, merge with the narrative constructed in sacrifice to powerfully scaffold people's memories. Through this process, the inchoate sensation of pain becomes articulated with a wider semantic network of meanings, so that individual pain and suffering become constitutive of particular, strategically negotiated interpretations of ongoing social relations. In the case of the rebellion, we might imagine that the ritual took pain, as a pure form of affect, and rendered it into loss, regret, and mourning, tying these emotions to people's understandings of a set of historical events. The affect produced in sacrifice enabled this process because it meant that people were committed to reading the possible meanings of certain events in a particular way as they sought to make their pain intelligible through the means of a larger shared narrative. But the very affect that made the ritual scaffolding of memory persuasive also meant that it remained incomplete. After all, memory is not pure cognition; not only are there many nonlinguistic ways that the past lives on in the present, but as I have sought to show, sensual, bodily experiences play into the construction of memory as well. People may have declared in their speech following the rebellion, "We didn't mean to hurt each other—it was all the government's fault," yet one wonders what other kinds of memories remain built into the structure of people's daily interactions.

Conclusion

Extreme pain, Elaine Scarry (1985) argues, "unmakes" the world. Following this assumption, we perceive pain as entirely negative, and we respond by trying to rid ourselves of it, to assuage it, to mask it. In addressing the question of how ritual heals social pain, my approach contributes to an understanding of this process. Yet the approach I have offered is also one that views pain, as a form of affect, as potentially productive. In contrast to those who argue in favor of either the imposition of meaning or the persuasiveness of practice, I have offered an alternative account: that ritual efficacy works by scaffolding individuals' memories, through the fusion of pain, a form of affect, with a strategically produced narrative.

And yet the question remains as to why the rituals that people performed following the rebellion of 1947 did not entirely work and why people seemed so overwhelmed by their painful memories when they remembered the rebellion during the election of 1993. I can only answer this question with regard to my specific case, but I believe that my answer has relevance for this dilemma with regard to other kinds of ritual healing, not least among them contemporary forms of psychotherapy (see, e.g., Frank 1973; Schafer 1983). My answer is this: while these rituals drew painful affect into the production of memory, they could never entirely control it, both because something as unstable as bodily affect evades total control and because life moved on, providing new kinds of conjunctures. In turn, this tells us something else about the nature of ritual healing. If the work of healing is about bringing together the physical, affective elements of experience and welding them to a particular kind of narrative, then historical contingency is also a fundamental part of ritual healing; the relationship between narrative and affect has to be renegotiated continually.

But if the rituals held after the rebellion did not totally erase pain, they did transform it into a pain of a different kind, moving the events that caused pain from ones that were endured to ones that were potentially transformative. The outpouring of memories that occurred during the elections caused distress, and people felt both fear and remorse as they talked about the events. But this outpouring was not unstrategic. What I noticed as I watched people recall the events of 1947 was that they were aimed largely at trying to influence the outcome of the elections by shaping who it was that younger people would vote for (see Cole 1998). Without delving into the complex politics of the situation, suffice it to say that most of the older people who had lived through the events believed that they were caused by a political party's efforts to contest the power of the colonial state. Having experienced considerable violence in their lifetime, these elders preferred to vote for the party in power because they hoped that it would keep state interference at a minimum. By contrast, several members of the younger generation wanted to cast their votes for the candidate they thought would lead them in the opposite direction. In response, older people used their painful memories, recast as public, normative discourse, as a political strategy to influence the outcome of the election: never again, they said, will we become involved in state politics. What seems to have happened is that from the time the rebellion took place, the meaning of the events had changed. From a source of unmodified grief, it had transmogrified into an important part of one generation's moral architecture, a moral architecture that became a part of their political strategy as they tried as best they could to pass their experience on to their children. As Kierkegaard (1983[1849]) reminds us, "[Y]outh has the illusion of hope; the adult has the illusion of recollection."

Notes

1. In two recent articles, Pamela Reynolds (1990) and Sansaka Perera (2001) address the role of ritual in post–civil war Zimbabwe and post–civil war Sri Lanka, respectively. However, to my mind these examples, while clearly highlighting the importance of ritual, do not adequately address the question of how ritual works, nor how it intersects with larger questions of ideology.
2. Throwing dogs in water is in fact the customary Betsimisaraka "burial" for dogs (it is taboo to bury them). Thus attaching a human body to a dog

symbolically as well as physically degrades the victim by equating them with dogs, the lowest form of animal life.

3. SHAT, Dossier 8H176, Note de Service, Juillet 1947.
4. ARDM, Série D872, D873, D879.
5. CAOM, Série IID 129, Rapport Politique, 1949.
6. Ibid.
7. Based on my experience of the region around Mahanoro, this is an extraordinary number of sacrifices. I attended over 25 sacrifices while I was there, but even assuming that I never heard about a portion of the sacrifices that took place, I would guess that there were not more than 150, if that.
8. CAOM, Série IID 129, Rapport Politique, Mahanoro 1949.
9. By "incidental remembering" I mean that remembering the colonial past was not in fact the goal of Zakatiana's ceremony; rather, through the process of reworking his relationship to his ancestors, Zakatiana also incidentally reworked memories associated with the colonial past. I develop the idea of incidental versus intentional remembering more fully in Cole 2001.
10. See CAOM, Série IID, Rapport Politique, 1948.

References

Archival Documents

Archives de la République Démocratique de Madagascar (ARDM), Antananarivo Affaire Politique, MDRM "1947"

Série D872, Affaires "Rébellion Malgache"

Série D873, Poursuites contre le MDRM et Ses Membres "Attentat à la Suréte de l'Etat"

Série D879, Déposition des Temoins, 1947

Centre des Archives d'Outre Mer (CAOM), Aix-en-Provence

Série IID, Rapports Politiques et Economiques des Circonscriptions 129, Mahanoro

Services Historiques de l'Armée de Terre (SHAT)

Série 8H176–177, Deuxième Bureau

General References

Allen, P. 1995. *Madagascar: Conflicts of Authority in the Great Island.* Boulder, Colo.: Westview Press.

Bloch, M. 1998. "The Resurrection of the House amongst the Zafimaniry of Madagascar." In *How We Think They Think.* Boulder, Colo.: Westview Press, 85–99.

Cole, J. 1998. "The Uses of Defeat: Memory and Political Morality in East Madagascar." In R. Werbner, ed., *Memory and the Postcolony: African Anthropology and the Critique of Power*. London: Zed Books, 105–125.

———. 2001. *Forget Colonialism? Sacrifice and the Art of Memory*. Berkeley: University of California Press.

Csordas, T. J., and A. Kleinman. 1996. "The Therapeutic Process." In C. F. Sargent and T. M. Johnson, eds., *Handbook of Medical Anthropology*. Westport, Conn.: Greenwood Press.

Durkheim, E. 1995 [1912]. *The Elementary Forms of Religious Life*. Trans. K. E. Fields. New York: Free Press.

Erikson, K. T. 1976. *Everything in Its Path: Destruction of Community in the Buffalo Creek Flood*. New York: Simon and Schuster.

Feeley-Harnik, G. 1980. "The Sakalava House." *Anthropos* 75: 559–585.

Frank, J. D. 1973. *Persuasion and Healing*, rev. ed. Baltimore: Johns Hopkins University Press.

Geertz, C. 1973. "Notes on the Balinese Cockfight." In *The Interpretation of Cultures*. New York: Basic Books, 412–453.

Huntington, R. 1988. *Gender and Social Structure in Madagascar*. Bloomington: Indiana University Press.

Kierkegaard, S. 1983 [1849]. *The Sickness unto Death*. Trans. H. V. Hong and Edna H. Hong. Princeton: Princeton University Press.

Kleinman, A. 1999. "Experience and Its Moral Modes." In G. B. Peterson, ed., *The Tanner Lectures on Human Values*, vol. 20. Salt Lake City: University of Utah Press.

Kleinman, A., and J. Kleinman. 1999. "The Moral, the Political and the Medical: A Sociosomatic View of Suffering." In Y. Otsuka, S. Sakai, and S. Kuriyama, eds., *Medicine and the History of the Body*. Tokyo: Ishiyaku EuroAmerica, 141–153.

Lévi-Strauss, C. 1963. "The Effectiveness of Symbols." In *Structural Anthropology*. New York: Basic Books, 186–205.

Massumi, B. 1996. "The Autonomy of Affect." In P. Patton, ed., *Deleuze: A Critical Reader*. Oxford: Blackwell, 217–239.

Nietzsche, F. 1923 [1887]. *On the Genealogy of Morals*. Trans. H. B. Samuel. London: Allen and Unwin.

Perera, S. 2001. "Spirit Possession and Avenging Ghosts: Stories of Supernatural Activity as Narratives of Terror and Mechanisms of Coping and Remembering." In V. Das et al., eds., *Remaking a World: Violence, Social Suffering and Recovery*. Berkeley: University of California Press, 157–210.

Reynolds, P. 1990. "Children of Tribulation: The Need to Heal and the Means to Heal War Trauma." *Africa* 60(1): 1–37.

Roth, M. 1989. "Remembering Forgetting: *Maladies de la Mémoire* in Nineteenth-Century France." In "Memory and Counter-Memory," ed. N. Z. Davis and T. Laquer. Special issue, *Representations* (Spring): 49–68.

Sandkuhler, J. 2000. "Learning and Memory in Pain Pathways." *Pain* 88(2): 113–118.

Scarry, E. 1985. *The Body in Pain: The Making and Un-Making of the World.* New York: Oxford University Press.

Schafer, R. 1983. *The Analytic Attitude.* New York: Basic Books.

Scheper-Hughes, N. 1992. *Death without Weeping: The Violence of Everyday Life in Brazil.* Berkeley: University of California Press.

Schieffelin, E. L. 1985. "Performance and the Cultural Construction of Reality." *American Ethnologist* 12: 704–724.

Suárez-Orozco, M. 1992. "A Grammar of Terror: Psychocultural Reponses to State Terrorism in 'Dirty War' and Post–'Dirty War' Argentina." In C. Nordstrom and J. Martin, eds., *Paths to Domination, Resistance and Terror.* Berkeley: University of California Press, 219–259.

Tambiah, S. J. 1977. "The Cosmological and Performative Significance of a Thai Cult of Healing through Meditation." *Culture, Medicine and Psychiatry* 1: 97–132.

———. 1985. "The Magical Power of Words." In S. J. Tambiah, ed., *Culture, Thought and Social Action: An Anthropological Perspective.* Cambridge, Mass.: Harvard University Press, 17–59.

Thomas, P. 1998. "Conspicuous Construction: Houses, Consumption, and 'Relocalization' in Manambondro, Southeast Madagascar." *Journal of the Royal Anthropological Institute* 4(3): 425–444.

Turner, V. 1967. "A Ndembu Doctor in Practice." In *The Forest of Symbols.* Ithaca, N.Y.: Cornell University Press, 359–393.

Tronchon, J. 1986. *L'insurrection Malgache de 1947.* Paris: Editions Karthala.

Response:
Collective Memory as a Witness to Collective Pain

Stanley Tambiah

Memory is of course a vast subject; so is pain. I want to remark on how pain is interpersonal and collective, beyond the individual, and how pain itself can be transformed.

From a social, cultural, and anthropological point of view, we know that various forms of collective memory are evoked and enacted in ongoing communal life. Such genres as cosmologies, myths, and narratives are all part of collective memory and are remembered, misremembered, enacted, recited, and performed at particular sites in the present, on public occasions. We know that these myths, narratives, or cosmologies are never static but always change when they are transmitted. They are therefore very mixed, according to the interests of the reciters, the positions they occupy, and so on.

Foundational myths that are said to be representative of the past actually change in a historical process over time, as do religious doctrines with all their variants. Although in communal life people want to relate the present to a past that is thought to be foundational and unchanged, in actual fact that foundational story is reworked again and again in terms of ongoing circumstances and processes.

Jennifer Cole's account of the collective experience of the 1947 Malagasy rebellion is an illustration of this. The interesting point of her story is that the experience of the rebellion is transformed from its colonial contours, a war of independence from colonial domination by the French, and it becomes a foundational memory that is reworked into the present postindependence era, restoring the ancestors as guardians of national life.

The sacrifice to the ancestors becomes a central act to effect their return, to purify, and to settle disputes as an integrative mechanism. But an interesting issue is raised, which I think anthropologists face all the time. Although the official ideology portrays the sacrifice as a mechanism for coming to terms with the ancestors when disputes and differences occur, nevertheless at the operative level of practice the performance of these mechanisms in public life enacts disputes and tensions that are not totally integrative. The sacrifice itself is in one way a divisive mechanism because it shows up the inegalitarian aspects of society in considerations such as who can sacrifice, who is invited, or how many buffaloes are sacrificed. So we are left with the question: How is this kind of reworked memory woven into actual life? To what extent does it transform and integrate pain? And to what extent, realistically, does it also work to produce the internal division and disputes that are part of our human condition?

In discussing the relationship of past to present, of foundational myths to present experience of pain, Roman Jakobson's notion of duplex structures is helpful. Jakobson (1971) said that duplex structures could be seen as having two kinds of manifestations. One is what he called "code to message." We can reinterpret code as a paradigmatic memory of an occurrence, which is the message or context. So code to message is the passage of meaning from a paradigmatic conception to its relationship to the present context, the indexical message. The reverse manifestation is where the messages of present-day contexts are related backward to the paradigmatic occurrence.

As an example of the message to code form, I want to mention particular circumstances relating to a paradigmatic foundational story. Among Shi'ite Muslims, the Muharram is a staging of the Karbala story, what some would call an unabashedly tearjerking account of the martyrdom of Husain, grandson of the prophet and son of Ali. This particular narrative of assassination is a foundational story for Shi'ite Muslims, how they painfully separated from the Sunni, and it also relates Islam to the present international context.

Its most important recital is on the tenth and final day of mourning in the month of Muharram. The first phase, called the *rouza,* refers to the assembly at the fateful tomb, when moral lessons are preached. The imam gives a long sermon, elaborating what present-day Shi'ite Muslims are suffering, their daily world, their relationship to Sunni Muslims, the relationship of Muslims to the West, and so on. The whole past of the struggle is worked into this sermon, which is very much indexed to the people in their present world assembled there. This first phase sets the stage for the next, final phase, the recitation of the battle at Karbala when Husain was slain. This is the phase that induces lamentation, the weeping and tears that are a sign of religiosity and moral purification.

The point is that the current trials and tribulations of the congregation are given focus and assimilated to a paradigmatic foundational occurrence. The foundational narrative is an understood collective memory of focal stories. The Muharram grieving brings some relief, no doubt, to the present day; but at a deeper level, there is also an understanding and realization and acceptance of the ongoing human condition of suffering.

This relates to the work done by anthropologist Patricia Lawrence (1999, 2000) on the current conflict in Sri Lanka between the Tamil insurgents and the Singhalese army. Her study is about how the Tamils, over the last two or three decades, have been periodically subject to the army's abduction of young men. Some are taken to camps and tortured and then let free. Others are taken and killed and are never heard from again. Once these young men are taken, their families can't go for relief or any explanation of what has happened to the police or army, because they are the inflictors. So what happens is that there is an intensification of the existing local mother goddess cults. The mother deities give prosperity and health and also act as punitive agents when people transgress morally. The mother cult is intensified and takes a new form, which addresses itself to the terrible pain of disappearances and torture, when the grieving mothers, whose sons have been taken away and whose husbands can't intervene, go to the temple.

Here the oracle comes in. Judith Becker's discussion of trance consciousness is very relevant to this. The oracle is a vessel of the deity and feels all the pain of the deities. They ask questions of the oracle: "Where is my son? Will I find him again?" At the same time, the oracle enacts the very pain of torture that the prisoners are supposedly undergoing in front of the mothers. The oracle then makes a pronouncement as to whether the mother will find him. Some of the messages are very clear: "You will never find him; he's dead."

The point is that the whole performance becomes an enactment of collective memory, because a number of mothers and witnesses each retell similar stories. This collective telling and collective pain is the formation of a collective memory. Second, the trance performance of the oracle gives a final, ritual closure to a painful experience by determining whether the young man is gone forever or may return in the future. This closure cannot occur as long as they don't know.

The mothers of those who will return from torture have to take a vow to do voluntary penance. Likewise, people who were tortured or maimed and then returned say that when they were being tortured, they took a vow to the mother goddess to do penance if she would take care of them. The penance to the goddess is pain in the form of fire walking, putting spikes through the cheek, and so on, that is voluntarily undertaken in order to bring closure and transform a situation of involuntary pain.

Undertaking voluntary pain to bring closure, and to move from the terrible pain of mangling and torture to another state, is another aspect of collective memory as a witness to collective pain and the attempt to transform it through ritual. Elaine Scarry (1985) has talked about torture as a silencer. There are instances here of people who have lost the faculty of speech as the result of torture and are brought to the oracle in hopes of regaining their speech.

References

Jakobson, R. 1971. *Selected Writings.* Paris–La Haye: Mouton.

Lawrence, P. 1999. "The Changing Amman: Notes on the Injury of War in Eastern Sri Lanka." In *Conflict and Community in Contemporary Sri Lanka,* ed. S. Gamage and I. B. Watson. New Delhi: Sage Publications.

———. 2000. "Violence, Suffering, Amman: The Work of Oracles in Sri Lanka's Eastern War Zone." In *Violence and Subjectivity,* ed. V. Das, A. Kleinman, M. Ramphele, and P. Reynolds. Berkeley: University of California Press.

Scarry, E. 1985. *The Body in Pain: The Making and Un-Making of the World.* New York: Oxford University Press.

Discussion:
Pain, Healing, and Memory

SARAH COAKLEY: I have a question for the anthropologists. I'm not sure quite how the sacrifice works in the different cases you've presented to us. The sacrifice is so laden with encoded meanings that it's very hard for an outside culture to get the meaning of it. Is it possible that rituals of closure to alleviate pain could be created in a culture that is highly secularized and unfamiliar with ritual activities? I'm thinking of something like the Lockerbie disaster, which was extremely traumatizing for the people who lost loved ones and also for Lockerbie town, where bodies were falling out of the sky and bits of flesh hitting the ground. What sort of ritual could be enacted to heal memories in a case like that, or would a fiat without an existing set of encoded religious practices be unsuccessful?

JENNIFER COLE: I don't see in principle why you have to have rituals in place to make a new one successful. As I mentioned, there is an obvious parallel to what people did with the Truth and Reconciliation Commission in South Africa to what happened in Madagascar after the rebellion. In addition to the private cattle sacrifice rituals that I was focusing on, the French set up big tribunals and emphasized how great it was that everybody confessed what they had done wrong. So I think you *could* create rituals of closure in situations like Lockerbie. They would probably be rituals of remembrance more than rituals of forgetting.

COAKLEY: That's an interesting paradox. Questions have already been raised implicitly about the relationship between forgetting and remembering. It seems that sometimes you have to remember in order to forget; it's not that you're creating a disjunction between them.

COLE: In terms of how the ritual works, people create the verbal master narrative in the context of incredibly heightened emotion. It's well known that emotion makes memory labile. What the Malagasy are doing really is rewriting their memories by drawing in the whole group who jump up and down with them, saying, "That's right, that's right, that's right."

CLIFFORD WOOLF: The molecular mechanisms that underlie many of the processes responsible for pain are almost identical to those responsible for memory. The similarity is incredible, to the extent that many drugs that were used to treat pain had to be abandoned because they caused amnesia. I think the evolutionary development of pain and memory go hand in hand, and that may be important when we look at pain in the wider context.

COLE: Painful memories are related to what Voloshinov (1976) calls the "unofficial conscious." Voloshinov argued that what actually distinguishes the conscious from the unconscious is not the difference between two kinds of reality; because both are ultimately expressed through words, which are fundamentally social, both are aspects of consciousness. Rather, the difference between the conscious and the unconscious lies in the degree of ideological sharing. The unconscious is guided by inner speech, which is a relatively idiosyncratic ideological realm, because it has not yet been completed in words, which finish complete thought and render it social. By contrast, consciousness is expressed in words that are part of ideologies. They're shared openly with others. Voloshinov renamed the social unconscious of inner speech the unofficial conscious.

This notion of the unofficial conscious differs considerably from a Freudian concept of the unconscious, which is usually conceptualized as the location of presocial psychic drives. As the existence of individual memories of 1947 makes clear, the memories of the rebellion have not been erased, nor would I say have they been repressed in the psychodynamic sense of the word. Rather, through the articulation of social and individual memory that takes place through sacrifice, memories of 1947 have been socially suppressed. They've been pushed into the background against which the work of constructing an official social narrative plays out.

In the contemporary literature that specifically addresses the question of how ritual transforms collective pain, one possible model that addresses sacrifice ritual is found in Godfrey Lienhardt's (1961) classic discussion of symbolic action. Lienhardt argued that sacrifice as a healing ritual works by symbolically removing the patient's weakness in using words and symbolically replacing that weakness with something strong. The effect, Lienhardt suggested, was to detach weakening from strengthening elements within the rite and the consciousness of the participants.

One of the most powerful contemporary accounts of how to deal with traumatic memories is offered by Judy Herman (1992), who argues that all trauma creates a generic, transhistorical, traumatic memory. She sees this as a special kind of memory, sealed off from everyday consciousness, which is nevertheless painfully lodged within the person's psyche. For Herman, healings occurs only by accurately gaining insight into the actual cause of suffering and telling that story in a kind of insight therapy, literally re-membering it and integrating it into your narrative.

In contrast to the focus on remembering, so central to these accounts, where memory is implicitly—and we know wrongly—assumed to entail an accurate portrayal of the past, the mnemonic work of sacrifice seems to me to be a systematic effort at forgetting in order to heal. It is as if the painful memories were responsible for making one sick, and the state of health is achieved by asserting, "Yes, painful events did happen—" or in some cases, "Yes, I did wrong—but this is not the way things should be." The ritual thus works to create a kind of directed forgetting. Although Betsimisaraka[1] clearly believe that forgetting requires ritual work, there is also evidence that it is often easy to forget. As Laurence Kirmayer has noted, it is quite easy to forget when there is a tacit agreement not to remember.

Perhaps the work that takes place in sacrifice bears the closest resemblance to what hermeneutic psychoanalyst Roy Schafer (1994) argues occurs in psychotherapy. Schafer focuses on how, in clinical interactions, the analysant gradually learns to revise the narrative that shapes his or her experience. Though Schafer doesn't focus on memory, his account of what happens seems to me to bear a striking resemblance to what takes place in sacrifice. People going through psychoanalysis tell the analyst about themselves and others in the past and present. In making interpretations, the analyst retells these stories. In the retelling, certain features are accentuated, while others are placed in parentheses. Certain features are related to others in new ways or for the first time. Some features are developed further, perhaps at great length.

What occurs in sacrifice is more dramatic and has many more performative elements than the psychoanalytic analogy allows, and it also works very evidently to involve a wider community of people in the new narrative. Nevertheless, it seems to me that perhaps Betsimisaraka and certain psychoanalytic practitioners have found different routes to a common truth: that excising painful experience by changing the story can also work as a means to re-inhabit a painful world. The anthropologist Gananath Obeyesekere (1990) used the phrase "the work of culture" to refer to the ways in which painful motives and affects, such as those occurring in depression, are transformed into a publicly accepted set of meanings or symbols. In light of the present example, we might extend this and call it "the work of memory."

ARTHUR KLEINMAN: I think this session and the music session are very provocative because they bring into the domain of pain the collective, which is almost routinely left out of the laboratory or clinical setting. It's crucial to see how they instate that. In the music session, we saw music as a mediator between the cultural world and the body. In this session, we have an argument from Tu Weiming about the deep cultural structure that informs experience and that links the world to the person through ideas and practices of cultivation, and a conceptual system involving a medium of energy that exists not just in the individual but in the social world and in nature itself.

I thought it was extremely important that, in the example we just heard from Jennifer Cole and Stanley Tambiah, we see the moral as a mediator. What is at stake locally in moral meaning is carried in memory, whether it's repressed, forgotten, or expressed through the experiences of individuals, and it ties the moral to the emotional. That's why we have to talk of the "somatomoral" dimensions of pain.

Note

1. The term "Betsimisaraka" refers to the peoples who inhabit the central east coast of Madagascar, ranging roughly from Mananjary in the south to Vohemar in the north. The name means literally "the many who will not be sundered" and originated in a political federation formed during the nineteenth century in the north of what is now Betsimisaraka country. Later, the name was codified and applied by both Merina and subsequent French colonizers to some southern areas of the east coast as well.

References

Herman, J. 1992. *Trauma and Recovery.* New York: Basic Books.

Ingalls, D. H. H., J. Masson, and M. V. Patwardhan, trans. 1990. *The "Dhvanyāloka" of Ānandavardhana with the "Locana" of Abhinavagupta.* Cambridge, Mass.: Harvard University Press.

Lienhardt, G. 1961. *Divinity and Experience.* Oxford: Clarendon Press.

Obeyesekere, G. 1990. *The Work of Culture: Symbolic Transformation in Psychoanalysis and Anthropology.* Chicago: University of Chicago Press.

Schafer, R. 1994. *Retelling a Life: Narration and Dialogue in Psychoanalysis.* New York: Basic Books.

Voloshinov, V. N. 1976. *Freudianism: A Marxist Critique.* Trans. I. R. Titunkik. New York: Academic Press.

Pain as Isolation or Community?

Literary and Aesthetic Representations

Among Schoolchildren

The Use of Body Damage to Express Physical Pain

11

Elaine Scarry

One day long ago I was in the midst of looking at paintings in a museum when a sweet voice (but quite loud and belonging to no one I could see, for it came from beyond the doorway) suddenly spoke: "Now, children, I want you to go into the next room and sit in front of the painting that has the most physical pain in it." A second later, a large crowd of seven-year-olds came tumbling through the doorway, and for a while, as they milled around the large gallery and I went back to looking at paintings, I lost track of them. But before long, their motion and murmuring subsided; the room was still; the disarray of children had coalesced into two coherent gatherings. Half of the children sat huddled together on the floor beneath Rubens's *Prometheus Bound;* the other half (actually, a little more than half) sat silently beneath Pacecco de Rosa's *Massacre of the Innocents.*

Prometheus, bright white with pain, is naked and upside down. His face and arm fill the lower right-hand corner; his bare chest, groin, thighs, and feet proceed upward on a diagonal. He is held in place by a giant eagle whose outstretched wings are wider than Prometheus is long. Because the colors of the feathers—painted at Rubens's request by Frans Snyders, a leading painter of birds—merge with the swirling tree above and cliff below, the raptor seems vaster still, as though encasing the big-bodied man. The eagle resides on the same tilting diagonal as Prometheus, but because he is buoyant and right side up, he is at ease and in his element. He has slammed the man to the ground and yet seems somehow almost to be carrying him through the air.

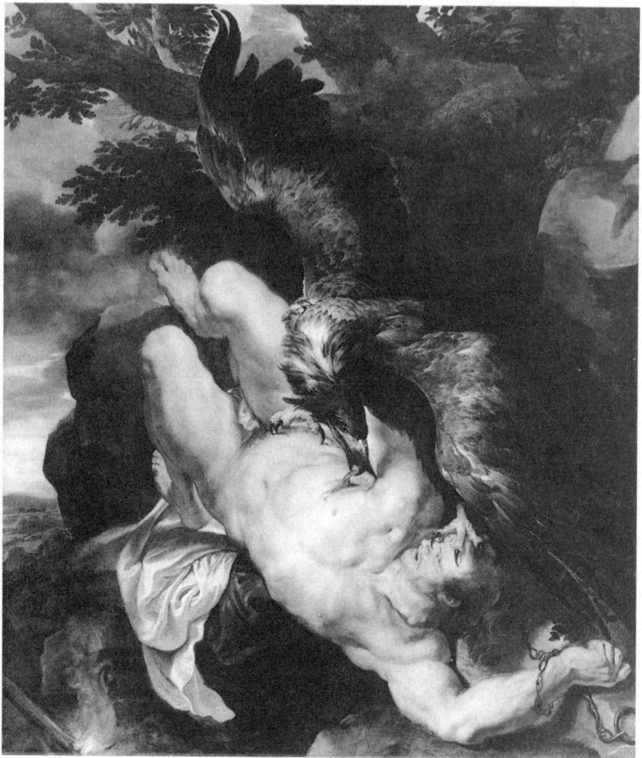

Figure 11.1. Peter Paul Rubens, *Prometheus Bound.*

The bird overpowers the man as the painting overpowers those who stand or sit below it—"A sudden blow"; "a feathered rush."[1] Talons rest lightly on Prometheus's nostril, temple, belly, and groin, poised to penetrate the moment the man resists or pushes up against his assailant. But he has already been penetrated: the eagle's beak has sliced open a neat cut below one breast through which he fishes out the tip of an organ, a ghastly tonguelike projection that occupies the center of the canvas. Our eyes, the eyes of the bird, and the eyes of the man are gathered together around this central event.

Depicted in *Prometheus Bound* (Figure 11.1) are both the agent of injury (the raptor) and body damage (the exposed organ); and it is probably through these two elements that the museum children have inferred that the man is in pain. The equally overwhelming *Massacre of the Innocents* (Figure 11.2), where swords flash and babies bleed, similarly depicts both the weapon and body damage, and it is probably again these two elements that let the museum children sense the presence of pain. How body damage enables us to perceive pain and yet sometimes also greatly confuses our perception is the subject of this chapter.

Because the existing vocabulary for pain contains only a small handful of adjectives, one passes through direct descriptions very quickly and (as noted in Medvei 1949, 40) almost immediately encounters an "as if" structure: "it feels as if . . . : it is as though. . . ." On the other side of the ellipse there appear again and again (regardless of whether the immediate context of the vocalization is medical or literary or legal) two and only two metaphors, and they are metaphors whose inner workings are very unstable. The first specifies an external agent of the pain, a weapon that is pictured as producing the pain; and the second specifies bodily damage that is pictured as accompanying the pain. Thus a person may say, "It feels as though a hammer is coming down on my spine" even where there is no hammer; or "It feels as if my arm

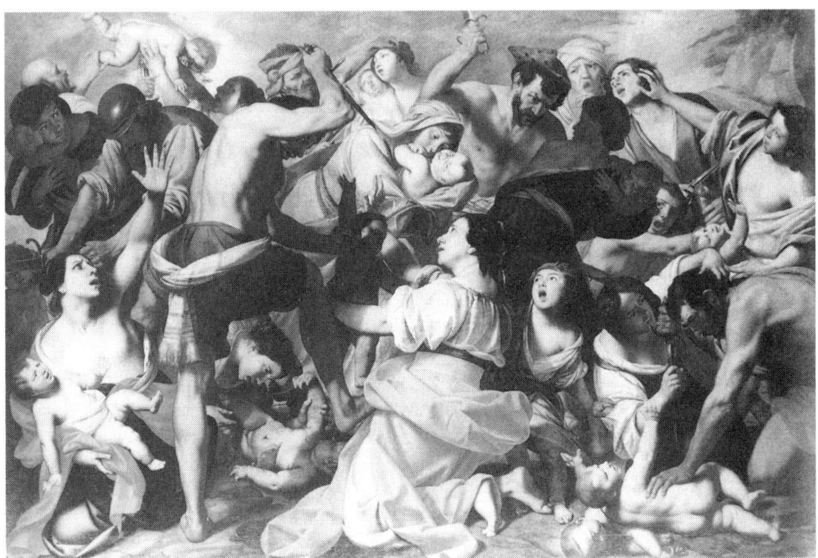

Figure 11.2. Pacecco de Rosa, *Massacre of the Innocents.*

is broken at each joint and the jagged ends are sticking through the skin," even where the bones of the arms are intact and the surface of the skin is unbroken. Physical pain is not identical with (and often exists without) either agency or damage, but these phenomena are referential. They have observable material features of shape, weight, and color; consequently we often call on them to convey the experience of the pain itself.[2]

In order to avoid confusion here, it should be noted that it is of course true that in any given instance of pain there may actually be present a weapon (the hammer may really be there) or wound (the bones may really be coming through the skin); and the weapon or wound may immediately convey to anyone present the sentient distress of the person hurt. In fact, so suggestive will they be of the sensation of hurt that the person, if not actually in pain, may find it difficult to assure the companion that he or she is not in pain. In medical case histories of people whose pain began with an accident, the sentences describing the accident (the moment when the hammer fell from the ladder onto the person's spine) may more successfully convey the sheer fact of the patient's agony than those sentences that attempt to describe the person's pain directly, even though the impact of the hammer (lasting one second) and the pain (lasting one year) are obviously not the same (and the patient, if asked whether she has the feeling of "hammering" pain, might correct us and say, "No, it is knifelike").

The central point here is that insofar as an actual agent (a nail sticking into the bottom of the foot) and an imagined agent (a person's statement "It feels as if there's a nail sticking into the bottom of my foot") both convey something of the felt experience of pain to someone outside the sufferer's body, they both do so for the same reason: in neither case is the nail identical with the sentient experience of pain; and yet because it has shape, length, and color, because it either exists (in the first case) or can be pictured as existing (in the second case) at the external boundary of the body, it begins to externalize, objectify, and make sharable what is originally an interior and unsharable experience.

Both weapon (whether actual or imagined) and wound (whether actual or imagined) may be used associatively to express pain. To some extent the inner workings of the two metaphors, as well as the perceptual complications that attend their use, overlap because the second (bodily damage) sometimes occurs as a version of the first (agency). The feeling of pain entails the feeling of being acted upon, and the person may either express this in terms of the world acting on him ("It feels like a knife") or in terms of his own body acting on him ("It feels like the bones are cutting through"). Ordinarily, however, the metaphor of bodily damage entails a set of perceptual complications wholly distinct from those which characterize the language of agency.

The Body in Pain concentrates on the language of agency and shows the perceptual and political complications that accompany it. The problems it creates are grave. On the one hand, it is, as was noticed a moment ago, a potentially benign resource. If someone can say to a physician or a friend "It feels as though a huge beak is cutting open my breast," it may begin to confer some picturable features on the pain and assist the physician or friend in comprehending the immensity of the otherwise invisible experience. The virtue of the pictured beak is that it can be pushed outside the boundary of the body, carrying out there some of the attributes of the pain with it. Pain clinics sometimes invite a person in pain to confer an object form on the sensation of hurt and then push it outside the body.

But that objectification and separability from the body—though themselves great advantages—can also become great disadvantages: the knife that can be lifted away permits all the attributes of pain to be lifted away and bestowed on something else. The features of extreme pain, such as its totalizing, world-destroying power, can be lifted away from the person in pain and conferred on the regime that tortures, so that it is now not the person's pain but the pathetic torturer that appears to have world-destroying power.

The unanchoredness of the image of the weapon lets it be torn away from the referent: the cascades of weapons drifting across television and film images seldom work to direct thoughtful attention to people in pain. In those situations where a weapon *does* elicit compassionate attention, the weapon is usually yoked to the person in pain so that the referent of pain remains steadily visible. This yoking can take many different forms. Christian iconography, for example, makes it difficult to decouple the weapon (the cross) from the pain of Christ because the weapon and the body of Jesus are affixed to one another and do not easily undergo any spatial separation, as they might if the story centered on a different kind of weapon.

The problems that come from the language of agency, then, come from the ease with which it can be separated from the sufferer; and the benign potential comes by holding the referent steady and not letting the spatial separation take place. The problems that come from the language of body damage are exactly the opposite: the image of the body damage often sits on top of and blocks our access to the person in pain. The benign potential of the body damage metaphor requires a solution that is the precise opposite of the one needed in the case of agency: now it is spatial separation, or a willed act of doubling, that seems to assist us in carrying out an act of sympathetic attention.

It may be helpful to back up a step and begin by underscoring the association between the felt experience of pain and body damage. William Breitbart (1992), citing the classic definition of pain from the International Association for the Study of Pain, described it as "an unpleasant sensory and emotional experience that we associate with tissue damage or describe in terms of tissue damage."[3] Thomas Szasz reports that so much is physical pain felt as a mutilation that patients sometimes do physically mutilate their bodies in order to bring the actual body image "up to date" with the felt experience (1957, 138). Paul Schilder stresses that pain is felt as a wound or opening into the body (1950, 89). (This observation corresponds with the fact that pain is depicted in both medical advertisements and the visual arts as a turning of the body inside out.) So associated are pain and damage that when H. K. Beecher published *Measurement of Subjective Responses* in 1959, he felt it necessary to state that in combat there is no coherent relation between the size of the wound and the amount of the pain, contrary to all intuition on this subject (1959, 165, cited in Melzack 1973, 30).

The problem with expressing pain through the metaphor of body damage is the nonseparability of the two: the body in pain is the same body whose surface is broken, and the overwhelming visual spectacle of that broken surface may either repel attention—causing the onlooker to wince, recoil, and turn away—or may instead be suggestive of the attributes of pain, but the obscenity of the hurt may drown out our apprehension of the nonobscenity of the person beyond.

This phenomenon is familiar in the need for the continual reminder (in both the medical and everyday world) that it is the disease, not the person, that is the enemy. As it is the work of the disease to annihilate the person, so it is the work of the disease to eclipse the person in our field of vision so that the person disappears. Odysseus abandoned Philoctetes because the grotesque features emanating from the wound—the pus, the smell, the vocalized shrieks—were to him obscene: Odysseus believed no prayers could be directed to heaven on their ship with Philoctetes aboard.

The perceptual path along which body damage eclipses our recognition of the person in pain is something like this: the graphic characteristics of the wound may transcribe the felt experience of the pain but may give a misleading account of the person in pain; the red rawness of the sore may correctly suggest the felt-red rawness of the pain beneath, but it simultaneously and wrongly makes the person in pain seem red and raw. Like Philoctetes, the person himself now smells and is pus filled. It is as though the person is a template of pain rather than a person in pain. The bodily mutilations presented in the rapid fire of media images are no more invitations to sympathetic identification than are the weapons streaming past our eyes. The person—the potential object of our attention and concern—has been buried beneath the overlay of wounds.

Virginia Woolf complained about the absence of a language for physical pain and observed that if there were such a language, it would have to be obscene. The metaphor of body damage provides the missing form of expression—but one that, as Woolf predicted, is obscene. We have so far argued that the obscenity of body damage correctly expresses the obscenity of pain but wrongly makes the person in pain seem obscene, or alternatively, creates a surface to which we have such a strong visceral aversion, that we do not even notice that there is a person back in behind that flamboyantly broken skin.

Someone at this point in the argument might complain that while it is brutal to perceive a person as obscene, it is also brutal to perceive body damage as obscene. But the word is being used here descriptively, not normatively. The visceral aversion we have to seeing the inside of the body, or things coming out of the body (or to quote the *Cambridge Encyclopedia of the English Language*, "substances exuded by the body" ([Crystal 2003, 172]), is what the word "obscene" means. The word registers the objection, the swift swerving away of the self, from any uninvited display of the interior of another person's body, whether it is the tip of the liver erupting out through a slash or everyday "substances exuded" like saliva, urine, ear wax, or excrement. There is a small subset of places or substances inside the body whose display we simultaneously desire (and they may elicit a powerful conflation of attraction and aversion); but most interior bodily facts are greeted with aversion—or more accurately, they are facts from which we withhold any greeting, not just with small clucking noises of disapproval but with an overwhelming visceral "no," as though one's whole torso turned away to spare the senses that are located on the forward positions of face and form. What makes the medical profession, or any act of caretaking, remarkable is that its practitioners must override this visceral "no" and greet—place the face close to—the uninvited display of another person's liver or excrement. The unfortunate way this generous confrontation with the interior of the body may work to eclipse the caretaker's attention to the person who exists on the other side of that exposed interior is part of what we are trying to comprehend. And there are, of course, some wounds from which even highly practiced physicians pivot away. St. Christopher hospices are known to have originated to help people whose ghastly cancer tumors caused physicians to shun them (Dermit 1992).

The way in which body damage correctly transcribes the obscenity of pain but in doing so repels humane attention to the person is illustrated by the paintings of Francis Bacon. His work is often identified as having physical pain for its subject but is not usually understood as inviting compassionate attention to pain, despite the frequency with which Bacon himself spoke of "the poignancy" of his paintings, of wanting to make a given image "more poignant, more near" (Sylvester 1988, 12, 72). Human figures and faces have been violently damaged in these paintings, as though flayed, their features shoved out of symmetrical planes, melted, or turned inside out. Bacon described himself as pushing "the figurative" not in the direction of "damage" but in the direction of "abstraction"; but in the living world, our bodies and faces acquire what he is identifying as the quality of abstraction only when they have suffered some terrible disease, accident, or act of cruelty.

Bacon's vocabulary of "abstraction" implies a departure from the material plane, whereas his announced intention (as well as the manifest quality of the canvases themselves) was to make unnegotiable the viewer's commitment to the material plane, to "bring the figurative thing up into the nervous system more violently," to "[come] across directly into the nervous system" (Sylvester 1988, 12, 18).

In Rubens's *Prometheus Bound,* the uninvited tip of the organ, its hard-to-escape location at the center of the painting, is counterbalanced by the vast portion of the canvas in which the man and his world remain intact. The protruding liver, cut, and beak together comprise approximately one-fiftieth of Prometheus's body surface and less than one-two-hundredth of the full canvas. Upside down, the man is in jeopardy but also intact. Even if, like the Philadelphia schoolchildren, one does not know that he stole fire from heaven on humanity's behalf (memorialized at the bottom left corner of the painting in the torch that has dropped from his hand—still clenched but now in pain), he is self-evidently a large actor in a large conflict with a large opponent.

But what if we now reverse those proportions? Say, the eagle were to keep pulling the entrails up through that small, neatly cut wound, eventually piling up stomach, pancreas, liver, intestines before us, until the space that could now be accorded to personhood were only as large as the tiny space that Rubens formerly accorded the wound. Then we would exactly have arrived at the central panel of Bacon's *Three Studies for Figures at the Base of a Crucifixion* (Figure 11.3) in which a small residue of personhood, a recognizable human mouth (that may be smiling or speaking or screaming), is affixed to a naked, unencased, freestanding intestine. Here body damage, as Bacon intended, acts directly on our nerves, delivers a blow, but unlike the blow delivered to the children sitting beneath *Prometheus Bound* or the *Massacre of the Innocents,* there is no center of consciousness to hold on to.

Can one locate inside oneself, as one looks at this painting, a seed of compassion that, if nourished, might grow? Compassion toward what? Toward whom? The world of the canvas has been emptied of almost any personhood that we can recognize or reach. Does not the mouth simply lead to more insides? Would one find in there a recognizable human face and limbs out of which one might begin to fashion a decent response?

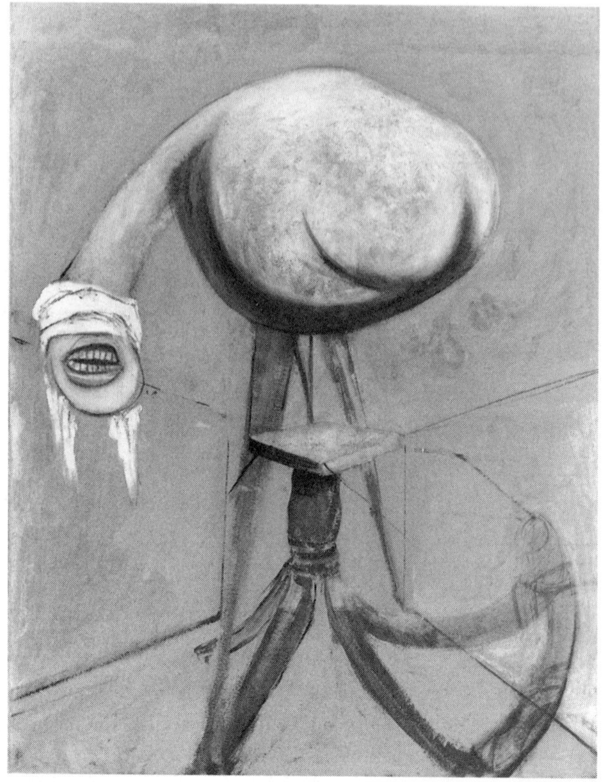

Figure 11.3. Francis Bacon, *Three Studies for Figures at the Base of a Crucifixion* (1944), central panel.

The reversal in the ratio of organ to person when we go from Rubens to Bacon is not just an exercise in the viewing of paintings.[4] The scale of the wound, as Beecher noticed, has no necessary relation to the scale of the person's pain; but the scale of the wound does have some coherent relation to the onlooker's capacity for sympathetic attention. So difficult is the act of nursing in burn clinics—where a vast portion of the outside covering skin has sometimes been taken away from the person and the inside exposed—that nurses may elect to undergo a form of education called "staying" in which they try to reverse the impulse to vacate their post, try to overcome their inability to make ongoing contact with the person who lives on the other side of a vast wound.[5]

The difficult labor of "staying"—the ease of vacating the canvas of personhood—is relevant to many parts of the medical profession, even where the visible harm is less totalizing than in a burn clinic. Even if only the tip of the liver has intruded itself into the physician's midst, the physician must, in order to treat the medical problem, bring his face so close to the organ that it may begin to take up as much visual space as in Bacon's rendering. How can a physician do what he or she must do if he or she pays attention to the full stature of the person, some parts of whom extend all the way up into the treetops, and other parts extend deep into the cliffs below? The edge of the canvas ceases to be the outermost inch of the painting and becomes instead any part of the painting not contained inside the narrow circumference of the wound.

The tendency of body damage to isolate attention has been further magnified by the general shift from general practitioner (or family doctor) to specialist. The general practitioner used to know the patient's cliff-to-treetop stature, having routinely measured him each year, and knew as well his antecedent life story, including the aspiration for firelight that preceded, and may have contributed to, his current liver trouble; the specialist, interested in the liver alone, does not even notice that the patient is upside down or, noticing that, thinks this must be the way Mister (what was his name again?) Promiseus has all his life carried himself through the world. The physician can no more imagine that the liver, or the bearer of the liver, actually invented the lights under which he is now operating than we can suppose that Bacon's creature endowed us with some other widely shared gift.

The surprise is that *if* one *can* suppose that—*if* one *can* imagine that this gaping, blindfolded intestine is the originator of, say, the art of painting—one then at once feels dawning within one the recognition of the creature's physical pain, the immense sorrow of it and the immediate need to eliminate it, not just the disgusting aversiveness of it. If, in other words, one can grasp a personhood as immense as the visible body damage is immense, the two together make the recognition of pain possible.[6] This doubling is, as has long been recognized,[7] the imaginative strategy at work in Sophocles's *Philoctetes,* whose hero is endowed not only with an immense wound (which began in his foot but has now festered through the full canvas of his body, so

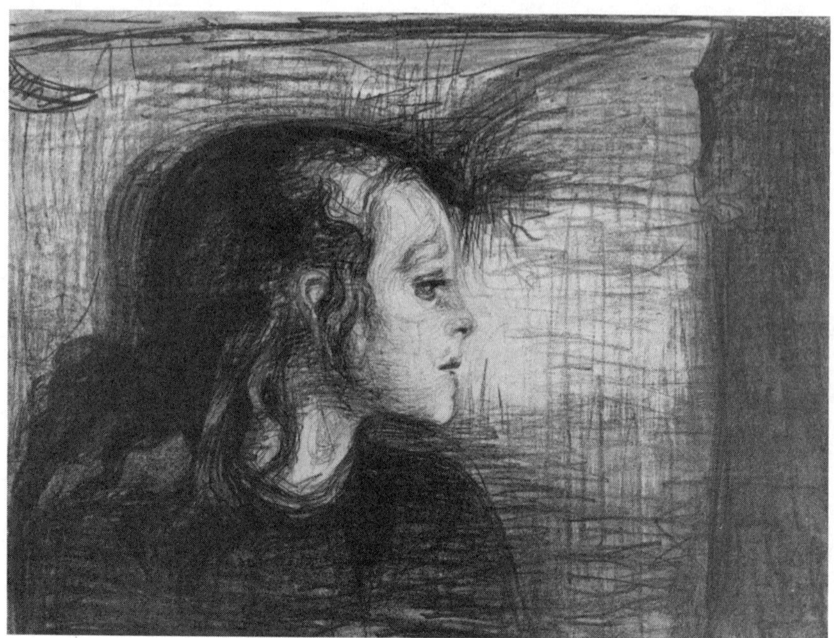

Figure 11.4. Edvard Munch, *The Sick Girl,* lithograph.

that he now seems to onlookers a bundle of pus-filled rags) but with an equally immense gift—the bow without which the Trojan War cannot be won. The Trojan War is interrupted while its participants stop to contemplate the nature of pain, but they can contemplate pain only by taking notice both of the monstrously aversive damage and of the wound bearer's unique position in the line of transmission that carries forward the essential tools of civilization.[8] Most human beings have not stolen fire from heaven on behalf of humanity, have not invented the art of painting, and do not possess the key tool that will enable their civilization to survive: do these absences place their pain beyond the reach of other human beings? But those immense gifts are simply a way of telegraphing, in condensed and rapidly comprehended signals, the density and immensity of personhood that every person has.

How close do we get to another person's pain when there is no visible body damage, no uninvited eruption of the person's interior into our midst? Edvard Munch's *The Sick Girl* (Figure 11.4) provides an occasion for contemplating this question, for in its comeliness, its seemliness, the image exists at a far remove from the obscenity and unseemliness of Bacon's painting or of Sophocles's hero. What is "seemly" is not only what is seen (what, because it stands before us, "seems") but what we have agreed to see, for the word is cognate with the Old English word *som,* meaning "agreement" or "reconciliation."[9] What, in contrast, is unseemly is not, as we might at first suppose, what is unseen but what we have not agreed to see, what has appeared before us without our consent. In this respect, the unseemly has a coercive presence that coincides with the coercive, or unconsented to, nature of pain and illness.

How then does a comely image—one to which we readily assent—communicate the coercive character of pain or illness? Unlike Prometheus, who is upside down, or the Smiling Intestine, who is inside out, the child in Munch's lithograph is outside out and upside up: in fact, art critic Dieter Buchhart, noticing the stark uprightness of her head against an equally upright square pillow, observes that her verticality is at odds with any notion of illness.[10]

We might, as though looking at a succession of stills in a film, look across many versions of *The Sick Girl,* for Munch returned many times to the image in paintings and lithographs made between 1886 and 1928. We might then glimpse the dire bodily events that imperil her, for she seems to toss and turn (her profile now to the right, now to the left), to alternate between chills and fever (the prints are sometimes tinted blue, sometimes red),[11] to be vividly present, then to drift away (her profile sometimes strongly marked, and other times, as Buchhart observes, nearly erased). So, too, we might infer her jeopardy by the response of others: in the painted versions of the image, a woman sits beside her with head so bent over that her face is parallel to the floor, as though the girl's death is inevitable, so inevitable the woman has adopted the posture appropriate to its already having occurred. Or we might infer her jeopardy from Munch's own obsessive attention to her, the sheer number of times he returned to the image and his open statements about its origins in the childhood years he and his sister shared until she died. In other words, if we cannot sense her jeopardy, we can—looking across multiple versions—sense that others sense it, and in this way see that it is so.

But the paintings and lithographs are not stills from a moving picture, and ordinarily we see only a single lithograph or painting at a time. The one reproduced in Figure 11.4 is from the Fogg Museum and resides there without any of its companions. Still, if we can sense her imperilment at all—and it is not clear to me that we can—it is because the motion that can be glimpsed across multiple versions (the motion of tossing, moving through different temperatures, ebbing and flowing) is *almost* discernible in any one of the lithographs or paintings in isolation. Motion makes evident the fact of aliveness; minimal motion, the fact of being just barely alive, the hairline divide between being and no longer being. Munch believed he had registered this minimal motion, the motion of trembling:

> I re-painted that image many times during the year—erased it—let it emerge from the paint—And tried time and time again to hold on to that first impression. The *trembling* mouth—the transparent, pale skin—upon the canvas—that *trembling* mouth—those *trembling* hands.
>
> Finally, I gave in—exhausted. I had retained much of that first impression. That *trembling* mouth—that transparent skin—those tired eyes. But the colors were not finished. (Tøjner 2001, 54, emphases added)[12]

Trembling is a dyadic motion (the lips or fingers flash rapidly back and forth between two nearly indistinguishable points); trembling reenacts, within an exquisitely small radius, the right-left dyad of tossing and turning, the cold-hot dyad of fever and chills, the coming in, going out of now present, now almost gone. For Munch, trembling or quivering or wavelengths or wave lines were the condition of sentient aliveness: he saw it in the landscape ("earth vibrates"), in the air ("quivering in the air"), in colors ("the quivering on the yellow white facade, the colors dancing"), in flowers ("flowers whose character, type and vibration are determined by joy and pain"), in himself ("I hear the blood roaring in my ears . . . My skin tingles"), in vision ("what we see are light waves that affect the retina"), in audition ("what we hear are wavelengths, received by the eardrum") (Tøjner 2001, 63, 91, 118, 136). Most of all, he saw it in *The Sick Girl,* as the fourfold repetition of "trembling" suggests. Soon after the passage about his small sister's hands and mouth, he directs our attention to his own quivering, wavy-line presence in the work:

> I was also aware that my own eyelashes contributed to my impression of the image. I made reference to them as shadows over the painting. In some way the head became the image. Wavy lines appeared—peripheries with that head at the center. I came to use those wavy lines in many later pictures. (Tøjner 2001, 64)

In the Fogg lithograph, the shadowed upper and lower horizontal bars register the presence of his lashes, which open onto the horizontal corridor that contains her bright face. Munch wrote that painting was not a transcription of the world but a transcription of the brain: "Painting is the perception of the brain, filtered through the eye" (Tøjner 2001, 136). Unlike the painting of Bacon or even of Rubens, *The Sick Girl* contains no transgressive display of the interior of the body, but it does carry us close to the interior, for we look from inside Munch's eyes, through his eyelashes, up to, and even through, her thin hair and translucent skin.

Across the paintings and play we have so far been looking at, we can begin to see how our ability to make contact with another person's pain is assisted by the fact of body damage, but only if there is simultaneously an act of doubling, so that body damage and personhood are given, as it were, two separate locations of equal magnitude. If only extreme damage is depicted, then we must imaginatively supply a separate narrative of personhood, as we did in the case of Bacon's Smiling Intestine whom we credited with the invention of painting; if instead only extreme seemliness is depicted, then we must undergo the imaginative work of finding in the acuity of the lines the registration of the distress the painter's title tells us is there. We could not, at first, carry out the labor of compassion toward the creature in the Bacon painting because there was no locus of personhood to which to attach any such feeling; and we could not, at first, carry out the work of compassion toward Munch's sick girl because, though the image at once conveys personhood and so at once inclines us toward sympathy, we are again stranded and puzzled: Sympathy about what? Is something wrong?

The insistent requirement for a double location is not, as was noticed earlier, a description of what happens to perception only in the presence of paintings or plays but what seems to take place widely in the living practice of medicine. As inadequate as our present culture may be in the treatment of pain, some advances over earlier eras have been made, and almost all of them entail accepting a separable location, or platform of address, for the body that is hurt and the person who hurts. Childbirth often now involves one person attending to the birth of the child and another person explicitly dedicated to sitting face to face, meeting eyes with eyes, matching breath to breath with the person undergoing labor. So, too, many hospitals (such as Boston's Beth Israel) now have, in addition to and distinct from the physicians who attend the patient's organic disease or damage, pain teams who address the person's sentient distress. Star Bright, the program for hospitalized children in extreme and ongoing physical pain, is also structured on the principle that two separable forms of address must be made to the young person.

It may be that in a much earlier time the two-part division of labor between physician and nurse provided such a double location, but unless nurses are given the power to prescribe pain killer and are themselves accorded salaries and status equal to the physician who addresses the body damage, it seems implausible that the arrangement can solve the ongoing problem of untreated people in pain. The importance of doubling needs to be stressed because our intuitions tell us that medical practice should aspire to "wholeness," "oneness," "integrity," "integration"; whereas in the sphere of pain, the aspiration toward "oneness" has instead contributed to the failure to assist those in pain. The absence of visible body damage makes it hard for physicians or nonphysicians to credit the reality of the patient's pain; the presence of visible body damage may either repel or receive the onlooker's attention, but in either case it sits on top of, and obscures, the person in pain.

The pronounced act of doubling in an array of other paintings and novels illustrates how consistently the principle operates across different artistic styles. Both visual artists and verbal artists interested in expressing physical pain spatially separate the person's wounded bodily surface from the depiction of a consciousness in pain.

Throughout her works, German graphic artist Käthe Kollwitz calls attention to the suffering of unrepresented people. In the lithograph *O Nation, You Bleed from Many Wounds*, the suffering of the person in the center is in part conveyed by the triptych of bodies in postures suspended between pain and mourning (Figure 11.5). The alert, still

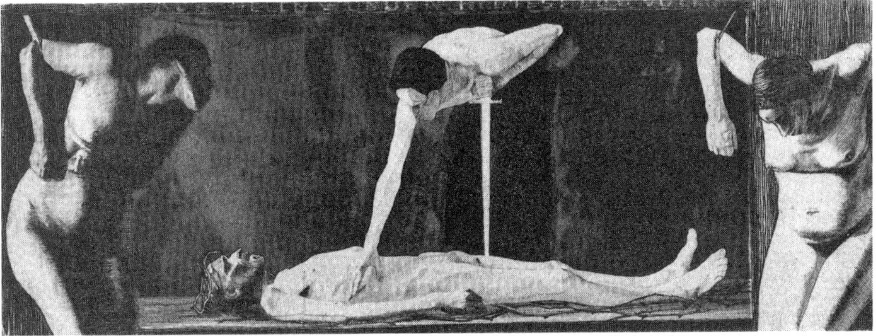

Figure 11.5. Käthe Kollwitz, *O Nation, You Bleed from Many Wounds* (Aus vielen wunden blutest du, o volk).

alive sufferer on the left and the hovering protector figure both direct our attention to the one in greatest peril at the center. This central sufferer has no wounds that mutilate the surface integrity of his body (though he is so emaciated that the interior of his body threatens to break through his skin in sharp cheekbones and a rib cage so protruding the protector can close her whole hand around it).[13] The title, however, inscribed directly onto the picture surface and running the full length of the man, acts to register the unpictured fact of the wounding in its lament, "O nation, you bleed from many wounds." The bodily image and the micronarrative work side by side in an act of doubling. The written registration of the interior of the body is evocative of pain, and the unscathed surface of the man provides an unoccluded site for the reception of our concern.

The Downtrodden (Figure 11.6), made by Kollwitz four years later, is so intimately connected to *O Nation, You Bleed from Many Wounds* that one might momentarily suppose it to be the same work. The pain and mourning co-present in the two lateral figures in the first print now appear in more highly differentiated right and left panels: on the left, the open hand of the man and exposed face of the unconscious child make visible the vulnerability of the laboring poor; like the man on the left, the crucified woman on the right holds her eyes as though grief-stricken, and the extended hand of her companion reiterates the man's expression of frank need. The central figure, more rigid than the figure at the center of the earlier work (his sharp chin and illuminated feet spiking upward and outward), is more certainly dead than the earlier

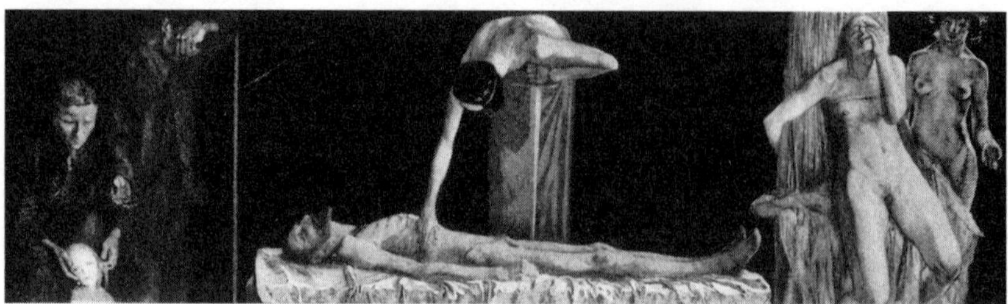

Figure 11.6. Käthe Kollwitz, *The Downtrodden.*

figure and—as though the painting were an official autopsy report—the cause is certainly hunger: now it is not cheekbones and ribs alone that threaten to break through the skin but knees, knuckles, wristbones, and ulna. The guardian, who protects the corpse (but has not successfully protected the living person), is herself emaciated, as sharp shoulder blade, spine, and forearms attest.

A crucial change in the transition from *O Nation, You Bleed from Many Wounds* to *The Downtrodden* is the removal of the wounds from the inscribed title and a positioning of them inside the picture image itself. But Kollwitz does not locate the wounds on the surface of the body, where they might make the person what the poet Shelley called "a monstrous lump of ruin"; she instead places them on the cloth beside the body. The detail of the central panel (Figure 11.7) makes evident the wounds in the cloth that are like orifices into the body, outlined the way lips or nostrils sometimes are, and therefore expressive of sensory acuity as well as pain. Kollwitz in the two triptychs allies the pain of the poor with the tribulation of Christ, as the inclusion of cross and thorns suggest, and the way she has sorted out the perceptual complications of depicting pain recalls the strategy used in a particular painting of Christ by the Renaissance artist Mantegna, where the wounds, like lipped openings, are at the periphery of the body, hands and feet, about to cross over onto the draped cloth (Figure 11.8).

This perceptual strategy of doubling can be recognized in the visual arts even when it takes place in a radically different style. Aubrey Beardsley shares Kollwitz's commitment to line over color (he was himself an ardent devotee of Mantegna), as well as her astonishing ability to expose, through line, the inner life of the body. But he comes to the body through the fin de siècle decadence he helped to create rather than through her social conscience and religious compassion. His untitled poster (Figure 11.9), made to advertise Fisher Unwin books,[14] might be titled "Girl, Wounded Tree, and a Book Shop," for it is derived from an earlier drawing the publishers much admired that Beardsley had titled "Girl and a Book Shop" and that had contained a wounded tree, an inclusion whose strangeness contemporaries both commented on and complained about.

The wound to the tree is perceptually attributable to the woman because the two are striking visual analogues. The young tree and young woman stand in the same visual space. Each is primarily characterized by the exaggerated rigidity of the spine, as well as by the shared flourish at the top: the outflowing hair and hat of the woman and the leafy boughs of the trees, which touch and penetrate one another. The base of the splint that supports the tree visually penetrates the base of her spine, even requiring the lower part of her torso to sway back to let this occur. Her body is stressed—made emphatic—by being stressed (put under some invisible pressure), as though it were, like the tree, encased. The pressure is also registered in the stiffness of her arms, palms turned back, rather than in toward the body. Although her own body surface is uninterrupted by any visible wound, the emphatic analogue heightens

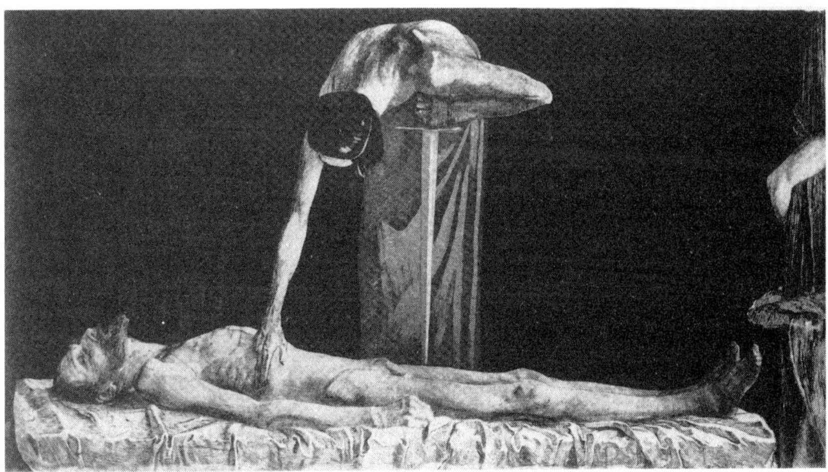

Figure 11.7. Käthe Kollwitz, *The Downtrodden,* detail.

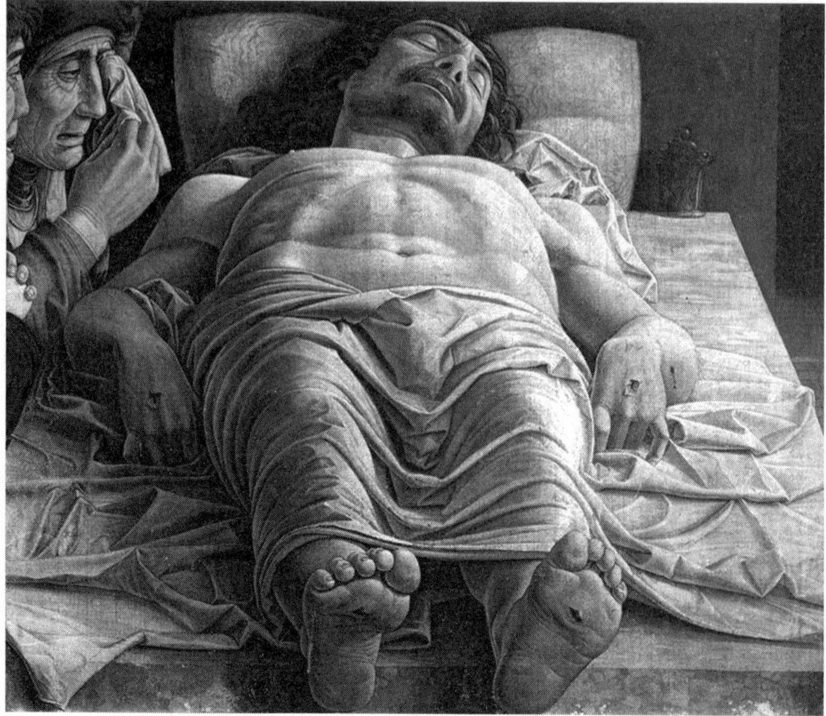

Figure 11.8. Andreu Mantegna, *The Lamentation over the Dead Christ.*

our sense of her discomfort until the pressure on her spine so turns her torso that one might come to believe her head is on backwards.

The colors of the poster magnify the kinship: the red-orange splint is the same color as the woman's vibrant dress, and like that dress, the splint is high-waisted. The trunk is black, as is her waistband; and the tree's bandage is white, as are her undergarments and skin. Tree and woman rhyme: they are both red, black, and white. The only non-shared color is her golden hair and the tree's light green leafy top; thus analogous parts of them are alike in being given an exceptional color. Beardsley said he used the "flat tints" of his posters as if he "were colouring a map" (Sturgis 1999, 212).

Inside and outside change places in this map: in the center of the tree's bandage, the white gives way to small spots of red as though the tree is bleeding, just as the woman's innermost slip is transparent, letting through small drops of red, but now the red belongs not to her blood but to her artful stocking. Yet even as we look at the stocking the sense of wounding reemerges because, like the tree, she stands on a single leg.

Of central concern here is Beardsley's reliance on doubling, his way of getting us to perceive someone's extreme discomfort by a wound, but a wound that is spatially separated from the person. But what inside the

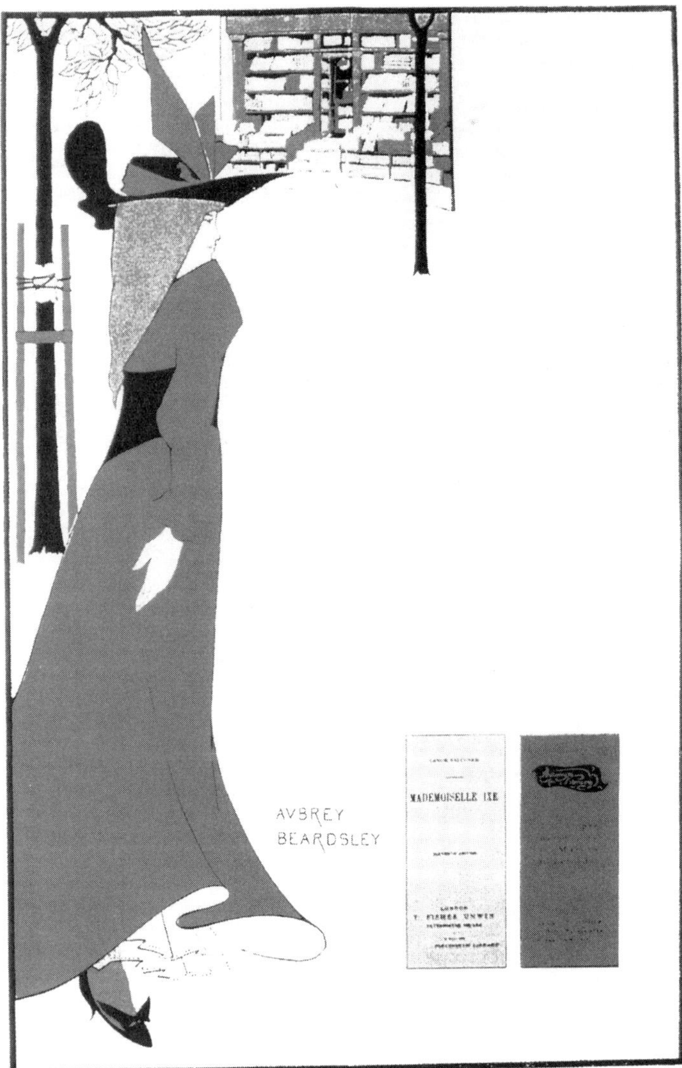

Figure 11.9 Aubrey Beardsley, "Girl, Wounded Tree, and a Book Shop" (my title).

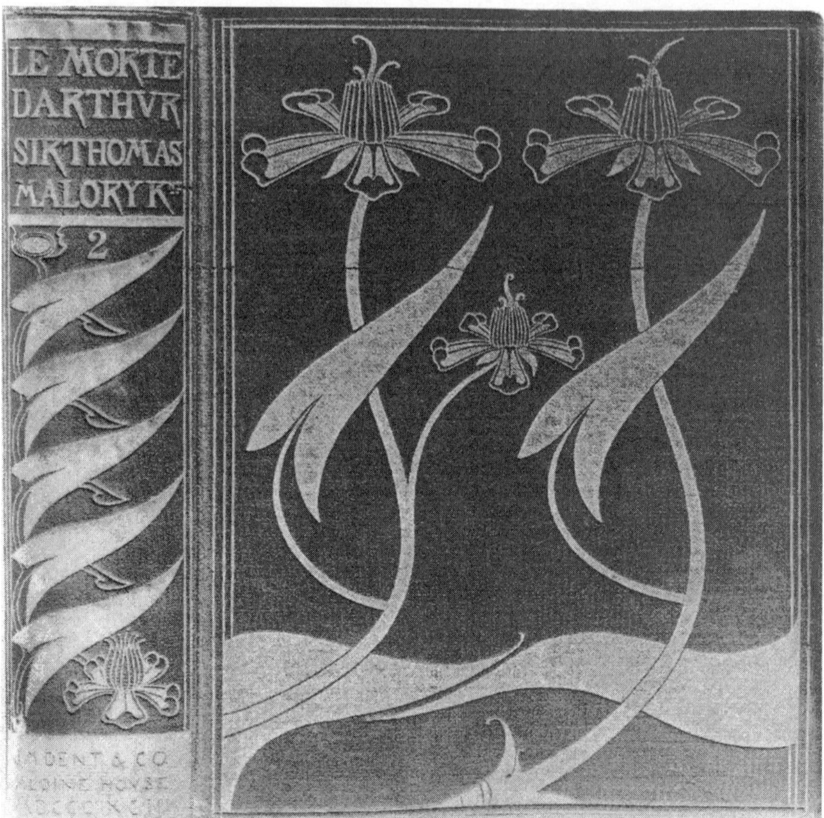

Figure 11.10. Aubrey Beardsley, cover and spine, *Morte D'Arthur.*

sensation of distress struck Beardsley? Is the poster a structural pun? Was he, who so ardently loved books, thinking about the fact that trees, persons, and books all have spines? Throughout the 1890s, until his death at the age of twenty-five, he created lavish designs not just for the front covers of books but for their spines (Figure 11.10 shows the cover and spine of his *Morte D'Arthur;* and Figure 11.11 a letter in which he maps the placement of his picture of Balzac on a book's spine). Books, trees, and women all also have leaves: books and trees certainly, and the woman is, if not leafy, at least many layered in the breezy swirl of her skirt, slips, and stocking. The woman's erect hat, reaching into the treetop, also makes its way up the steps of the elegantly curved, two-dimensional book shop (itself as flat as the page of a book or the paper of a poster). As the poster reverses in and out, so it toys with top and bottom. The two book covers at the bottom of the poster reproduce the color of her hair and hat, and there in the lower corner, the flamboyant shape of her hat reappears around the title "The Upper Berth."[15]

Beardsley's act of designing himself (or an elegant proxy) into the

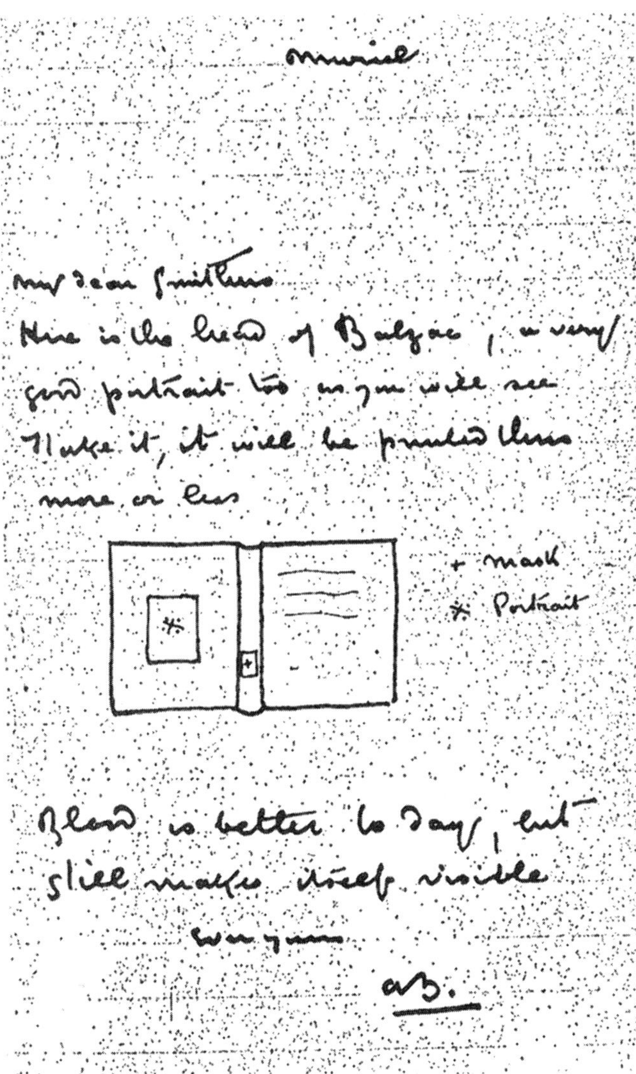

My dear Smithers

Here is the head of Balzac, a very good portrait too as you will see. Make it, it will be printed thus more or less

Blood is better to day, but still makes itself visible

Ever yours

AB.

Figure 11.11. Aubrey Beardsley, letter with cover design for Balzac's *Père Goriot*, showing placement of Balzac's portrait on spine of book.

stiff-spined cover of a book—like Yeats's wish to leave behind the body and become a mechanical bird—is pulled forward by his adoration of books and pushed from behind by his own ever-intensifying illness. In his five-sentence letter to book publisher Fisher Unwin, three sentences are about the poster, two are about his own bodily distress (Maas, Duncan, and Good 1990, 78), and this ratio often reappears in his quick, energetic letters. Indeed the letters, as though splashed with blood, record the pace of his constant hemorrhaging:[16]

> Quite an exciting flow of blood on Tuesday night, I thought I was in for another bad illness. Luckily we had a splendid hemorrhage prescription at hand; and the bleeding was stopped in an hour. There has been no return, and I feel wonderfully well considering all things and in good spirits.[17]

> On Friday afternoon I broke down again and have stained many a fair handkerchief red with blood. Perfectly beastly. I don't believe I shall pull through the winter.

> Words fail to describe the horrid state I have been in. Today is my first of any respite from blood spouting.

> Blood is better today, but still makes itself visible.[18]

> New alarms! The blood having stopped coming from the lung begins to flow from the liver in considerable quantities via the bum. Perfectly beastly is it not? (Maas, Duncan, and Good 1990, 148, 157, 196, 274, 278)

"Once out of nature, I will never take my shape from any natural thing." The white sheets of Aubrey Beardsley's correspondence with artists and publishers almost seem like the white pages displayed on the shelves of "A Book Shop" at the top of the poster. Perhaps with a magnifying glass large enough, one might see on them the same tiny drops of blood that show through the tree's bandage and the woman's slip.

But of course the white poster as a whole is the analogue for the handkerchief marked with red. Beardsley's way of describing his drawings is not far from his way of describing his hemorrhages. Here is how, at the age of twenty, he described his illness and his art to his former housemaster at Brighton Grammar School:

> My dear Mr. King, I've been horribly ill this year, and for the first few months of it I had to stop my drawing altogether. In the spring however I set to work again and struck out an entirely new method of drawing: Fantastic impressions treated in the finest possible outline with patches of "black blot." (Maas, Duncan, and Good 1990, 37)

The letter anticipates the account he later gave to W. B. Yeats: "I make a blot on the paper, and I begin to shove the ink around and something comes" (Sturgis 1999, 121). Beardsley's biographer, Matthew Sturgis, questions the literal accuracy of this description, saying that there is little evidence that Beardsley worked directly with ink in this way. But that makes it seem all the more likely that there is a blurring in his mind between the marks he made on paper and the marks he made on the handkerchief into which he coughed. It is relevant to notice that reviews of his drawing style that were made in complete ignorance of his tuberculosis underscore structural features of the work that place it close to Beardsley's own private descriptions of coughing blood. Here is one parody of Aubrey Beardsley (sometimes called Awfully Weirdly by his contemporaries) in *Punch:*

> Take a lot of black triangles,
> Some amorphous blobs of red;
> Just a sprinkling of queer spangles,
> An ill drawn Medusa head,
> Some red locks in Gorgon tangles,
> And a scarlet sunshade spread:
> Take a 'portière' quaint and spotty,
> Take a turn-up nose or two;
> The loose lips of one 'gone dotty',
> A cheese-cutter chin, askew . . .
> Take an hour-glass waist, in section,
> Shoulders hunched up camel wise;
> Give a look of introspection
> (Or a squint) to two black eyes.[19]

One may recall our earlier definition of "obscene" as the uninvited presentation of the interior of another person's body, and our definition of "unseemliness" as that which comes before us without our consent. All the more striking, then, is the artful transformation that could make us willing and even admiring onlookers of his bleeding lungs—not that Beardsley ceases to be obscene, but that he teaches us something before we come to our senses and look the other way.

And Beardsley buys time, I have been arguing here, in part through the principle of doubling: by severing the obscene spectacle of body damage from the site of personhood, he steers us toward his heroine and persuades us to stay long enough to feel, if not compassion, then interest, or if not interest, at least "sensation," strong sensation. Though the poster "Girl, Wounded Tree, and a Book Shop" is not among the most frequently reproduced of his works, it was well known in his own day. Asked to provide a brief biography to W. Palmer, his former schoolmate and editor of *Havell's Annual*, Beardsley wrote a dense paragraph mentioning positions (such as art editor of the *Yellow Book*) and major works (such as the 300 illustrations for *Morte D'Arthur*). But in the final sentence of the letter, he dashes off a final suggestion to W. Palmer: "You might just mention my posters that made rather a sensation. Avenue Theatre and Pseudonym Library" (Maas, Duncan, and Good 1990, 76). The poster for the Pseudonym Library is the one we have here been identifying by the pseudonym "Girl, Wounded Tree, and a Book Shop."

What social realist Käthe Kollwitz does by the spatial separation of body and cloth, what fin de siècle Aubrey Beardsley does by the spatial separation of body and tree, we again discover when we move from the visual arts to the verbal arts. Two instances are available in the magical-realist novelist Miguel Asturias and in the decadent, fin de siècle writer Joris-Karl Huysmans. (As in the visual arts, a deep commitment to the body can be arrived at by the path of realism, or instead by the path of aestheticism).

The fact that we turn to the Guatemalan writer Asturias for an extraordinary account of pain is not accidental, for Asturias (and more generally, the twentieth-century Central and South American novel) attends to the body not only in the dimension of sexual desire and mortality (subjects found in the Anglo-American and European novels) but also in hundreds of other dimensions: the weight of one's own eyelids, the phenomenology of exhaustion, the felt experience of opening and closing the hinge joint at the elbow or the hinge formed by the back and upper legs, the feel of the moist earth beneath the feet, the state of having hiccups, what it feels like to place one's hand on the part of an animal that is fat. Miguel Asturias's *Men of Maize* is incantatory physical writing—even when the novel describes a relatively neutral somatic event, such as walking down a path in a forest; more so, when we enter, as we often do, the beauty or the aversiveness of human sentience.

Men of Maize is about the resistance of Guatemalan Indians to Spanish colonists who cut down the forest and turn their sacred plant into a cash crop. It starts with the tale of Gaspar Ilóm, an Indian leader whose capacity to protect his people from injury is nearly absolute. Does his capacity to protect others come from his unusual size or muscular strength? Asturias never says so. Instead, Gaspar Ilóm's prowess is attributed to his perceptual acuity: he is a genius in the realm of sensory attention. He moves as a warrior and revolutionary through the forest, disguising himself in the scent of flowers, rosemary, heliotrope, and gardenia to bring his own scent to the precise point of neutrality where it disappears, just as his own eyelids become continuous with the leaves of the shade forest in sleep, and his ears with the magnified sensory surfaces of vegetable and animal realms, sunlit ears of rabbits, ears of corn (Asturias 1975, 10 and passim).

But in the early pages of the novel, the Spanish invaders do, in fact, distract Gaspar Ilóm from his guardianship over his people, and they do it in the only way a person with a genius for attention can possibly be distracted: they put him in excruciating physical pain. Pain is the only event in the world that could ever have distracted Gaspar Ilóm from his stewardship.

But how can Asturias convey the pain that Gaspar Ilóm is in? How can he convey it in all its totalizing obscenity so that we will understand not only why that pain constituted a diversion but why it could not possibly not have acted as a diversion? How, most important, can he do that without eclipsing the very ground of personhood that is the basis of our regard for Gaspar Ilóm as a sentient being? Asturias solves the problem by an act of doubling, by taking all the visible body damage that expresses the fact of pain and transferring it to another surface, the body of a dog. ("I have given a name to my pain," says Nietzsche [1974, 249], "and call it 'dog.'")

In the book's opening pages, a dog suddenly runs into the center of the town square, wheeling and howling, his penis erect, urinating, vomiting, hurling himself about; open red ringworm sores cover his hairless skin and anus. Here is unseemliness: the dog is revolting to himself and to us. Uninvited substances from his interior are placed in front of us, as well as the onlookers lounging in the public square. The horrifying description is elaborated and sustained over four pages. Even the agent of the dog's pain—ground glass laced with poison—is temporarily withheld from us so that no avenue of comprehension is afforded us; we have no way to distance ourselves, even one inch, from the second-by-second unfolding display.[20] The dog is a wildly mobile form of Bacon's blindfolded Smiling Intestine, something dreadfully alive yet having no location free of obscenity that might enable us to feel compassion for him, let alone devise a strategy to assist him. "Life," Asturias writes, "clings hardest to the basest parts of the body" (1975, 12).

But the baseness of pain is not permitted to cling to Gaspar Ilóm's body because when, a short time later, the Indian hero is himself subjected to the same pharmacological mix of glass and poison, Asturias—having already conveyed the obscene, reeling horror of pain—need give us only one terse paragraph: Gaspar Ilóm dives down to the bottom of a lake, swallowing all its water as he descends. Drowning in pain, he willfully drowns himself to rinse out the poison, then emerges, still alive.[21] The vision of a human being triumphing over pain lasts only a moment, for pain is now, as always, the winner: the Spanish have taken advantage of his absence, his profound inattention, to slaughter his village. That slaughter makes visible the true work of pain. Gaspar Ilóm a second time drowns himself, this time without reemerging.

Our compassion—or simply, our regard—does not go to the dog who disappears in the thick matter of his own display, a creature hurled across the pages of the book. The immensity of what is suffered carries over to the stately portrait of Gaspar Ilóm and the annihilation of, first, his mental world (his capacity to have any object of perception present to his mind other than the felt fact of pain), and then his material world (his family, his village, the ground of his being). Pain decontextualizes: it breaks the sufferer away from all other dimensions of his world, including his own body. This is what makes the dog's pain obscene: there is no context for any of the events transcribing themselves on the surface of his body (his erection, for example, has nothing to do with desire) nor any context between himself and the outer world (he zooms through the public square, carrying the intimate interior facts that have no place, not the smallest accommodating corner, in the public world). The swift power of pain to decontextualize—to make a fatal break between the sufferer and his world—is what we again witness in the case of Gaspar Ilóm.

Our inability to attend compassionately to the dog and our ability to attend compassionately to the man do not turn on the fact that one is a dog and the other is a human being. Asturias could have reversed this outcome by making the human being act as the porter of horrifying body damage and the animal the location of living embodied consciousness. Nor does the difference turn on a discrepancy in the degree to which the two are embodied: Gaspar Ilóm's body is described as fully as the dog's, but we see him in the exquisite precision of his sensory acuity and the delicacy of human tissue that precision implies. Asturias provides an extraordinary instance of the way the phenomenon of doubling and spatial separation can be used to coax the reader's consciousness into a deepening comprehension of pain. But the phenomenon is visible in other books as well, and one in particular, Huysmans's fin de siècle masterpiece *Against Nature* (1959).

It is not surprising that when an artist uses the technique of doubling—spatially separating the site of body damage and the locus of suffering—the artist usually chooses to make a human being the locus of suffering and to make some nonhuman creature or thing the surface on which body damage is displayed. Most of us sympathize with the man, not the wounded cloth, in Käthe Kollwitz's *The Downtrodden;* the girl, not the bandaged tree, in "Girl, Wounded Tree, and a Book Shop"; and with Gaspar Ilóm, not the damaged dog, in *Men of Maize.*[22] But, as was noticed a moment ago, it is just as possible for human and nonhuman to reverse locations in this structure of perception, and *Against Nature* provides an instance, for here the human being carries out the loud display of body damage and a giant tortoise acts as the unlikely recipient of our sympathetic attention.

This is a small point, but a point worth noticing. Otherwise, we might mistakenly believe that the reason the human being is usually our locus of sympathy is that we have a natural concern for human beings in pain. But in fact the record over many centuries suggests that the opposite is the case: we have as a species an astonishingly consistent record of ignoring other people's pain if there is no body damage or no weapon to make it visible. By watching Huysmans toy with the direction of our sympathies, we see how plastic and versatile this structure of doubling is, and (most important) we recognize the crucial role it is playing in eliciting our concern for human beings in those cases where we do manage to care for them.

Chapter 4 of *Against Nature* folds together two stories—the story of a man's toothache and the story of a reptile's death (Huysmans 1959, 53–61). The chapter ends with the account of an excruciating toothache that sends our hero and narrator, DesEsseintes, fleeing from his body, pacing up and down his room, "blundering into the furniture in his pain." Yearning to have the offending source of his pain pulled out, he sets aside his usual obsession with class and runs to a semi-trained puller of teeth whose staircase and doorway are covered with "great splashes of blood and spittle." The excruciating removal of the tooth is built up out of four elements: a rapid conflation of pain, fear, and shame; a description of sensory details inside the head ("cold metal against his check . . . a whole galaxy of stars . . . the loud crack of the molar"); a high-handed registration of the patient's ungainly, prelinguistic noises ("stamping his feet and squealing like a stuck pig"); and comic exaggeration that accurately records the way events inside the body seem vastly magnified (the dentist "bore down on him as if he wanted to plunge his arm into the depths of his belly"). Finally, the dentist grasps his pliers around the tooth and lifts DesEsseintes up in the air; gravity pulls the patient's body back down into the chair, and as his body drops, the "blue tooth tipped with red" tears away from his mouth and looms in the air.

The tooth that looms in the air looms large in our imaginations, in part because the shrieking pain it caused was large, and in part because DesEsseintes, before beginning the tale of the toothache, has given us an elaborate synesthetic account of the mouth as a musical instrument—a pipe organ—on which a symphony of the tastes of liqueurs can be played: "dry curaçao, for instance, was like the clarinet with its piercing, velvety note; kummel like the oboe with its sonorous, nasal timbre; crème de menthe and anisette like the flute, at once sweet and tart, soft and shrill." Trombones, trumpets, cornets, tubas, cymbals, violins, violas, violoncello, and harps are all discovered to reside there, until the open mouth acquires the scale of a yawning (concert shell), open to the air. It is this big thing that is put in pain when the pain comes.

Moving quietly across the story of the tooth—coming before it and coming after it—is the second story that dominates the chapter, the story of a giant tortoise. The tooth has a hard enamel shell and soft tissue inside, full of bright pain. The tortoise also has a hard outer shell and soft tissue inside, though not until the last split second of the story does it occur to DesEsseintes that the soft interior of the turtle might, like his own, be in jeopardy. The tortoise has been purchased by DesEsseintes for his aesthetic amusement or, more precisely, to display and validate his exquisite aesthetic refinement, for he possesses an "oriental carpet aglow with iridescent colors," and he imagines that a dark object lumbering back and forth across its silvery surface will "set off these gleaming tints." When the dark lumbering object fails in its aesthetic mission, DesEsseintes has its shell "glazed with gold" until "the reptile blazed as brightly as any sun." When even that fails to bring out the tints of the carpet, he has the tortoise "encrusted with precious stones"—after first sorting through the flashing colors of cymophanes and sapphirines, opals and hydrophanes, aquamarines and rubies. But the tortoise, suffocating under the weight of this artifice, stops moving, and only after DesEsseintes finishes with his story of his tooth does it occur to him that the dark object in the corner of the room is dead.

The striking juxtaposition of tortoise and tooth subverts DesEsseintes's theoretical position. He believes nature (like the tortoise) is dark and dull, and artifice (like the oriental carpet and the reptile's flashing carapace) is dazzling and bright. But the recollection of his tooth pain and tooth extraction is the reminder that the blue-and-red-tipped interior of the body is unsurpassed in its terrible vivacity. The dental assistant offers to wrap his extracted body part in a newspaper—suggesting that all the artifice we wrap around nature (including carpets and encrusted jewels) is merely black and white and smudged by comparison with the bright fact of aliveness at the center.

But this feat of theoretical repositioning is secondary to the sheer feat of sensory cross-referencing that occurs between the primeval tortoise and our late flower of civilization, DesEsseintes; for the elaborately transcribed interior sensitivity of our hero is repositioned onto the tortoise, despite the fact that we are never, until the last second, invited to speculate about the interior of the tortoise's own body and barely see even its exterior because it is dark and shadowy at the outset and increasingly obscured by layers of gold and stones as the story progresses. Like the other visual and verbal works looked at here, *Against Nature* reverses inside and outside, while also reversing figure and ground. It was not the carpet but the tortoise that was secretly "aglow" and whose "silvery glints" at last reach our eyes.

We have seen across paintings, lithographs, posters, plays, and novels how often a compassionate insight into the pure fact of another's pain, or into some previously underappreciated aspect of that pain, relies on the visible presence of body damage, but body damage that is then distinctly separated from the site of sympathy because personhood and wound vary greatly in the ratio of space dedicated to them (Rubens's *Prometheus Bound*), because the two are given two obsessively distinct locations on a single person (Sophocles's *Philoctetes*), because one of the two is located in a space distinct from the person (the inscription and the person in *O Nation, You Bleed from Many Wounds*; the wounded cloth and the person in *The Downtrodden*), or because the two may actually be located in different sentient beings (the tree and the woman in Beardsley's poster, the poisoned dog and the poisoned man in Asturias's *Men of Maize,* the blundering man and the lumbering tortoise in Huysmans's *Against Nature*).

And this perceptual structure of emphatic separation, I have argued, helps us understand why it is that in medicine, where repairing body damage and diminishing the pain are both goals, these goals are better achieved where arrangements permit a deliberate doubling of address by two sets of caretakers. The solution may be the Rubens's ratio solution, as when a general practitioner knows his patient many years before the ghastly wound appears and therefore can hold the spectacle of the wound within the large frame of richly understood personhood; the inspired cancer doctor who meets the patient for the first time once the cancer is under way but, in addition to chemotherapy and surgery, dedicates hours each week to learning the patient's psychic interior is also following the Rubens solution.[23] The Sophoclean model of a double location (one address to what is borne on the sufferer's foot, another to what is carried in his hand) is emulated in childbirth practices where one person stands near the mother's womb to assist the potentially perilous passage of the child into the world and another person sits with his or her face close to the mother, sharing the work of breathing exercises. The unusual hospital that tries to have "a resident humanist in the emergency room"[24] is also following the Sophoclean model. The Kollwitz-Beardsley-Asturias-Huysmans model of two separate sentient surfaces is visible in those hospitals that have a pain team distinct from the medical team that addresses the patient's body damage: though there is a single patient, the two teams routinely carry out their work during two distinct visits at two distinct hours of the day, as though there were two distinct patients time-sharing a single bed.

So much do we value a vocabulary of "unity" and "oneness" that the vocabulary or practice of intentional doubling may (as noticed earlier) at first seem strange, but its efficacy is repeatedly validated both in art and in medicine, not only in the pockets of medicine already cited but in others that appear more odd or anomalous. Children who, in response to physical brutality, create multiple personalities sometimes assign one specific personality the task of feeling the physical pain, thereby relieving the other personalities from having to feel or even know about it: one child, when asked who Molly was, replied, "She feels pain for us."[25] In such a case, the child herself (rather than the medical community) initiates the Kollwitz-Beardsley-Asturias-Huysmans model of a double location. The principle of doubling may also help us to understand why victims of terrible physical brutality—such as the Jews in World War II—sometimes delay the period of beginning to speak about the event: scholars have recently shown that the Holocaust begins to be persistently mentioned in Jewish American literature only in 1957, 1958, and 1959 (see Greif 1997; Novick 1999). The delay may be explained in part by the need to wait until survivors have collectively had time to create a tangible, visible site of personhood separate from the injury so that they can speak about the obscene body damage without themselves feeling in danger of being once more eclipsed by it.

It is part of the argument here that we do not at present have enough instances of deliberate acts of doubling in medical contexts where people with visible body damage are being cared for. Increasing their number might lead to a more successful elimination of physical suffering, the standard by which the practice of medicine must always be judged.[26] Doubling and spatial separation need to be more widely present not only in the treatment of individual sufferers but in medical education more generally. If humanities courses were given a place in the curricula of medical schools (distinct from, but as emphatic as, courses on the treatment of body damage), would the ability of physicians to see and comprehend pain grow more acute and more capacious? At the very least it would give physicians time to walk through art galleries and stop and stand among schoolchildren.

Notes

1. The phrases are from Yeats's "Leda and the Swan," describing Zeus's rape of Leda.
2. This paragraph and the three that follow originally appeared in Scarry 1985, 15–16. The book attends to the perceptual complications that arise from the image of the weapon, whereas the present chapter attempts to sort out the perceptual complications that arise from body damage. The complications of the weapon most often arise in political frameworks; and the complications of body damage, in medical frameworks.
3. The conflation of pain with body damage is not limited to the definition given by the International Association for the Study of Pain. According to Jean E. Jackson, "most definitions of pain take as a core meaning an association with body damage" (2000, 5).
4. The lineage from Rubens's *Prometheus Bound* to the paintings of Bacon can also be seen in *Painting 1946* in the Museum of Modern Art. This work, which Bacon tells us originated in his mind with the image of a black bird landing in a field (Sylvester 1988, 11), depicts a buoyant black umbrella open in the presence of a huge hanging carcass of meat, as one might see in a meatpacking room.
5. "Staying" was described by a nurse in a lecture to the "Research Group on Suffering," Hastings Center, New York, 1983.
6. For some viewers, the title of the painting—*Three Studies for Figures at the Base of a Crucifixion*—may provide a location of personhood as large as the location of injury because it conjures up the story of Christ. (I argue below that when Käthe Kollwitz inscribes a title on one of her lithographs, it brings about just such an act of doubling.) But in Bacon's case, it is hard for the word "crucifixion" to work this way because, in his own paintings of the crucifixion, he subverts the external countenance of Jesus into an intestinal image. In his extended interviews with David Sylvester, Bacon tells us he thinks

of Cimabue's *Crucifixion* as "a worm crawling down the cross," a conception that influences his own painting (right-hand panel of *8*), which, were it not for the rib cage and leering mouth, could indeed be accurately described as a worm, or as an intestine, slithering down a cross or vertical surface.

7. I am thinking here of Edmund Wilson's famous essay on the play in *The Wound and the Bow* (1947).
8. In terms of the story line, the bow acts as the lure to bring Odysseus and Neoptelemos back to Philoctetes, whom they would otherwise leave unregarded on the island where Odysseus originally abandoned him. But this just means that unless one can see the features of personhood on the other side of the wound, one cannot hold on to why it is that one ought to care about his or her pain. When they are informed that they cannot win the Trojan War without Philoctetes's bow, they are also being informed that they cannot win the Trojan War without taking account of the nature of physical pain.
9. See Onions 1995, s.v. "seemly"; and Barnart 1988, s.v. "seem." As the unseemly is that which comes into our presence *without* our consent, the obscene is that which comes into our presence *against* our consent. Most etymological dictionaries state that the etymology of "obscene" is unknown; the *Oxford Dictionary of English Etymology* specifies that it was "originally a term of augury" and meant "ill omened, abominable, disgusting."
10. Dieter Buchhart, in Schröder and Hoerschelmann 2003, 249. Buchhart is here describing the 1886 painting titled *The Sick Girl,* but the verticality is equally descriptive of all the later paintings and lithographs of this image, many of which are reproduced in this book.
11. The observation of chills and fever in the shifting colors is Dieter Buchhart's, in Schröder and Hoerschelmann 2003, 50.
12. As one might expect of the artist of *The Scream,* Munch uses the word "pain" frequently throughout his written notes; and sometimes one senses in Munch the same lineage from Rubens that one perceives in Bacon: "A bird of prey is clinging to my soul / Its claws have ripped into my heart / Its beak has driven itself into my chest and / the beating of its wings has darkened my sanity" (Tøjner 2001, 71).
13. The thorns encircling the body and the sword near the groin work, in conjunction with the protruding bones, to remind us of how close we are to the ripping of skin and stark opening of the body. Kollwitz's weapons (thorns and sword) show the same thoughtful handling as her depiction of, or restraint from depicting, body damage: as stressed earlier, the problem with the weapon as an expression of pain is that it can be too easily severed from its referent in the body; here the weapons are held steadily adjacent. It is also the case that, like the sword held by the protector, the encircling thorns seem to keep away any who would violate the body.
14. Specifically, their "Pseudonym and Autonym Libraries." See Sturgis 1999, 164, 212.

15. As Matthew Sturgis observes, though Beardsley stressed the sexual power of women, he also always pictured them as "intelligent," repeatedly depicting them holding or standing in close proximity to a book (1999, 216). The association between the woman (or persons generally) and books or writing is also evident in one contemporary critic's complaint about the drawing "Girl and a Book Shop": though the bookstore, in his view, is "well designed," the woman is too "calligraphic" (163).
16. Beardsley was first diagnosed with tuberculosis in 1879 when he was seven years old; the bacterium was first identified in 1882 and until that point was thought to be hereditary (Sturgis 1999, 15).
17. Beardsley is here twenty-four. This and the following two quotations are from his letters to Leonard Smithers (whom Sturgis describes as a classical scholar, book seller, art lover, and collector of erotic materials), on August 6, August 31, and November 5, 1896. Beardsley also mentions his hemorrhages to other correspondents, but in a slightly more formal or medical language (see, for example, his letters to W. Palmer and to André Raffalovich, in Maas, Duncan, and Good 1990, 76, 150).
18. This is one of three sentences in his letter about placing the head of Balzac on the book's spine, reproduced in Figure 11.11. It and the following quotation are from the letters to Smithers on March 13 and March 16, 1897. Beardsley is now twenty-five (the age at which he dies).
19. "Art Recipe," in *Punch,* quoted in Sturgis 1999, 226–227. Satirists in America called him "Jim Smears" (p. 227 note), a name presumably intended only to refer to the quality of his prints and containing no allusion to the blood-smeared handkerchiefs, yet evokes them for anyone familiar with the letters.
20. Anna Henchman has examined Thomas Hardy's way of giving us the sensory features of an event before identifying it in order to let us feel the full impact of the sensory. She calls this process "deferred identification." See her unpublished paper, "Deferred Identification in Thomas Hardy."
21. Asturias does, immediately prior to this event, ask us to imagine an unspecified human being suffering body damage by including a terse account of a prophetic dream: the mother of Gaspar Ilóm's infant dreams that an unidentified man drinks amber liquid containing the reflection of two white roots; then he "fell writhing to the ground, feeling as though his intestines were ripping him open, his mouth foaming, his tongue purple, his eyes staring, his nails almost black against his fingers yellow in the moonlight" (1975, p. 20). The brief passage reanimates the extended account of the dog without requiring the recitation of its many horrifying details.
22. Needless to say, we are not limited in the number of objects with which we may sympathize (and people may feel sympathy toward both cloth and man, tree and woman, dog and man). If we only sympathize with a single site, it is because, as reiterated at many points, visible body damage repels or eclipses sympathetic attention.

23. Cancer physician Eric J. Cassell (1985) speaks at length and over time with patients about their dreams, work, aspirations, family, and illness during the period when he is also giving them, for example, chemotherapy. Cassell comments on his own "surprising" insistence on doubling but explains: "This is a medical story, an illness story, and illness stories are different from other stories because they almost always have at least *two* characters to whom things happen. They always have at least a *person* and that person's *body*" (1985, vol. 2, 15).
24. I was myself once invited to occupy this newly created position by a physician at the Hospital of the University of Pennsylvania. Philip Roth, to whom I described the incident, includes in *Anatomy Lesson* (Roth 1983) an invitation to Zuckerman to become a resident humanist in the emergency room. Despite the fact that Zuckerman and I both declined our invitations, the aspiration for such an arrangement seems an inspired one.
25. Patricia Jones (1985), citing cases in Lasky (1978), Kluft (1984), and Bliss (1980). The last of these articles describes a child, one of whose personalities was assigned the chore of "crying" for the others, because the act of crying tended to result in swift punishment by a parent (p. 1389).
26. Cassell (1985) identifies the diminution of suffering as the act by which medicine stands or falls.

References

Asturias, M. A. 1975. *Men of Maize*. Trans. G. Martin. New York: Delacorte Press.

Barnhart, R. 1988. *Dictionary of Etymology*. Bronx, N.Y.: H. W. Wilson.

Beecher, H. K. 1959. *Measurement of Subjective Responses: Quantitative Effects of Drugs*. New York: Oxford University Press.

Bliss, E. L. 1980. "Multiple Personalities: A Report of 14 Cases with Implications for Schizophrenia and Hysteria." *Archive of General Psychiatry* 37: 1388–1397.

Breitbart, W. 1992. "Pharmacological Approaches to Suffering in Cancer Pain." Paper delivered at the conference *Pain and Suffering: An Interdisciplinary Conversation*, the Pain Center and the Institute for Medicine in Contemporary Society, SUNY Stony Brook, April 24, 1992.

Cassell, E. J. 1985. *Talking with Patients,* vol. 1, *The Theory of Doctor-Patient Communication,* and vol. 2, *Clinical Technique*. Cambridge, Mass.: MIT Press.

Crystal, D. 2003. *Cambridge Encyclopedia of the English Language*, 2nd ed. Cambridge: Cambridge University Press.

Dermit, S. 1992. "Chronic Pain Programs: Problems and Opportunities." Panel at the conference *Pain and Suffering: An Interdisciplinary Conversation*, the Pain Center and the Institute for Medicine in Contemporary Society, SUNY Stony Brook, April 24, 1992.

Greif, M. 1997. "The American Transformation of the Holocaust, 1945–65." Honors thesis, Harvard University.

Huysmans, J. K. 1959. *Against Nature*. Trans. R. Baldick. Baltimore: Penguin.

Jackson, J. E. 2000. *Camp Pain: Talking with Chronic Pain Patients*. Philadelphia: University of Pennsylvania Press.

Jones, P. 1985. "She Feels Pain for Us: The Relationship between Multiple Personality and Child Abuse." Unpublished manuscript.

Kluft, R. P. 1984. "Multiple Personality in Childhood." *Psychiatric Clinics of North America* 7: 121–134.

Lasky, R. 1978. "The Psychoanalytic Treatment of a Case of Multiple Personality." *Psychoanalytic Review* 65: 355–380.

Maas, H., J. L. Duncan, and W. G. Good, eds. 1990. *The Letters of Aubrey Beardsley*. Oxford: Plantin Publishers.

Medvei, V. C. 1949. *The Mental and Physical Effects of Pain*. Edinburgh: E. & S. Livingstone.

Melzack, R. 1973. *The Puzzle of Pain*. New York: Basic Books.

Nietzsche, F. 1974. *The Gay Science*. Trans. W. Kaufman. New York: Vintage.

Novick, P. 1999. *The Holocaust in American Life*. Boston: Houghton Mifflin.

Onions, C. T. 1995. *Oxford Dictionary of English Etymology*. Oxford: Clarendon Press.

Roth, P. 1983. *Anatomy Lesson*. New York: Farrar, Strauss, Giroux.

Scarry, E. 1985. *The Body in Pain*. New York: Oxford University Press.

Schilder, P. 1950. *The Image and Appearance of the Human Body: Studies in the Constructive Energies of the Psyche*. New York: International Universities Press.

Schröder, K. A., and A. Hoerschelmann, eds. 2003. *Edvard Munch: Theme and Variation*. Ostfildern, Germany: Hatje Cantz.

Sturgis, M. 1999. *Aubrey Beardsley: A Biography*. New York: Overlook Press.

Sylvester, D. 1988. *The Brutality of Fact: Interviews with Francis Bacon*, 3rd ed. New York: Thames and Hudson.

Szasz, T. S. 1957. *Pain and Pleasure: A Study of Bodily Feeling*. New York: Basic Books.

Tøjner, P. E. 2001. *Munch: In His Own Words*. New York: Prestel Verlag.

Wilson, E. 1947. *The Wound and the Bow: Seven Studies in Literature*. New York: Oxford University Press.

The Poetics of Anesthesia

Representations of Pain in the Literatures of Classical India

12

Martha Ann Selby

The primary question that I wish to address during the course of this chapter is one of continuity: what do our earliest medical texts in Sanskrit, the *Caraka-saṃhitā* (ca. first century CE) and the *Suśruta-saṃhitā* (ca. second century CE; see Basham 1976, 21; Wujastyk 1998, 39–41, 104–105), have in common with texts on poetics, as well as poems themselves, when it comes to readings and representations of pain, suffering, and grief? My work is currently taking what I think, at least, is an interesting turn. I spend much of my time reading, translating, and analyzing poetry from the three classical languages of South Asia—Old Tamil, Sanskrit, and one of the literary Prākrits—and I constantly look for the medical embedded in the poetic. I have found that early medical ideas that concern sexual and dietary behavior (driven as they are by yearly cycles, geography, and climatic change) are very clearly reflected in certain poetic genres. Although we find these ideas in greatly transmuted and aestheticized forms, they are most definitely present as evidence of lived, embodied practice.

Likewise, I constantly look for the poetic embedded in the medical. I am stubbornly committed to a reading of classical medical texts in Sanskrit with the same eyes through which I read poetry—that is, through the eyes of a semiotician deeply concerned with issues of voice, empowerment, cultural history, aesthetic practice, and the production of knowledge. When taken as a whole, what do these diverse genres tell us about pain and the suffering body? What I would like to state at the outset is that in the classical Indian context it is not about "the

Lie," as Susan Sontag (1979, 8) might say; it has nothing to do with a flat denial that death, suffering, and pain exist. Instead, the representations of pain and dying that I have come across during the last few months while thinking through this essay have to do with issues of suspension: of breaking or deadening points of contact between the observer and the observed. I want to look at two different medical narratives and take the issue of "voice" into account. Then I want to examine Indian aesthetic theory from two classical traditions (Sanskrit and Old Tamil) to see how poetics might well be remaking the medical in terms of understanding the body as it suffers in pain, in longing, and in grief.

There are two logical points of entry in the medical literature in Sanskrit from which we might speak of pain. These are found in the fifth section of the *Caraka-saṃhitā* titled the *Indriya-sthāna* (literally "The Section on the Organs of Sense" but more precisely, "On Prognosis"), in its discussions of how to know if a patient's death is imminent, and in the same text's fourth section, the *Śārīra-sthāna* ("The Section on the Body"), in its lengthy narratives of pain related to labor and childbirth. In the opening *sūtras* of the *Indriya-sthāna*, we find ways that have been devised to tell if a patient's death is near by the color of his complexion and, more important, by the way he sounds. We must note that it is not what the patient is saying that is important here but the very *quality* of his voice that is of prognostic importance to the physician. As far as the complexion is concerned, pallor is bad, especially when it appears on the entire body or on precisely half of it, as are "flower-like signs in the nails or teeth, a muddy coating on the teeth . . . abnormal color in the lips and extremities . . . or black moles, freckles, and streaks that appear suddenly on the face."[1]

A healthy voice "resembles that of a goose, a *krauñca* bird, the felly of a wheel, a kettle-drum, a sparrow, a crow, a pigeon, or a *jharjhara* drum." The abnormal voice "resembles that of a sheep, and is feeble, subdued, indistinct, choked, faint, poor, and stammering."[2] The text goes on to explain that a sudden onset of an abnormal type of voice, a presence of various types of one voice, or a multiplicity of voice types is highly suspect and inauspicious. There is nothing in this passage that addresses the issue of content, of what the patient has to say about his condition, but the focus is on what is observable to clinically trained eyes and ears. In general, the authors of the classical Indian medical texts do not seem to remark on the pain of the patient; rather, they have found it more expeditious, perhaps, to frame everything in terms of learning how to read the outer surfaces and emanations of the body in terms of signs, symbols, and omens as the patient approaches his dying moment. There is one very interesting exception, however, and the *sūtras* that I am about to read do suggest the context of a sort of "clinical interview." But note that there is nothing to indicate that death itself is painful but instead a profound inversion of life. The following *sūtras* enumerate a plethora of reversals and inversions that, when read as a whole, create a world that is literally reversed and stood on its head and where we might suppose the voices of actual patients emerging. These lines are culled from *Caraka-saṃhitā, Indriya-sthāna* 4.7–26:

> 7 He who sees the sky as solid as earth, and the earth as empty as the sky is sure to die.
>
> 9 If one stands in clean water and doesn't have a net but sees one, his life will be snatched from him.
>
> 10 If one is awake and sees ghosts, assorted demons, or other astonishing things, he will be unable to live.
>
> 12 If one sees rays of light without clouds, or clouds and lightning when there are no clouds in the sky, he is sure to die.
>
> 13 If one sees the sun or the moon as if they are clay plates overstretched with black cloth though they are clear and pure, he will not live.
>
> 14 If one is sick or not and sees a solar or lunar eclipse when there is none, it is a sure sign of death.
>
> 15 If one sees the sun at night, the moon in the daytime, sees smoke in the absence of fire or fire without spark at night, he is sure to die soon.
>
> 20 One who hears sound when there is none or hears no sound when there is should be regarded as nearly dead.

23 If one reverses hot and cold, rough and smooth, and soft and hard, he is about to die.

25 If one perceives an object correctly with an organ of sense that is no longer functioning, it is a sign of death.

Again, these are all indicators of confounded perception, not acute pain or even, it would seem, a fear of dying. Nor is the voice of the dying patient ever replicated. It is instead hammered into the flat, descriptive narratives of the observing physician. However, in the narratives that describe the ideal pregnancy, labor, and birth experiences in the *Śārīra-sthāna,* the patient's voice must necessarily emerge, because in these passages female experience is being described by male medical authorities. We can easily see that there was a dialogue between women and medical men in explicit and implicit ways. At times, physicians are explicitly urged to consult "authoritative women," and at certain junctures in these passages when medicine is indistinguishable from ritual, women and brahmins are unusually lumped together as sources of knowledge and advice. But what about the implicit dialogue between men and women? This is far more difficult to formulate, and I have tried to think about this myself in terms of the outer and inner surfaces of a woman's body, what men can describe through a sort of clinical lens, and what can only be described by a woman herself, as she undergoes the deep and subtle changes in her innermost, darkest, and most secret of contours—those dark, subtle experiences of opening, quickening, tightening, and loosening that only a woman could feel and describe with any degree of accuracy.

In a list of pregnancy symptoms, we find items that any observant man could see and describe with no input from a woman; the drooling, the vomiting, the swelling, and so on. But then there are symptoms that only a woman could possibly describe: a vague heaviness in the limbs, that subtle sense of "opening" that one feels in early pregnancy, the heartburn and awkward discomfort of later pregnancy. There seems to be a true sharing here of knowledge, of a meeting of the divisions between public, male clinical description and a private female narration, that has gone into the making of these texts. What are the details that a clinical male eye can see, and what are the details that could only come from a woman's own experience? From the labor and childbirth passages, we might compare "a tired look about the face" or "a vacant look in the eyes" with the very specific and painfully accurate simile invoked to describe that special onset of fetal loosening, "a feeling as if a bandage has been removed from the chest," as well as pains that are described as "quickening" or "piercing." There is a marked difference in description in these particular narratives that retain the flat style of the descriptive clinical "report" but simultaneously allow the voice of the female patient to emerge. To me, this indicates a manifestation of a fusion between male and female ways of knowing the female body according to its public and private, or rather, its visible and invisible, surfaces.

What happens when we move from the physical world of medical description and look at issues of pain and suffering in the worlds of Sanskrit and Tamil aesthetics? In early Sanskrit theories of representation, which first emerged in a text on dramaturgy from the second century BCE[3] (Bharata's *Nāṭyaśāstra*), we find this notion of *rasa,* a formulation concerned with the experience and appreciation of dramatic performance and, as an extension, literature in general. *Rasa* appears in the medical literature as well. In both worlds, the word means "taste," "essence," "sap," "juice," or "flavor." In the realm of physical, sensory experience—in the medical, bodily realm—*rasa* comes in six flavors: sweet, sour, salty, pungent, bitter, and astringent. In the world of aesthetics, there are eight (and sometimes nine) types of *rasa:* the erotic, the comic, the compassionate, the cruel, the valorous, the terrible, the abhorrent, and the miraculous (the debated ninth *rasa* is that of tranquility). Each *rasa* is matched with a corresponding *sthāyibhāva* (literally, a "permanent feeling"). For example, the erotic is matched with passion, the compassionate with grief, the terrible with fear, and so on. The erotic *rasa* is the aesthetic experience of the erotic evoked by a representation of passion in either a poem or a play. The compassionate *rasa* is the aesthetic experience of compassion evoked by a representation of grief, and so on. There are many elements in plays and poems that can produce *rasa*—in the erotic context, a lover and his beloved can evoke *rasa,* for instance. But what is interesting about this system, as empathic as it might seem, is that *rasa* is something tasted or experienced. It is never "felt." Daniel Ingalls has explained this beautifully: "*Rasa* is not simply the apprehension of another person's mental state. It is rather a supernormal relishing based on an involved sympathy."[4] Ingalls is describing an important aesthetic distinction that can be understood through the act of comparing Sanskrit textual prescriptions with similar concerns in Tamil texts for the ways in which poetry should properly be appreciated. A "distancing" should occur between what is represented by a text and its audience or appreciator. *Rasa,* in fact, acts as a kind of baffle; it provides "padding" between the elite observer and what he is observing. *Rasa* converts not just portrayals of passion but also scenes that disgust or terrify into items for delight and relish. Many of the early rhetorical texts claim that portrayals of events that are too close to reality will destroy *rasa* and leave the audience in a state of despair, and when the goal of a performance is that of delight, lesser forms of representation are undesirable. They are termed *anaucitya,* or "inappropriate." Pain is recognized in this system, to be sure, but it must be portrayed in such a way that will not cause even a glimmer of distress to an audience. In the medical narratives that I discussed earlier, suspension is achieved through the clinical observation of visible surfaces, then by refashioning these surfaces into coherent systems of symbols and omens. Suspension in Sanskrit poetics is achieved through connoisseurship and expertise in portrayal—the trick is to experience the "feeling of a feeling," in a way, and never enter into the world of the feeling itself. Even in love poetry when the lover jilts his woman, readers implicitly know that there will always be a reunion eventually; if there is no reunion, the erotic *rasa* is destroyed or is transmuted into another unmatched *rasa,* such as that of compassion.

In Sanskrit erotic poetry, we find an interesting reversal of Susan Sontag's formulation of disease befitting the romantic (Sontag 1979, 42–48). In the Sanskrit poetic tradition, love causes illness; illness does not attract love. There is, in fact, an oscillation between the two poles of illness and health: the poles of pain and joy. Languor in love causes neurosis and real physical illness. There are countless examples in the erotic tradition of emaciation, swooning, and anorexia-in-love when a woman is left on her own, as in the following example from the *Amaruśataka,* a seventh-century anthology of erotic poetry:

Amaruśataka 92 (a lovesick heroine to her friends)

Sighs parch my mouth.
My heart's torn out by the roots.
Sleep won't come.
I can't see my darling's face.
Day and night I cry,
and my limbs have withered
since I ignored my lover
who had fallen at my feet.

Friends,
what good were you counting on
when you made me be angry
at that dear man?

There are also instances in poems from this same anthology in which the suffering heroine's luster and health are instantly restored upon her lover's return. Here is an example:

Amaruśataka 88 (a lover muses to himself)

Her face faded, pale,
   starved,
   pinched from starvation,
   tired,
   curls all slack

found its luster again
   the instant
   I'd returned
   from abroad
   unexpected.

I just can't describe
that slim girl's proud mouth,
its wonderful taste
at the time we made love
and what I reverently drank from it.

Rasa quite literally "essentializes" emotion, turning it into something to savor. Ingalls has described the perception of *rasa* by a Sanskrit audience as "sympathetic." I would add the words "indirect," "intellectualized," and "removed" to round out a list of characterizations. In a late addition to the earliest extant text on Tamil grammar and poetics, the *Tolkāppiyam,* we encounter an obvious attempt "to incorporate the Sanskritic *bhāvas/rasas* into Tamil poetics."[5] Although this is a clear case of borrowing from Sanskrit aesthetic theory, there is a vast difference in the way in which *rasa* was "read" by Tamil poeticians, who seemed to be unaware of the essential difference between *bhāva,* or "raw emotion," and *rasa,* or the savoring of an emotion (Cutler 1987, 61). A Tamil reader's response to a poem has been traditionally understood as empathetic and direct. One gets the sense that responding to a poem or to a dramatic work was a "given" and that aesthetic response was something that did not require much mental reflection or intellectual articulation: no "supernormal relishing," to reiterate Ingalls here.

Rasa never became central to a Tamil understanding of poetry. Rather, the Tamil poets and poeticians developed a system incorporating two genres and fourteen distinctive landscapes, or *tiṇai*s. It is this system that became the hallmark of Tamil literary convention. As I have written earlier, *rasa* theory essentializes love and agony; medical discourse views pain from a fragmented distance. Tamil poetics also engages in psychic suspension, but in this particular world, this suspension is achieved via a process of externalization by transmuting love, anger, and grief into a topography within which emotional pain is remade through allegory. The body itself is seen as a terrain, and the geophysical world—and everything that grows within it—has emotional meaning foisted upon it. The world is carved up into the two permeable, shifting genres of *akam* and *puṟam*—the genres of love and war, of the private and the public, of the interior and the exterior. Each of these genres is subdivided into seven *tiṇai*s; each *tiṇai* is imbued with an unchanging emotional mode.

What I would like to explore in the remainder of this essay is the permeability of love and war, for it is within this borderland that the strongest and most troubling of emotions find expression. Naccināṟkkiṉiyar, a fourteenth-century commentator on the *Tolkāppiyam,* describes the relationship between love and war as being "like the inner palm of the hand and its back" (quoted in Zvelebil 1973, 108). As

Susan Cole would put it, the interdependency between love and war is a phenomenon of "spatial doubling," a "superimposition of one world upon another," resulting in a poetics of violence and loss that is spatially fluid and drifting and that underscores the profoundly disruptive natures of physical longing and death, blending them into one in a single, blurred gesture of poetic symbolization (Cole 1985, 19).

Because of the ways in which Tamil convention forges correspondences between *tiṇai*s across the generic boundaries of love and war, we are presented with a powerful tautology in trying to speak of emotion in these poems. The implicit reciprocities between the landscapes of love and war tend to *elide* all the actual pain and suffering. We do get hints of violence, bloodshed, and pain in passing, but in war poetry, it is almost offhand. War poems are like love poems; love poems are like war poems: the tears brought on by the agonies of love are transformed into bloodshed on the field of battle. It may come as no surprise that the Tamil words for love are formed from verbal roots that mean "to slay," "to kill," "to obliterate," "to negate," to "unbecome."

To illustrate these elisions and tautologies, I want to return to the issue of voice, particularly the voice of the mother. Tamil literary convention dictates that the mother is the only female character in poetry who can legitimately cross the boundary between love and war. In the love contexts, the one *tiṇai* in which the mother's voice is heard is that of *pālai,* the landscape of the desert, full of thorny scrub, sand, dying animals, and white-hot sun. *Pālai*'s twin *tiṇai* in war is *vākai,* the landscape of victory in battle. When the mother speaks in these two paired contexts, she laments and grieves over her absent children: her eloping daughter in love, her fighting son in war. Here are examples of each: the first from *Naṟṟiṇai*, an anthology of love poetry from the second century CE, the second from *Puṟanāṉūṟu*, a fifth-century war anthology:

Naṟṟiṇai 110 (what a mother said)

I held in one hand
a pot of burnished gold
full of sweet milk,
white and tasty,
mixed with honey.

I ordered her to eat
and as I beat her,
raising a small rod
with a soft tip
wound round with cloth,
she toddled away,
her golden anklets clattering
with their fresh-water pearls inside.

That little prankster
who ran under a canopy
so that the good, old nurses
their hair gray and thinning,
would slow down and stop in their tracks,
where did she learn this knowledge,
these manners?

As her husband's family grows poor,
she doesn't think once
of the rich rice her father used to give
and more pliable
than fine black sand
under running water,
she eats when she can,
that little one
with such great strength.

Let us see how the mother's grief over her daughter is transformed into anxiety for her son in the twin *tiṇai* of *vākai,* victory:

***Pu̱ranā̱ṉū̱ṟu* 312 (what a mother said)**

To bear him and bring him up
is my duty.
To make him honorable
is his father's duty.
To provide him with well-honed spears
is the blacksmith's duty.
To train him in good conduct
is the king's duty.

To kill in a good fight with a glinting sword,
to dismember bull elephants
and to come home again:

that is the duty of my son.

There are also stunning parallels between *neytal,* the *tiṇai* of jilted women who lament when their lovers leave them (and contrary to the dictums of Sanskrit propriety, separation in Tamil poetry is often permanent—there is no such thing as implicit reunion), and the *tiṇai* called *tumpai,* that of "battle frenzy" in the war contexts. *Neytal* poems are based on seashore imagery. The salty pools of tears, the marshy, infirm land, and the female form emaciated and dying from love in the romantic contexts are all transformed into the pools of blood and the gore-soaked battlefields of war, littered with the bodies of the male fallen. The following poem is from *Kuṟuntokai,* an early *akam* anthology. This particular poem is perhaps the best example of the violence that love can wreak:

Kuṟuntokai 290 (what the heroine said)

Those who tell me
to bear my love:

Don't they know about love,
or are they that strong?

Since I can't see my lover,
my heart swells
with hidden sorrow
and like a flood in spate
turning to a streak of foam
as it dashes against stones,

slowly,
slowly, I turn to nothing.

Here is a contrasting poem from *neytal*'s twin *tiṇai,* in the *puṟam* context, *tumpai.* The poem here is not spoken in the mother's voice but instead describes a mother's behavior upon hearing that her son had behaved like a coward on the field of battle:

***Puṟanāṉūṟu* 278**

The old woman had protruding veins,
dry, thin shoulders;
her waist a thorny twig.

When some said,
"Your son was afraid in battle
and turned tail,"

she said,
"If he broke down in the throng,
I'll slash these breasts which fed him,"
and, angered, sword in hand,
she picked the red field over,
turning over fallen bodies.

Seeing the place where her slain son lay,
scattered in pieces,
he pleased her more
than on the day he was born.

I have analyzed three different contexts in which there are attempts to represent textually ranges of physical and emotional agony. To place all of this within Elaine Scarry's framework as detailed in her extraordinary book *The Body in Pain: The Making and Unmaking of the World*, and to paraphrase her somewhat, these three groups of textual materials represent the "forcing of pain itself into avenues of objectification" by inventing and imagining linguistic structures that will accommodate its expression (Scarry 1985, 6). I have discussed the phenomenon of suspension in all three contexts in which experience is externalized and made material. Pain is elided in the clinical voice except when absolutely necessary; pain is disallowed in classical Sanskrit aesthetics; pain is grafted onto objects in the geophysical world in Tamil convention. Pain lives in the world of metaphor and symbol—all this language, after all, is a poetics. We cannot forget that the "medical" always resorts to the "metaphorical": the pregnant body is a pot; the dying body is a "flowering" one that ripens to fruit and rots. Agony, whether in love or war or in death, must be made spectacle—forced outward for all to see—before a language can be made for it, and it will therefore always dwell in the lands of elision, of distance, and in Elaine Scarry's phrases, along the devastating borderlands named "as if" and "as though."

Notes

1. *Caraka-saṃhitā, Indriya-sthāna* 1.8–12. All translated quotes from Sanskrit and Tamil sources used in the text are my own. Other resources, including translations to English, are noted in the References.
2. Ibid., 1.15–16.
3. This appears to be the most widely accepted date. P. V. Kane places the composition of this text between 100 BCE and 300 CE (Kane 1971, 424).
4. See Ingalls's introduction in Ingalls, Masson, and Patwardhan 1990, 36–37.
5. *Bhāva,* in this context, means "emotion" or "feeling," as opposed to *rasa,* "the feeling of a feeling," "sentiment."

References

Amaruśatakam. 1983. With the Sanskrit commentary "Rasikasañjīvinī" of Arjunavarmadeva. New Delhi: Motilal Banarsidass.

Basham, A. L. 1976. "The Practice of Medicine in Ancient and Medieval India." In *Asian Medical Systems,* ed. C. Leslie. Berkeley: University of California Press.

Caraka-saṃhitā. 1994. 4 vols. 3rd ed. Trans. and ed. P. Sharma. *Jaikrishnadas Ayurveda Series* 36. Varanasi: Chaukhambha Orientalia.

Cole, S. L. 1985. *The Absent One: Mourning Ritual, Tragedy, and the Performance of Ambivalence.* University Park: Pennsylvania State University Press.

Cutler, N. 1987. *Songs of Experience: The Poetics of Tamil Devotion.* Bloomington: Indiana University Press.

Foucault, M. 1994. *The Birth of the Clinic: An Archaeology of Medical Perception.* Trans. A. M. Sheridan Smith. New York: Vintage Books.

Ingalls, D. H. H., J. M. Masson, and M. V. Patwardhan (trans.). 1990. *The Dhvanyāloka of Ānandavardhana with the Locana of Abhinavagupta.* Cambridge, Mass.: Harvard University Press.

Kane, P. V. 1971. *History of Sanskrit Poetics,* 4th ed. New Delhi: Motilal Banarsidass.

Kuṟuntokai. 1967. *The Interior Landscape: Love Poems from a Classical Tamil Anthology.* Trans. A. K. Ramanujan. Bloomington: Indiana University Press.

Naṟṟiṇai Nāṉūṟu. 1976. Repr. 3rd ed. Ceṉṉai: Tirunelvēli Teṉṉintiya Caivacittānta Nūṟpatippu-k-Kaḻakam, Ltd.

Nāṭyaśāstra (of Bharata Muni). 1894. Ed. P. Śivadatta and K. Pandurang Parab. *Kāvyamālā* 42. Bombay: Nirṇaya Sāgara Press.

Puṟanāṉūṟu. 1985. Repr. 6th ed. Ed. with commentary U. Vē. Cāminātaiyar. Tañcāvūr: Tamiḻ-p-Palkali-k-Kaḻakam.

———. 1999. *The Four Hundred Songs of Wisdom: An Anthology of Poems from Classical Tamil: The Puṟanāṉūṟu*. Trans. G. L. Hart and H. Heifetz. New York: Columbia University Press.

Scarry, E. 1985. *The Body in Pain: The Making and Unmaking of the World*. New York: Oxford University Press.

Selby, M. A. 2000. *Grow Long, Blessed Night: Love Poems from Classical India*. New York: Oxford University Press.

Sontag, S. 1979. *Illness as Metaphor*. New York: Vintage Books.

Suśruta. 1963. *An English Translation of the Suśruta Saṃhitā Based on the Original Sanskrit Text*. Trans. K. K. Bhishagratna. 3 vols. Varanasi: Chowkhamba Sanskrit Series Office.

Suśruta-saṃhitā of Maharṣi Suśruta. 1995. 2 vols. 9th ed. Ed. K. A. Śāstrī. Kashi Sanskrit Series 156. Varanasi: Chaukhambha Sanskrit Sansthan.

Tolkāppiyaṉār. *Tolkāppiyam: The Earliest Extant Tamil Grammar Text in Tamil and Roman Scripts with a Critical Commentary in English*. Trans. P. S. Subrahmanya Sastri. Parts 1–3, "*Poruḷatikāram*: Tamil Poetics," 1959, 1952, 1956. Madras: Kuppuswami Sastri Research Institute.

———. 1963. *Tholkāppiyam in English with Critical Studies*. Trans. S. Ilakkuvanar. Madurai: Kural Neri Publishing House.

———. 1985–1986. *Tolkāppiyam: Poruḷatikāram*. Ed. Ku. Cuntaramūrtti. 3 vols. Aṇṇāmalainakar: Aṇṇāmalai-p-Palkalai-k-Kaḻakam.

Wujastyk, D. 1998. *The Roots of Āyurveda: Selections from the Āyurvedic Classics*. New Delhi: Penguin Books.

Zvelebil, K. 1973. *The Smile of Murugan on Tamil Literature of South India*. Leiden: Brill.

Response:
Doubleness, *mātam,* and Muharram Drumming in South Asia

Richard K. Wolf

As an ethnomusicologist, I thought it would be appropriate to respond to Elaine Scarry's and Martha Selby's intriguing essays by suggesting ways in which music and other aspects of ritual performance can externalize and materialize pain—in this case, that pain associated in Shī'ī Islam with the memory of a historical event.[1] Muharram commemorates the battle that was fought in 680 CE over spiritual and political leadership in the Islamic community. Husain, grandson of the Prophet Muhammad, willingly sacrificed himself on the battlefield of Karbala (present-day Iraq), refusing to pay fealty to the corrupt Ummayad ruler Yazid. The suffering of Husain and his party of martyrs is the point of departure for Shī'ī emotional religiosity and soteriology. In India and Pakistan, the ethnographic focus of this essay, Muharram attracts participation from multiple communities, each bringing to it a variety of interpretations (see, e.g., Korom 2002; Masselos 1982; Pinault 2001).

Indians and Pakistanis have extended the observance from the traditional ten days (the first to the tenth of the month of Muharram in the Islamic calendar) to two lunar months and eight days. Each of the first twelve days is imbued with a particular significance drawn from the narrative of the battle of Karbala and the martyrdom of Husain and his companions. Shī'ī piety is grounded, in part, on the idea that a certain kind of pain is good. As Mahmoud Ayoub put it, "[T]he suffering of *Imām* Husayn has been taken by the Shī'ī community to be a source of salvation through the interiorization and emulation of that suffering by the community" (1978, 15). This pain is morally and physically articulated for the individual and the group through narrative and mimetic aspects of Muharram observance. Much of the ritual narration and activity places the subject on the Karbala battlefield and allows him or her to imaginatively relive the experience of fighting a principled battle for which mortal victory was not an option.

Although the repertoires and forms connected with Muharram that I shall consider here are not usually defined as musical by participants, they do exhibit musical qualities (melody and rhythm) that observant Shī'ahs apprehend affectively. Before moving into a discussion of these performance forms, I shall reflect on how issues raised in Scarry's and Selby's essays converge with those arising from field research I conducted on Muharram in India and Pakistan.

Externalizing, Materializing, Aestheticizing, and Doubling

Selby's ruminations on "breaking or deadening points of contact between the observer and the observed" find tantalizing parallels in Scarry's use of the idea of "doubling." Scarry locates artistic, social, and moral problems in the metaphor of pain as bodily damage, corporeal mutilation; this she opposes to the metaphor of pain as an external, invasive agent affecting the body. She finds the former problematic because the notion of "body," or subjective experiencer of the pain, cannot be removed from the representation of "pain" itself or of its cause. Such a metaphor leads to metonymic confusion between the disease and its host, or index with icon, so to speak. Scarry presents this slippage as a "problem" for which verbal and visual artists have sought a "solution" in techniques of doubling: these artists somehow project the suffering, the grotesqueness, some striking and viscerally apprehendable sign of the pain, onto another subject, thus diffusing it—they literally prevent the metaphor of pain from becoming fused, or confused, with the experiencing body.

Selby discusses a different kind of displacement or suspension with respect to three related phenomena: (1) Second-century Ayurvedic texts read not the pain of the patient but the "signs, symbols, and omens" of the patient's dying moment; (2) Sanskritic *rasa* theory distills and conventionalizes the nuances of aesthetic experience, allowing the cultured individual to savor these *rasa*s at a distance. Drama, music, and poetry become vehicles for rarified experiences including those that we might metaphorically term painful. (3) In Tamil poetics, emotions appear to be slightly less removed from the savoring subject; yet once again we find a kind of aestheticized remove in which five landscapes are imbued with distinctive synesthetic qualities.

Whereas Scarry probes the elision between the experiencing body and the metaphor of what pain feels like, Selby brings out a synesthesia among different kinds of pain—the pain of love and of mortal combat—which is enabled through a shared ethnogeographic poetics. Both essays engage with issues of elision and separation between and among different kinds of subjects and objects; and both probe the poetics of, to paraphrase Selby, "how pain is externalized and made material."

How might this phenomenology be apprehended in ritual performance? In particular, how might music serve as a kind of doubling, a kind of externalizing and materializing of pain? I wish now to turn ethnographically to the observance of Muharram in South Asia. By necessity I must focus on a very specific aspect of what is an extraordinarily complex event, which has vastly different meanings for different peoples in different places and historical periods. So debated and conflicted are subject positions in Muharram that they have led to some of the worst communal violence on the subcontinent (see, e.g., Hasan 1997); yet it has also been a context for temporary manifestations of intercommunal harmony, so much so that some Indian writers have argued for Muharram as a model for national integration (Hasnain and Husain 1988).

Muharram "Pain"

As I mentioned, the image of pain in Muharram is a salvific one. It emerges in several ways connected with ritual performance. I would like to discuss three virtual sites of "pain" in Muharram, where it can be attached and detached, embraced and projected, internalized and externalized among complex objects and subjects: (1) the imagination—pain created and fostered by vivid description and mimetic performance; (2) the body—*mātam,* ranging from gentle hand strokes on the chest to blows with swords about the head; (3) objects—musical instruments, floats *(ziyārats),* horse *(zuljina).*

To explain these potentials for registering and transforming pain, it will be necessary to examine a few features of Muharram in South Asia in more detail. Muharram observances are composed of several parts, some more public than others. Shī'ī Muslims observe what could be viewed as four broad kinds of practices, some of which take place throughout the year and others of which are concentrated in the Muharram period: (1) attendance at *majlis*es (mourning assemblies), (2) involvement in processions (large or small), (3) individual visitations of local worship halls (e.g., Imāmbārgahs) and shrines as far away as Iran and Iraq, and (4) household rituals (e.g., reciting miracle narratives, making vows).[2] I will focus only on aspects of the first two practices.

The *Majlis*

The broad framework of the *majlis* holds consistent across regions, although the order of some components may vary slightly from place to place. A preacher (*zākir* or *zākira* [f.]) is invited to lead an all-male or all-female assembly in a language appropriate for the community and region.[3] The *majlis* typically begins with an offering of blessings to the Prophet Muhammad and his family *(salavāt)*; it may optionally be followed by the exemplary tale of the cloak *(hadīs kissa'),* in which Muhammad proclaims five persons he embraces in his cloak (himself, his daughter Fatima, her husband Ali, and their sons Hassan and Husain) to be the most "pure" *(panjatan pāk).* Next, three performance genres of poetry are performed as follows (quoted descriptions are from Qureshi 1981):

1. *soz* — "Short lament, usually expressing one emotion intensely and concisely. Chanted solo with group providing a sung drone or support for the soloist"; often rendered in classical *rāga*s by trained musicians. Six-line verse; rhyme scheme *aaaabb.*
2. *salām* — "Salutation or eulogy" whose mournfulness is mitigated by discussion of the Prophet's and his family's virtues. "Often reflective or didactic in character,

consisting of couplets with refrain. May be chanted as is *soz,* or without group participation." Couplets with refrain; rhyme scheme *aa, ba, ca, da,* etc.

3. *marsīyah* "Elegy or heroic narrative, often highly dramatic." Stereotypical sections: introduction, description of morning of battle and hero, departure for battlefield, recitation of genealogy, martial scenes, mourning, and so on. May be chanted to a melody *(tarz)* or recited dramatically *(teht-ul lafz).* 100–200 verses long; rhyme scheme *aaaabb.*

Following this, the first *sūrah* of the Qur'an is recited *(fāteha).* (Shī'ahs perform this reading outside of the *majlis* as well: both for auspicious occasions and in honor of the dead.) The *zākir* will then present a sermon (called *hadīs* or *majlis*) that relates themes from the Qur'an and other general Islamic sources as well as the Karbala narrative to participants' daily lives and current events; if the *marsīyah* is recited at length and without melody, however, the sermon portion of the *majlis* may be omitted. The congregation usually remains seated until the end of the sermon, at which time they all rise and recite *nauha*s (metric, martial, dirges) and beat their chests rhythmically. This is followed by another performance of chanted poetry *(ziyārat),* which invokes the twelve Shī'ī Imāms. Participants bow and turn toward Karbala (Iraq) and Mashhad (Iran).[4] Finally the *fāteha* is again recited, this time often in honor of deceased loved ones. This is one way in which the pain of individual loss is merged with the larger remembrance of suffering at Karbala.

Images of Pain I: The Imaginary

Pain, in the minds of pious Shī'ahs taking part in Muharram, adopts a variety of forms. Abbas, Husain's half brother, was the standard bearer in Husain's small party. His martyrdom is recalled in poetry and sermons, as well as in everyday life, through images of gruesome agony: Yazid's army has blocked off Husain's party from the Euphrates River, denying them water. Abbas struggles to fetch water for the thirsting children. After he fills a leather pouch with water, his enemies cut off his hands. The imagery is amplified in some tellings, producing a pitiful picture of the dismembered, dying man. In public processional contexts, Abbas's dual roles as a signifier of the battle as a whole (as standard bearer) and as altruistically loyal to Husain are embodied in two practices: (1) The carrying of *'alam*s (flag or other flat emblem attached to a pole) in procession; (2a) the fulfillment of vows by pledging children as water bearers; (2b) the provision of hot or cold drinks at stations *(sabīl*s*)* along a processional route.

Husain's murderer was said to have chopped Husain's head off, parading it on a lance for all to see. The more gory the descriptions of this in verbal performance, the more weepy the response among *majlis* goers; the skill with which orators speak, dramatize recitations, or add tuneful highlights to their texts are all evaluated by those who attend. Aesthetics are tied to religious feeling; the vicarious experience of the sufferer is never far away from the understood historical meaning of the Karbala story. And yet, like Sanskrit *rasa,* and "love, anger, and grief" "transmuted" and "remade" in the Tamil classical *tiṇai,* the experience of emotional pain in Shī'ī popular piety is to some extent distilled and aestheticized as an immediate object of its own. The emulation of Husain's suffering as a moral goal is stated succinctly in a bumper sticker from Hyderabad, Andhra Pradesh (India): "Live like Ali, Die like Husain."[5] While Husain's courage and spirit are inseparable from his pain, it is the image of bodily suffering that most effectively serves as a conduit for the larger moral message.

Husain's suffering is projected not only through verbal means but also through specific icons appearing in processions. For instance, important to South Asian Muharram processions are one or more highly decorated horses, called *zuljina* or *duldul,* which represent Husain's mount. Often, the steed is covered in artificial blood. The horse conveys a unique modality of pain: not only Husain's (conveyed by the blood) but that of his party, when the horse returned riderless, communicating by absence the demise of their leader. Unlike Selby's ayurvedic texts that read the omens of death in the patient, this sign is of death externalized and read after the fact. The horse achieves a paradigmatic significance as well: it is a metonym for war.

One of the most important items carried in procession is a float called a *ta'ziyah,* which represents Husain's tomb. In Iran, the same

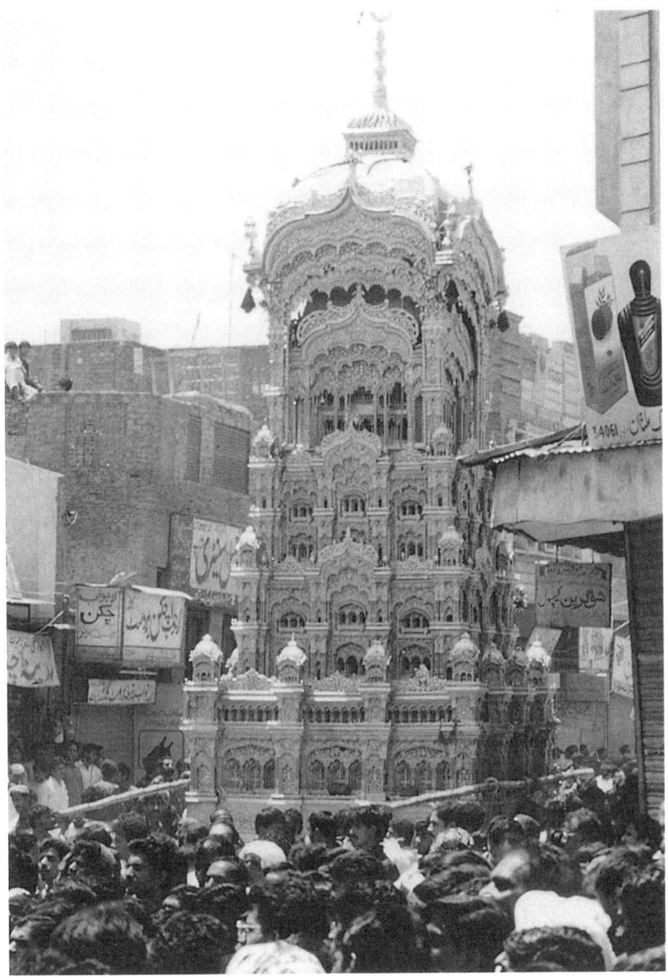

Figure R12.1. *Ta'ziyah* from procession on tenth of Muharram (Multan, Pakistan).

word is used for a passion play on the Karbala story (see Chelkowski 1979). The use of the same term for Husain's tomb in India and Pakistan condenses the imagery of the entire mimesis and anchors it in the commemoration of death. Some of the most elaborate *ta'ziyah*s are found in Multan, Panjab, Pakistan (Figure R12.1). In other cities, such as Hyderabad, Sindh, *ta'ziyah*s are not found at all. Instead, iconic elaboration is confined to large stationary *'alam*s (battle standards) (Figure R12.2).

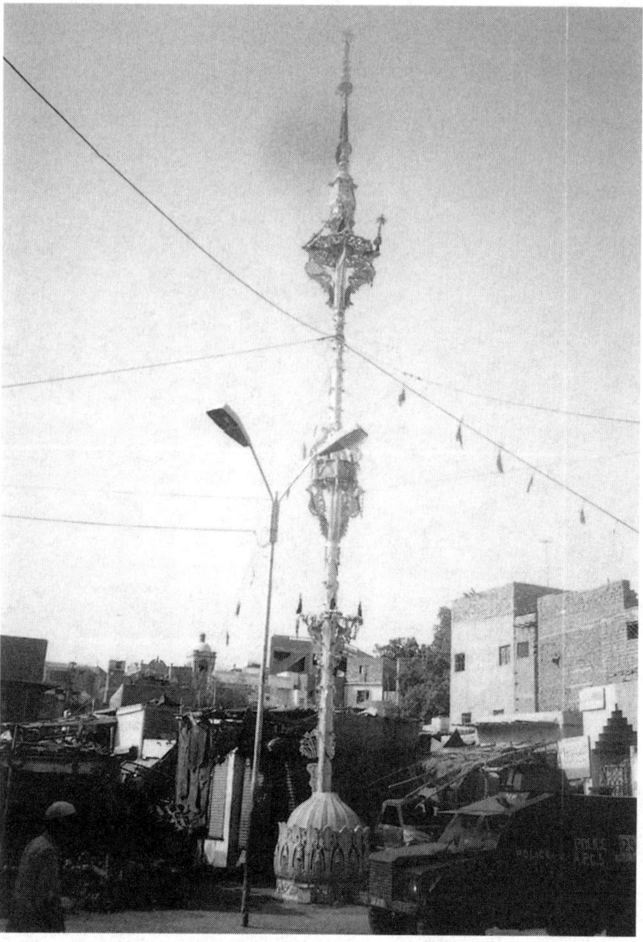

Figure R12.2. Stationary *'alam* from Hyderabad (Sindh, Pakistan).

Not all images of pain are bodily. Some of them arise from ironically tinged and emotionally mixed scenarios from the South Asian redaction of the narrative. For instance, Bano, mother of Husain's infant son, Ali Asghar, cradles her murdered boy in her arms and sings him a lullaby, described in the following "lullaby type" of *salām:*[6]

> Bano came to the slaying-ground saying
> Come sit in my lap, my Asghar

I'd sacrifice myself for the sight of your face
Come sit in my lap, my Asghar

With no one to beg water from,
nursing was a sad business[7]
You've slipped beyond my sorrowful self,
and been smitten with an arrow in your throat

The cradle's empty, whom shall I rock?
Whom shall I send to sleep with lullabies?[8]

Such lullabies are performed by women during *majlis*es, evoking not only the sadness of death but also the love of a mother for her child and her unwillingness to accept his loss. Just as *majlis*es are performed for virtually every important Shī'ī life-cycle event, subsuming personal victories and tragedies within the more substantial religious narrative, so too is a spirit of lamentation projected outward on to performance forms not normally considered sad. The wedding song is similarly affected by this process. In fulfillment of a vow Husain had made to his brother Hasan, Qasim (Hasan's son) was made to marry Husain's daughter before setting off to die in battle. The seventh day of Muharram is reserved for the commemoration (if not partial reenactment) of Qasim's wedding, complete with band (its composition varies locally) (see Wolf 2000).

Pain is highly differentiated in the key scenes of the Karbala narrative described above. By saying that this pain exists in the devout Shī'ī imagination is not to denigrate it but rather to suggest that pain is a creative force: it is a persistent cognitive theme that is elaborated in vivid corporeal images and refracted through affectively complex performance forms. Externalizing the pain, extracting it from the imaginary and making it palpable, vivid, involves inflicting physical pain on the body.

Images of Pain II: The Body

One of the most spectacular features of public Shī'ī Muharram observances is the bloody self-flagellation called *mātam* (literally, "mourning"). A natural magnet for Orientalist attention, *mātam* has become one of the most theologically controversial Shī'ī practices (Ende 1978). It drew such negative attention to Islam that Sayyid Ali Khamenei, Iran's religious leader, issued a fatwa in 1994 forbidding the public use of

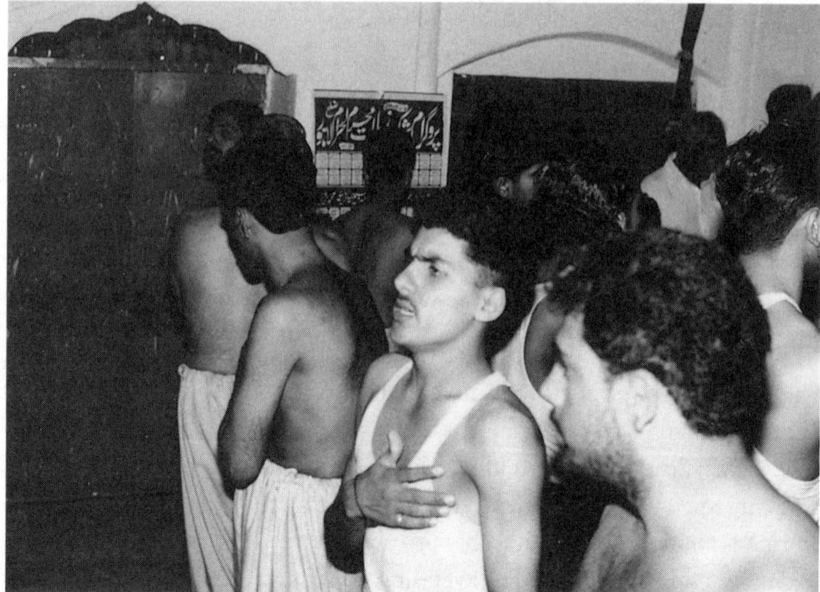

Figure R12.3. Row of men chanting *nauha* and performing *mātam* (Multan, Pakistan).

weapons to shed blood (Pinault 2001, 149). Indian and Pakistani Shī'ahs maintain direct links with Iran, largely through clerics who travel there for training. The Iranian fatwa has led to some discouragement of the bloody *mātam* on the subcontinent, but it nevertheless persists.

Mātam refers to a variety of practices. The simplest and most common is the gentle striking of the chest over the heart with the open right hand, a style that causes no immediate physical pain but is rather a sign of emotional pain: compassion for the suffering of Husain and his companions. More elaborate breast beating is performed with both hands in alternation. In both cases, participants may chant poetic couplets of the genre, *nauha,* in time with their arm movements (Figure R12.3). Men generally perform *mātam* more energetically than women, and save for certain communities of women (especially singers and dancers), men are the only ones to perform in public. One special style of *mātam* I observed in the Panjab involved an alternation between (1) an antiphonal tuneful recitation of *nauha* by two groups of men and boys, who beat their breasts slowly and deliberately, and

(2) rapid, extremely forceful, self-inflicted blows by a still different group, comprising two facing rows of bare-chested men. The latter declaimed their texts in a shouting rather than singing voice:

On the night of the sixth of Muharram in 1997 (May 14) in the area of Lahore's "old city" called Rang Mahal, a large crowd of Shī'ī men and women gathered in anticipation of the new *nauha*s that were about to be performed—this is the local tradition for the sixth of Muharram. A dozen or so handheld tape recorders were visible in the air near the small circles of men, who were reading the new texts off sheets of paper. Near me, one man said, "[let's do] *maiñ to chalā.*" He and a group of about ten to fifteen others wearing white *sālwār kamīz* began to recite the following refrain in a slow, waltzlike rhythm.

A	
maiñ to chalā hūñ marne	As for me, I'm off to die
sajjād tum rahōge	Sajjad, you shall survive
B	
qaidī banegī zainab	Zainab will be imprisoned
tum dekhnā safar se	You will see, come the month of Safar

Zainab is Husain's sister, who was marched off, ignominiously, to Damascus with the other remaining women and children after the slaughter of Husain's party. The speaker is Ali Akbar, Husain's eighteen-year-old son, addressing himself to Husain's other son Sajjad, who was ill and could not fight. Sajjad plays a special role in Shī'ī interpretations of *mātam.* It is said that just as Sajjad would have fought alongside his father Husain at Karbala, so too would all devout Shī'ahs have willingly sacrificed their lives (Pinault 1992, 105). In performing *mātam,* Shī'ahs identify with the Sajjad prototype.

In performance, the A section was repeated twice without moving to the B section. The B section here served as the rhyming portion in this *nauha* whose couplet form was *ab cb db,* and so on (a variant of the usual form *aa ba ca,* etc.). Following this repetition was a break in the singing. Another group composed of about fifty to sixty bare-chested men stood about twenty feet away: they were separated from the first group by a closely packed crowd of Shī'ahs who were listening, recording, doing *mātam,* or trying to learn the new texts and tunes.

These more serious *mātamdārs* (those who do *mātam*) were maintaining a loud, deep, and resonating pulse on their chests throughout the poetic recitation. Now they begin to shout repeatedly in a brisk duple meter the names of the two characters participating in this interchange: "Akbar, Sajjad." In the rhythmic notation below, each slash represents a strike on the chest. The rate is about eighty-four strikes per minute.

Ak . bar . . Saj jā d
/ . . . / . . .

Then the first group returns to its lyrical interpretation of the *nauha* text, aligning the words with *mātam* strokes in triple meter as before (about forty-two strikes per minute).

/	.	.	/	.	.	/	.	.	/	.	.
.	.	main	to	.	.	chala	.	hun	mar	.	ne
.	.	saj	ja	.	.	d	.	tumra	ho	ge	.
.	.	qai	di	.	.	bane	.	gi	zai	.	nab
.	.	tum	de	.	.	kh	.	nasa	far	se	.

Women also perform *mātam,* usually indoors or in secluded courtyards or neighborhoods. Their styles of *mātam* are generally less dramatic, but they too sing, often with great emotional fervor. Amy Bard (2002) describes women's *nauha* and *mātam* in Lucknow; the poetic text recounts the scene of Abbas attempting to fetch water:

> A middle-aged leader starts the *mātam* by intoning deeply and dolorously, "Husain Husain." A call and response evolves, with one group calling "Husain, Husain," and another repeating this after them at a slightly higher pitch. At this point, the word "Husain," is an almost angry cry, and the women's voices hold nothing of the sorrowful hysteria that characterized them at the end of the sermon. The call and response repeats, its speed increasing gradually, at least fifteen times, and then a lone voice, in this case a young girl's, starts off the first *nauhah:*
>
> This is the beginning of the Karbala story
> This is the beginning of the Karbala story
> O people, this funeral procession is that of Islam's founder
> This is the beginning of the Karbala story

Even the arms of the loyal Abbas will be severed
Even the arms of the loyal Abbas will be severed
Arrows will turn his waterskin into but a sieve
Arrows will turn his waterskin into but a sieve
This is the beginning of the Karbala story

This is the beginning of the Karbala story
O people, this funeral procession is that of Islam's founder
This is the beginning of the Karbala story. . . .

> Even before the nauhah fades out completely, the older women resume their "Husain, Husain," their voices contrasting stridently with the quick, high-pitched recitation of the ten- to twelve-year-old girls. However, they have a chance to chant the refrain only once before a group of somewhat older girls, their voices more robust than those of the first group, start a new nauhah. (Bard 2002)

This description of women's *nauha* and *mātam* practices conveys a sense of excitement and even competitiveness. Among men, competition is generated even more explicitly, especially among *mātam* guilds, which are organized according to performance-style preference, neighborhood, language use, kinship affiliation, and social preference.[9] The agonistic quality of *mātam* fits in with a broader Muharram theme of martialism that is often justified with reference to the Karbala battle, but it should be remembered that competitive display is also a common component of mourning ceremonies cross-culturally (Cannon 1989). The theme of violence becomes more pronounced when *mātamdār*s hold razor blades between their fingers and strike their bare chests. Others strike the tops of their heads with swords, or their backs with blade-laden chains *(zanjīr)*. All these methods require practice so that *mātamdār*s can maximize the flow of surface blood without causing themselves major injury. In some parts of India, rose water is sprinkled on the men to thin the blood and make it flow (and splash) more freely. Still another form of *mātam* involves fire-walking.

The activity of inflicting blows upon one's own body is valued for its pain-transformative function, which allows participants to "bind" (cf. Fernandez 1986, 45) the present with the past, placing the individual on the battleground of Karbala alongside Husain. And yet the psychophysiology of Shī'ī piety anesthetizes that pain. The very piety that Shī'ahs demonstrate by willingly inflicting wounds upon their bodies is said to be that which prevents them from being hurt by these wounds. Because the intention of this behavior is to cause pain, it is from a Shī'ī perspective inappropriate to view the subjective state of the participant as a form of "trance" (Hjortshoj 1977, 161, 176–77). The process of performing *mātam* becomes multiply transformative and in a way paradoxical: the intention of pain ameliorates pain.

The status of *mātam* as a form of materialization or exteriorization of pain can also be explored in its social performative dimensions: the more it is focused and intense, the more its participants are marked out as distinct from a larger processional population. Those who (as in the example above) line up in rows, bare chested, to perform *mātam* in an organized, styled manner stand out in small groups. Their bodies become instruments for sound and move in a fashion that has been criticized in some circles as too dancelike (Pinault 1992, 149–151). Those who perform bloody *mātam* may stand out as groups as well: at halting points in a procession, space will generally be cleared for the scattering of their blood and the reach of their implements. But these participants are more individuated in performance style than those performing coordinated hand *mātam:* I have never seen a line of men swing their chains in a stylistically coordinated manner, nor have I seen them chant. The least marked are those performing *mātam* in a casual, unstylized manner with their hands. They tend to blend in with the fray: they may chant *nauha*s, walk casually in procession, and perhaps coordinate their activities with the sound of drums or double-reed instruments if they are present.

Exteriorization extends a step further in a form of doubling in which *mātam* moves off the body completely onto musical or other sound-producing instruments.

Instruments of Sound

Muharram processions, particularly on the first and tenth of the month, still retain a flavor of those from the nineteenth and early twentieth centuries—the days of the Nawabs of Lucknow and the Nizams of Hyderabad—in which the splendid statecraft of the Shī'ī nobility was designed to embrace the diverse populace. Camels, elephants, bands of bagpipers, marching bands, and colorful regalia take to the streets in a colorful display of pageantry. The musical pieces sound to many like joyous, stately airs, but they are dirges, *nauha*s, which musicians have learned aurally from years and years of listening to Shī'ī men reciting them in processions.

Excepting a few branches of Sufism, Islamic legalists have tended to frown on the use of musical instruments for purposes other than public celebrations (weddings especially) or the military (Faruqi 1994, 6). Due to the significance of "the word" in Islam, poetry and sacred texts are not subject to musical prohibitions when they are melodically embellished.[10] Thus, *nauha, soz, salām,* and *marsīyah* are not proscribed unless they become too "musical."[11] Drums occupy a musically liminal position: when used to accompany "sensuous" music and dancing, they are as unacceptable as other musical instruments, but in certain functional capacities, such as the military and in weddings, they are acceptable.

A problem arises when drumming is performed during Muharram. Muslims take special pains to avoid all music at this time because, first, in highly charged religious contexts, Muslims would likely be more assiduous in their adherence to religious strictures. To drink alcohol might be a sin, but to drink it during the month of fasting would be a greater sin—so too with music. Second, out of respect for the fact that Shī'ahs regard Muharram as an occasion for mourning, many Muslims feel that music of all kinds—but particularly that which is joyful—should be avoided. Third, some Shī'ahs take a more antimusic stance than do Sunnis. One allegedly historical justification for this is that Shī'ahs revile the Prophet's wife, Aisha, who was said to be fond of music; therefore, they morally oppose music itself as well.[12] Lastly, drumming is specifically problematic for some Shī'ahs because it is said that Yazid's army beat the drums to announce and rejoice after they slew members of Husain's party.

Despite these objections, some participants in Muharram justify the use of musical instruments—especially drums and double-reed aerophones—because they understand them to articulate Muharram themes of salvific pain, sadness, martialism, aggression, and triumph (Figure R12.4). Although a range of participants attribute meaning to individual drumming patterns with varying degrees of specificity and

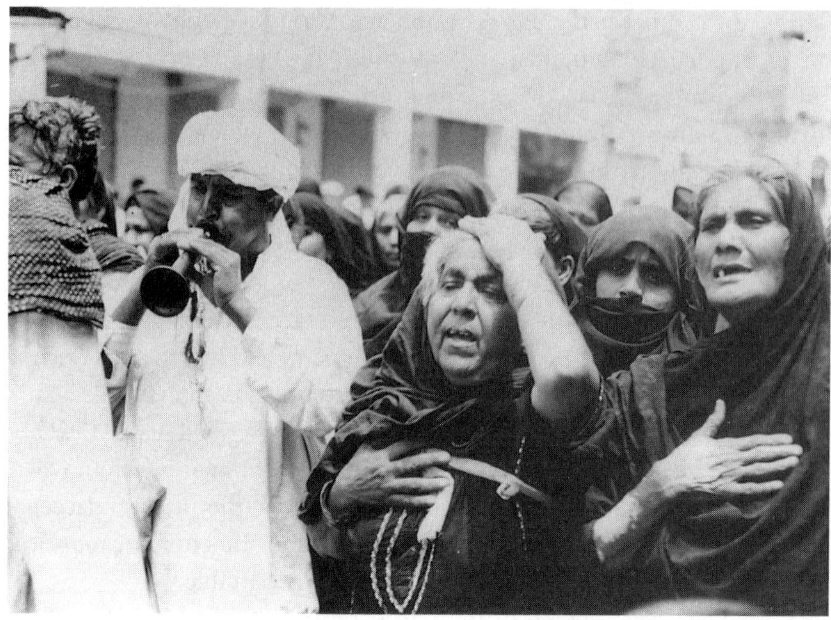

Figure R12.4. Women chanting *nauha* and performing *mātam* (Multan, Pakistan).

according to differing criteria,[13] one of the most consistent meanings is conveyed through a name: *mātam.* That is to say, for some participants beating the drums itself constitutes an act of mourning.[14] The idea I wish to emphasize is that the drums may act as a surrogate for the human body.

The interpretation of drumming becomes more complicated when we take into account the diversity of participants in Muharram and the changing political climate for its performance. I cannot treat this in any detail, but a few points are noteworthy. It is now rare to find Shī'ahs who drum or play any other instruments during Muharram; instead, Sunnis or Hindus perform these instruments. Due in part to Shī'ah–Sunni rivalries, Shī'ahs contend that Sunnis improperly rejoice during Muharram. They cite Sunni drumming—which they view as self-evidently joyous—as proof of their irreverence. It is neither true that all Shī'ahs, without respect to political motives, find Muharram drumming happy, nor is it true that all Sunnis express happiness at the martyrdom of Husain. In fact, Shī'ahs historically have performed the drums during Muharram—although few now know or admit to it—and there are still those who do, especially in pockets of the subcontinent that lack pronounced intercommunal tensions. Some Sunnis, on the other hand, demonstrate not happiness but respect for Imām Husain through their drumming. They believe that although the deaths at Karbala were tragic, Islam, in the end, emerged victorious. Instead of mourning, according to these Sunnis, Muslims should be morally triumphant during this holiday.[15]

The end result of this complicated game of transformed motives is that the aspect of drumming that signifies—or embodies or shows respect for or even mocks (in some contorted interpretations)—"pain" or "suffering" has often been twice doubled. It has first been removed from the body and resignified on the drums, and then it has been distanced from the central community of pious Shī'ahs and projected as a sign of otherness upon non-Shī'ī communities—most importantly Sunnis but Hindus too.

Conclusion

In this essay I have necessarily glossed over a great deal of detail and regional variation in order to emphasize three arenas in which pain is exteriorized during Muharram. I have argued that this exteriorization is spiritually useful because it helps Shī'ahs experience and contemplate pain in a manner central to their religious experience. First, narrative forms, processional components, and songs intensify the mental images of suffering associated with the battle of Karbala and, ideally, induce participants to weep. Second, forms of bodily mutilation (or gentle motions that stand for such mutilation) "double" this mental image of pain by inscribing it on the body; the salvific result of this action depends on the willful intention of the flagellant. Third, some of the emotional themes of mourning, pain and suffering among them, are exteriorized, however controversially, through the sound of musical instruments.

If this reworking of themes from Scarry and Selby has produced an academically generated "double" that leads us far afield from two fine originals, I hope that it nevertheless serves as a useful form of exteriorization and that it stimulates further reflection on the larger themes of pain and its transformation presented in this volume.

Notes

1. I conducted research for this essay in many cities and towns in India and Pakistan over twenty-eight months in the years 1996 to 1999. I am grateful to the American Institute of Pakistan Studies and the American Institute of Indian Studies for partial funding during this period. I wish to thank Amy C. Bard for her careful reading of this essay, for her correction of factual details, for her translation of Urdu passages (with my own slight modifications), and for allowing me to cite her data. She is not responsible for the interpretations I offer, however, which are my own.
2. Although Sunni Muslims may be involved in any of these activities as well (depending on the region and history of local communities), they tend to include only (2) and (3) and generally do not share Shī'ī views on the moral value of pain. Hindus also participate in activities (2) and (3), attaching their own meanings—sometimes, for instance, they view Husain as a deity.
3. In Lahore, Pakistan, for example, I noted assemblies in Urdu, Panjabi, and Saraikki. Sometimes famous preachers are invited from India for Urdu assemblies in Karachi, where there is a large immigrant *(muhājir)* community. Women can attend men's *majlis*es, provided they view them from a secluded area. Men cannot attend women's *majlis*es, however.
4. In Mashhad there is a shrine for Imām Reza.
5. Ali, Husain's father, was known for his intelligence and fairness.
6. Clerics and some Shī'ī laypeople hold that Rabab, another of Husain's wives, was historically Ali Asghar's mother and not Bano. *Majlis* poetry portrays both as possible mothers.
7. That is to say, Bano could not produce milk because she too was dehydrated.
8. Recorded at a *majlis* in Lahore Pakistan (1997) and translated by Amy Bard.
9. Pinault was told that there were some thirty-five to forty such guilds in Hyderabad, Andhra Pradesh, one of which traces its history back to the nineteenth century (Pinault 1992, 84–85).
10. The emphasis on the spoken and written word that is common to the Abrahamic religions is not a purely religious phenomenon; it is also cultural, probably stemming from ancient Arab beliefs in the power of poets and poetry (Shiloah 1995, 4).
11. The criteria for excessive musicality vary locally: they usually involve notions of melodic elaborateness or similarity to either classical or popular musics (Pinault 1992, 150; Wolf 2000).
12. See Shiloah (1995, 32) for traditions from the *hadīs* connecting Aisha with music. Shī'ahs revile her because she led the movement to overthrow Ali, the beloved first Shī'ī Imām (Rizvi 1987, I.37).
13. The details of these meanings cannot be explored here. See Wolf 2000.

14. In some regions, Shī'ahs beat their breasts in time with the drums. In others, musicians beat the drums independently of such flagellation.
15. Going one step further, one anti-Shī'ī cleric called for rejoicing on the tenth of Muharram (the day of Husain's murder) because it was auspicious for prophets from pre-Islamic times (Rizvi 1987, II.135).

References

Ayoub, M. 1978. *Redemptive Suffering in Islām: A Study of the Devotional Aspects of 'Āshūrā' in Twelver Shī'ism.* The Hague: Mouton.

Bard, A. C. 2002. "Desolate Victory: Shi'i women and the *Marsiyah* Texts of Lucknow." Ph.D. dissertation, Columbia University.

Cannon, A. 1989. "The Historical Dimension in Mortuary Expressions of Status and Sentiment." *Current Anthropology* 30(4): 437–458.

Chelkowski, P., ed. 1979. *Ta'ziyeh: Ritual and Drama in Iran.* New York: New York University Press.

Ende, W. 1978. "The Flagellations of Muharram and the Shi'ite 'Ulama.' " *Der Islam: Zeitschrift für Geschichte und Kultur des Islamischen Orients* 55(1): 19–36.

Faruqi, L. I., Al-. 1994. *Music: An Islamic Perspective.* Minna, Niger State, Nigeria: Islamic Education Trust.

Fernandez, J. W. 1986. "The Mission of Metaphor in Expressive Culture." In *Persuasions and Performances: The Play of Tropes in Culture.* Bloomington: Indiana University Press, 28–70.

Hasan, M. 1997. "Traditional Rites and Contested Meanings: Sectarian Strife in Colonial Lucknow." In V. Graff, ed., *Lucknow: Memories of a City.* Delhi: Oxford University Press, 115–135.

Hasnain, N., and A. Husain. 1988. *Shias and Shia Islam in India.* Delhi: Harnam Publications.

Hjortshoj, K. G. 1977. "Kerbala in Context: A Study of Muharram in Lucknow, India." Ph.D. dissertation, Cornell University.

Korom, Frank. 2002. *Hosay Trinidad.* Philadelphia: University of Pennsylvania Press.

Masselos, J. 1982. "Change and Custom in the Format of the Bombay Mohurrum during the 19th and 20th Centuries." *South Asia* 5(2): 47–67.

Pinault, D. 1992. *The Shiites: Ritual and Popular Piety in a Muslim Community.* New York: St. Martin's Press.

———. 2001. *Horse of Karbala: Muslim Devotional Life in India.* New York: Palgrave.

Qureshi, R. 1981. "Islamic Music in an Indian Environment: The Shiah Majlis." *Ethnomusicology* 25: 41–67.

Rizvi, S. A. A. 1987. *A Socio-Intellectual History of the Isna 'Ashari Shi'is in India: 7th to 16th Century* A.D., *with an Analysis of Early Shi'ism*. 2 vols. Canberra: Ma'rifat Publishing House.

Shiloah, A. 1995. *Music in the World of Islam: A Socio-Cultural Study*. Detroit: Wayne State University Press.

Wolf, R. K. 2000. "Embodiment and Ambivalence: Emotion in South Asian Muharram Drumming." *Yearbook for Traditional Music* 32: 81–116.

Discussion:
The Dislocation, Representation, and Communication of Pain

HOWARD FIELDS: I have a question for Elaine Scarry about representations in the brain and the issue of displacement of the location of the experience of pain. It's a thought experiment that comes out of a discussion that Arthur Kleinman and I had when we first met. If you were to image somebody's brain while they were undergoing pain, and you believe that neural activity in a particular part of the brain is responsible for the experience, how does that fit into this picture of displacement? What does that give to, or take from, the patient, and what impact does that sort of objectification of a highly personal experience have on your thinking?

ELAINE SCARRY: I suspect I probably don't intuit the full import of your question. Let's say that someone was in terrible pain that was centered at the base of her spine and that you were scanning her brain. I take it from the literature on the subject that rather extensive parts of the brain would be participating in that.

I guess it would be relevant to the specific procedures for representation that I was describing in this way: An artist might depict that pain by some terribly maiming distortion of both body and head that actually bore no resemblance to the physical reality. If you were standing by the person's bed, you would not see any maiming of their surface. Yet the representation would show that maiming even as it would try to preserve the integrity of the individual.

The versatility of pain has been shown in its ability to seek out new networks if you destroy or block some and in its ability to take over more and more of the bodily apparatus so every perceptual act is converted into one more experience of pain. In that sense, even if the pain occurred at a specific location in the back and in the brain, the truest representation would eventually show the person's full surface in some way maimed or mutilated by the felt experience.

LAURENCE KIRMAYER: That puts me in mind of a different kind of displacement. Some people who have survived torture describe having been able to go somewhere else in their head. It's not unlike hypnosis in the clinical context or aspects of meditation. In that other place they may have an out-of-body experience in which they can look back at their body and describe sensory qualities of the pain, but with a physical distance that can be relieving.

We also see the opposite of that in survivors of torture for whom their enduring pain has a memorializing function. It connects them to a story that they're very invested in, for example, because it's part of the reason they claim as a refugee for coming to a new place. That seems to perpetuate the pain for them. Rather than distancing it, they have to revisit it and live in that space.

If you transpose those positions back to neurology, they imply activity in other parts of the brain representing imaginal spaces that are somehow modulating activity in the somatosensory cortex.

FIELDS: Those would be *actual* displacements. The implication of this thought experiment—and I'd be interested in other people's opinion—is that the brain-imaging technique is not a counterfactual "as if," but it still lifts the experience into the object world, externalizes it, and allows it to be shared and understood. It somehow separates the displacement and the objectification and removes it from the counterfactual.

SARAH COAKLEY: It hardly separates it in the same way that doubling in ritual performance does.

FIELDS: No, it's the opposite.

COAKLEY: Exactly. One might argue that the PET or fMRI scan is a sad, secular relic of a culture that doesn't know how to double ritually any more.

FIELDS: I think we've got all our weapons on the table.

SCARRY: Now I understand better what you're saying. T. S. Eliot said in *A Love Song of J. Alfred Prufrock* that it's as though the nerves could be seen on a pattern on the screen, and that's actually come true. And I think that's a blessing in cases where physicians can't find an organic base and suddenly the PET scan or the fMRI shows it.

FIELDS: That's what I believe too.

SCARRY: The pictures assert the fact that there's something going on. The one thing they don't do is convey the fact of the *felt experience.*

ELIZABETH TOLBERT: Both Elaine Scarry's paper and Martha Selby's papers are talking about ways of representation. It strikes me that representation is always about displacement. Is there a special kind of displacement going on here? What makes the displacement of pain different than any other kind of representation?

Supposedly, if you watch somebody doing a movement, the same sensory motor map is activated as if you were doing the movement yourself. Would that overlap between a representation of something and your own internalization of it shed some light more generally on embodiment and representation? I do think there's a cultural reason why we can't talk about pain or emotions in the same way that we talk about other kinds of representation that seem obvious to us.

SCARRY: Is the taboo on expressing pain a cultural taboo, or does it come from the intrinsic difficulty of expressing it? Although there are lots of cultural taboos against it, I think that it goes way beyond cultural taboo. Even for people who devote themselves to this around the clock, like certain physicians or Amnesty International workers, it's hard to get it into language.

I think it differs from other events in the much greater urgency and difficulty in having person A, who's not in pain, know that person B is in pain. It's important, too, that romantic love be communicated, but there's no trouble communicating it—that's why we have 300,000 ways to say it. There's an awful lot of evidence that pain is not so easily communicated. That itself is a problem for people who are in pain, because the lack of objectification in the world contributes to the pain. If you can provide objectification to the person in pain, you diminish the pain somewhat. That's why the pain of a woman giving birth is in some way lessened by having someone share it with them.

ARTHUR KLEINMAN: I agree with your point in the case of acute pain, but I don't think it's generally true that we don't have language for chronic pain. Read Reynolds Price's (2000) or Bob Murphy's (2001) accounts of cancer in the spinal cord. I think they're brilliant statements about what the pain feels like. Another area that's most impressive is heart disease, where people have well described angina pectoris, pulmonary edema, or plural diffusions.

I agree entirely with what you say about metaphor. It isn't as if people are describing something in direct terms that don't require metaphor. There *is* a distanciation, an objectification, a throwing outward into the world in images. But it seems to me that in fact the language of pain *is* those metaphors. In the same way, scientists use other metaphors for pain.

I think you are more of a defender of the McGill pain questionnaire (see Melzack 1975) than I am. I find the questionnaire incredibly crude. It's like using a synonym finder to look for different terminology. Yes, there are some big differences between throbbing and burning, for example, but this strikes me as a poor way of getting at the meaning of pain, for which metaphors are more effective.

William Styron (1990) talks about depression as pain, saying it feels like a heated-up room that he can't get out of. I find that a very effective metaphor. The Chinese use the term *men* for depression, which gives the sense of something closing in or oppressing. They have plenty of terms for sadness, but they don't use them for depression. Clinically, the most common term is *men,* the character for which is the doorway radical with a heart within it. That feeling can be exquisitely portrayed by people using a very physicalist language.

I agree that tremendous, acute pain shatters language and destroys worlds. But with chronic pain, over time people develop metaphors that come close to how they feel the experience—and that can be remarkably communicative. So maybe it's important to distinguish kinds of pain in relationship to language.

SCARRY: Yes. My work has addressed the terrible pain of burns, cancer, and torture rather than more modest forms of pain where there are interludes of relief that allow one to at least recover some grounding and stamina to deal with the next moment of pain when it comes. I agree that in recent years there have been some really good attempts to describe various forms of chronic pain.

That has to be seen against the background of people endlessly reporting that when they were in pain, people didn't believe them. Or people reporting, for example, "I never understood what Aunt Mildred was talking about until the autopsy, when they found a tumor this big inside her head." That's a case where the body damage confers the reality of what the person experienced. I've overheard strangers talking to one another, saying, "It's so boring when he complains." In poetry, complaint, lament, and elegy have magnificent, elegant forms. Complaint as a speech act is, with very few exceptions, not a form that wins listeners. Country western music and reggae music are somewhat exceptional.

KLEINMAN: How about blues? I wonder if there isn't a Western bias to this inasmuch as Wittgenstein, in *Philosophical Investigations* (2002 [1953]), says that acknowledgment should be the first act in regard to pain, but it isn't, and instead we interrogate pain. Marshall Sahlins (1976) pointed out that this notion of interrogation might be one of the deep cultural structures in Western society.

Acknowledgment is common in other traditions as an initiating act. The first movement, routinely, is not to ask whether the pain is real but to acknowledge the experience of the person in pain. The Western response may have something to do with the distinctions we make between real and unreal, the importance we place on the idea that there's a single truth, which drives all other ideas to the side. This leads to an interrogation that's very much a part of medicine—the medical interrogation—but also part of everyday life. However, it undermines the act of acknowledgment of pain that seems to exist in many societies.

SCARRY: I have to say I disagree. I believe that the very heart of suffering is that it's so vibrantly real when it's happening that it takes away the object of every other form of perception. We say that you see stars when the dentist's drill hits a nerve; imagine that with no drill but prolonged, on and on and on. The difficulty of expressing that, and the benefit to be derived from someone actually being there for the person suffering, is not a matter of cultural stipulation. I don't believe that it has to do with the interrogating methods of Western medical culture but, rather, that it is part of something that's nonnegotiable.

LUIS GÓMEZ: I have similar reservations with the cultural interpretation. But I also felt that both papers were so eloquent that in some ways they belie the claim that pain is difficult to talk about. To phrase that as an honest question: How can you determine that the expression of pain is really more difficult than the expression of other extreme forms of experience such as intense joy or intense calm or mania or the emptiness of schizophrenia? What's the data that pain is more difficult?

SCARRY: First of all, people who have been in excruciating pain often say that they didn't understand what it was like not to be able to communicate the pain until they experienced it. But there's more general, external evidence. It's often said that other equally physical states like joy or the erotic are also hard to render in language. But a simple consultation of literature shows that pleasurable states are language building. Eating is a very physical act, but we've built dinner parties around it. We build colloquy around it, and that's not just specific to the United States. With physical love, it's true that people making love talk baby talk, which you could say is a degeneration of language. But they are also able to generate hundreds of magnificent narratives. There's almost no state, other than pain, that doesn't have full representation in literature.

GÓMEZ: It seems like the kind of question that could have an empirical answer. Do you have any kind of empirical data?

SCARRY: Arthur Kleinman says he's not impressed by the McGill pain questionnaire. But I've read reports that say that when patients are given the McGill pain questionnaire, their eyes fill with tears.

GÓMEZ: For that to be empirical data, there would have to be a control, like a joy questionnaire.

KLEINMAN: I've given hundreds of McGill pain questionnaires, and I haven't seen that experience. Quite the opposite. People say that they felt the language was dehumanizing.

NICHOLAS WOLTERSTORFF: Both sides seem compelling when they're expressed. Using the example of grief rather than pain, I think Elaine is absolutely correct that it's impossible for a person who hasn't felt the death of a child to imagine what that experience is like. In my own case, I thought I had imagined that and discovered that I was woefully unsuccessful.[1] Probably the same sort of thing is true for intense physical pain.

On the other hand, it may be that when two people have had the experience, then they can agree fairly well on the descriptions of it. I think it is a peculiar case in which people who have had the experience can judge the language effective, but the same language is singularly inept at communicating the experience. There is much language that is good at communicating concrete description: what a tree looks like, for example. But this seems to be different. If you haven't had the experience, the language won't communicate it.

CLIFFORD WOOLF: There's another interesting side to it. You're talking about whether someone who's never experienced pain can empathize with someone who has had pain. But if you ask patients to record their own pain in diaries, once they are out of pain, they find it very difficult to empathize with the pain they've already had. I think it's very difficult to record the pain when it takes over because it is such a total experience. But when it's no longer there, it's very difficult to recall that intense experience. Even self-empathy is a problem, never mind communicating it with other people.

KAY KAUFMAN SHELEMAY: I just want to throw one other parameter into the mix. As we talk about modalities of suffering and representation, we haven't talked about temporalities and the fact that the acute pain is ostensibly shorter term and chronic pain is longer term. This brings in process and temporality, and it may be where we begin to find oral epics and music intersecting with the bodily experience of either acute or, even more strongly, chronic pain, because there is time to embed yet another temporal process. I think temporality is part of the nature of the metaphor, not just the modality of the experience.

TOLBERT: I have a very similar point. You have an intense experience, but you can't actually remember it, so you have to create another intense experience that can be metaphorically mapped onto it. If you want to actually convey an experience, you do not describe it—you create another experience.

That was so striking with Martha Selby's examples. As she was talking about aesthetic distance, we were all crying. I think that's because an experience has been created here in this room that we can then metaphorically map onto another experience.

KIRMAYER: It strikes me both from looking at how clinicians deal with people in pain and from my own experience of persistent, severe back pain that the experience of acute pain is fairly universal. If someone says, "I'm in acute pain," we understand that at least in an abstract sense, but we don't want to revisit it. We certainly don't want to experience it for any duration. When you said that the drill makes us see stars, we all understood that, but the idea that it could be prolonged is an unimaginably terrifying possibility. I think that's what we're seeing: it's not that people could not describe the pain but that the description is so painful, so frightening, and so disturbing that people shy from it.

I was just at a conference on somatization in Australia, where the clinician's caricature of the chronic pain patient is very much about the clinician trying to distance himself or herself from the patient. The clinicians talk about the patients with a critical view as though they are dwelling on something that they could let go of. I think that our deepest hope and fantasy is that people are just dwelling on something they could let go, and we conspire to make it seem that way.

Years ago Hilbert (1984) wrote a paper on flawed reality construction and the notion of chronic pain in which he argues that we do not have good categories for chronic pain in our culture. I think the reason is exactly, as you say, that it goes beyond culture, because there's no place in the world where people really want to imagine the kind of pain that is totally derailing and disorganizing and leaves no room for thought.

STANLEY TAMBIAH: I want to raise an anthropological observation about communication of pain between persons. In this country, and I think in the West in general, there is a reticence, a certain privacy, almost a cultural taboo against talking to people about your disease, whereas in South and Southeast Asia, in Thailand or Sri Lanka, for example, people constantly talk to each other about the state of their illness. Second, in the West you have so medicalized and given such technical labels to suffering, whereas in that part of the world the old humoral theory still holds that herbal drugs are an extension of food. Many of their foods they eat every day also have medical properties, and the language of humoral theory is part of everyone's discourse about illness. These interpersonal dimensions certainly differ between societies and affect how one communicates pain and disease.

MARTHA ANN SELBY: As a rejoinder to that, and to Elaine Scarry's comment on representation in literature, I can offer a nice illustration. In writing my dissertation, I did a statistical count of the whole corpus of Tamil *Cankam* poetry to see how many poems were about pleasure and how many were about grief and suffering (Selby 1994). Suffering won by a landslide.

SCARRY: I doubt they would be direct descriptions of physical pain.

SELBY: In some cases; but they are mostly about grief, longing, and mourning.

SCARRY: By the way, I never meant to say that physical pain is somehow more important or worse than emotional pain, only that it involves a particular representational problem. The poems you quoted were amazing, and they managed to turn the body inside out by relocating perception while preserving the delicacy of personhood.

TU WEIMING: Pain is complex and sometimes very difficult to express, especially acute pain, which is a separate category. But I think there's a major difference between discourse about healing the body, which we talk about every day, and expression, which is intensely personal, though it may not be "private." Here the private and public domains must be clearly differentiated, even if they are perceived differently in different cultures.

Intensely personal experience is the most communicable experience because "intensely personal" means it is something that every other human being can understand sympathetically. But it's not necessarily private. The privatization of intensely personal feeling is culturally conditioned, and the private and public are in a dialectic interplay. I am private, but my family is public. As I talk to my family, I move from my privatized self to a personal feeling of sharing. Or, in some cultures, the family is private, and the larger community is public. Through the interplay, intensely personal feelings can be publicly accountable. In that case, communicability is very, very significant.

Another thought I had is very intriguing. Looking at pain neurologically, we can now pinpoint it very, very precisely. However, if you look at the human body as an interconnected, complicated system, with pain having a tremendous impact on many other kinds of emotions, it makes it very difficult to simply accept that specifically pinpointed link. This may also be related to the question of meaning. The meaning does not really lie in how to locate the specific place where the perceived suffering occurs but in the other linkages that affect the whole ethos or even other parts of the physical body. Meaning relates not just to interpretation but to all internal self-communication.

Here, then, is a way of seeing *locatable* "pain" diffusing into "suffering."

Note

1. Nicholas Wolterstorff's son Eric was tragically killed in a climbing accident (see Wolterstorff 1987). —*Eds.*

References

Hilbert, R. 1984. "The Acultural Dimensions of Chronic Pain: Flawed Reality Construction and the Problem of Meaning." *Social Problems* 31: 365–378.

Melzack, R. 1975. "The McGill Pain Questionnaire: Major Properties and Scoring Methods." *Pain* 1: 277–299.

Murphy, R. F. 2001. *The Body Silent: The Different World of the Disabled.* New York: W. W. Norton.

Price, R. 2000. *A Whole New Life: An Illness and a Healing.* New York: Scribner.

Sahlins, M. 1976. *Culture and Practical Reason.* Chicago: University of Chicago Press.

Selby, M. A. 1994. "Toward a Grammar of Love: A Comparative Study of Interpretive Modes in Classical Indian Poetry." Ph.D. dissertation, University of Chicago.

Styron, W. 1990. *Darkness Visible: A Memoir of Madness.* New York: Random House.

Wittgenstein, L. 2002 [1953]. *Philosophical Investigations,* 3rd ed. Trans. G. E. M. Anscombe. Oxford: Blackwell.

Wolterstorff, N. 1987. *Lament for a Son.* Grand Rapids, MI: William B. Eerdmans.

When Is Pain Not Suffering and Suffering Not Pain?

Self, Ethics, and Transcendence

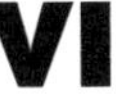

On the Cultural Mediation of Pain 13

Laurence J. Kirmayer

Some of the most dramatic expressions of cultural diversity and distinction are found in the meanings of pain and suffering. Indeed, there is a long history of exoticism and cultural voyeurism built on recounting feats of endurance, self-injury, mutilation, and extremes of asceticism and privation by religious practitioners and devotees. These are often taken—by those both within and without the culture—to demonstrate the hidden powers accessible through specific spiritual practices and, in a broader and more profound way, to warrant the truth and power of the whole tradition.

How can we understand the effectiveness of music, prayer, and symbolic action to alleviate pain? What are the mediators between the diverse rituals and religious practices found in most cultures and the dramatic transformations of the meaning and experience suffering? Can we build models that bridge the gulf between religious or aesthetic experience and our emerging understanding of neurophysiology? Do these models have any relevance to clinical work with patients suffering from acute or chronic pain?

One approach to these questions centers on the nature of embodiment—the many ways in which human experience emerges from our bodily being-in-the-world. The bodily givens of experience described by phenomenology reflect both the physiological machinery of the body and its cultural shaping through ongoing interaction with others across the lifespan. Physiology underwrites the stories that constitute the self, even as our self-depiction remodels bodily structures and reconfigures their functions.

Contemporary cognitive neuroscience understands mind and experience as phenomena that emerge from neural networks at a certain level of complexity and organization. There is increasing recognition that this organization is not confined to the brain but also includes loops through the body and the environment, most crucially through a social world that is culturally constructed. On this view, "mind" is located not in the brain but in the relationship of brain and body to the world (Bateson 1979; Henningsen and Kirmayer 2000). Thus, in psychosomatic and sociosomatic processes, there is no "mysterious leap" from mind to body but rather the cooperative dynamics of a hierarchical system in which the lower levels involve the cellular mechanics of gene expression, and the upper levels involve social processes of making meaning and configuring human aspirations for transcendence. In between are scores of mutually coordinated levels, which are often ignored by disciplinary perspectives that focus narrowly on one or a few levels of explanation and which are simply collapsed or conflated in popular metaphors for illness experience.

In this chapter, I explore some of the implications of a hierarchical systems view for our understanding of the interplay of social and neurophysiological processes in ritual and symbolic transformations of pain and suffering. In particular, I consider three important sites of metaphoric mediation where social theories meet up with contemporary cognitive neuroscience: bodily posture or stance, facial expression, and the experience of temporal duration. Each of these basic aspects of experience gives rise to bodily grounded metaphors that are deployed in cultural systems of meaning to shape the experience of pain and suffering. These metaphors, therefore, occupy a middle ground between the physiology and mechanics of the body and overarching cultural formations. An integrative theory that works outward from such metaphors to explore the links across levels of explanation can help us understand the cultural mediation of pain and suffering in religious practice, healing ritual, and aesthetic experience.

My interest in the cultural mediation of suffering is motivated both by my clinical experience working with patients with chronic pain and by my work in cultural psychiatry. Responding to some of the case studies presented in this volume, I will speak of ritual, but I have in mind not only formal religious and aesthetic events but also the everyday routines of clinical practice, the interactions of clinician and patient aimed at therapeutic efficacy that remain a site of the "sacred" in the secular world (Needleman 1985). The notions we have of how different traditions work with suffering are pertinent to this clinical context, just as experiences in the clinic can shed light on pivotal moments of transformation in other domains of experience.

Cultural psychiatry is engaged in understanding how cultural diversity shapes the experience of suffering and healing. At the same time, a comparative perspective allows us to examine our own clinical practice as a cultural construction, the better to uncover and challenge its hidden assumptions. The selective focus of academic disciplines that emphasize one or another level of description is not adequate for the clinician charged with helping people from diverse backgrounds understand and face their afflictions. Clinical ethnography makes it clear that privileging one level or type of explanation over another has practical and moral implications for patients and their families (Delvecchio Good et al. 1992; Jackson 1999; Kirmayer 2000). Similarly, explanations for pain have a threefold import for clinicians: they guide diagnosis and treatment; they provide a basis for empathic understanding of patients' experience; and they locate the moral significance of symptoms and suffering. The challenge in clinical settings is how to put our knowledge of physiology, psychology, and social interaction together to help patients transform suffering in ways that are consistent with their cultural worlds and commitments.

Strategies of Explanation

Given the detailed accounts of pain-related processes available to us from ethnographic fieldwork, religious testimony, and molecular biology, there are two basic strategies for identifying links between such disparate levels of explanation: the "bottom-up" approach uses lower-level mechanisms to explain higher-order phenomena, whereas the "top-down" approach identifies meaningful patterns at a higher level as a way of discerning the purpose of lower-order mechanisms.

The bottom-up approach involves looking for direct links between a specific physiological process and a social context or variable that can be experimentally manipulated or controlled. For example, the discovery that there is an endogenous pain control system in the brain that produces opiatelike substances (Basbaum and Fields 1978) provides a strategy to probe social situations to identify their physiological impact. This endorphin system contributes to the placebo effect elicited when someone takes a pill that they expect will have an analgesic effect (Levine, Gordon, and Fields 1978). Somehow the expectation for pain reduction activates the brain systems that modulate pain. An expectation or belief therefore has a specific physiological effect that can, in turn, account for the change in experience.

Of course, identifying this potential link raises many unanswered questions about mediation. We have very incomplete knowledge of what happens in other parts of the brain to link a suggestion to an expectation and an expectation to a change in the modulation of synaptic transmission in pain-control systems. Endorphin pathways account for only part of the placebo effect, which depends on other cognitive and emotional effects of expectation (Price et al. 1999; Villemure and Bushnell 2002). However, the possibility that some form of classical conditioning creates links between specific symbolic stimuli and physiological responses suggests that complex cognitive mediation may not be needed to produce elements of the analgesic placebo effect.

We might therefore assume that activation of the endorphin pain-control system is the mechanism for the apparent tolerance or control of pain in some religious rituals. This was the hypothesis of cultural psychiatrist Raymond Prince (1982), who studied the Tamil rites of Thaipusam in Kuala Lumpur. In this annual ritual, devotees pierce their cheeks and tongues with long skewers and carry large cages bedecked with flowers, pulled by hooks in the skin of their backs (Simons, Ervin, and Prince 1988). Ervin and colleagues (1988) attempted to measure endorphin levels of devotees preparing for these rites but were stymied by methodological problems. Nevertheless, with methodological refinements, this strategy could reveal links between social actions and events and endogenous modulation of pain pathways. Having pinned down an independent measure of a pain-related process, we can use it to examine how social processes or events modify physiological functions.

This sort of research strategy can reveal much, but it leaves unexamined what it is about the social context and meaning of the rites that activates the endogenous pain-control system. This requires more detailed analysis and measurement or control of psychological mediators. Indeed, there is evidence that many other forms of pain control do not rely exclusively on this mechanism. For example, hypnosis is sometimes dramatically effective in reducing clinical pain (Hilgard and Hilgard 1975; Holroyd 1996; Montgomery, DuHamel, and Redd 2000), and the analgesic effects of hypnotic suggestion are not exclusively mediated by endorphins (Price and Barrell 2000). Instead, a variety of cognitive interpretive, affective, and attentional processes seem to be involved in modulating pain through hypnosis.

In viewing the social world through the lens of a specific physiological process, the bottom-up approach runs the risk of crude reductionism: thus, meditation on—and public display of—the power and beneficence of the gods in Thaipusam is reduced to the release of endorphins; or the power of music to transform experience is reduced to some hypothetical synchronization of brain waves by an insistent beat or the activation of reward systems in the brain (Blood and Zatorre 2001).

The top-down strategy of the social sciences begins with the assumption that there are unique properties and dynamics to the social world and the cultural organization of experience. Hence, social and cultural processes require close exegesis and explication in their own terms. Explanations of the impact of ritual or religious practice on experience are found in the structural logic of texts or the social causes and consequences of discourse and practice. This approach is not aimed at reducing social phenomena to some lower-level dynamic—although some versions of psychological anthropology do invoke reductive psychodynamic explanations for complex social processes. More often, the interpretation is in terms of higher-order social processes and larger cultural contexts. While avoiding facile reduction, this approach may abandon causal explanation in favor of merely noting correspondences and so leaves a gap between experience and its underlying substrate.

The usual way to bridge this gap is to look for analogies or metaphors that can be used across different domains. Of course, parallelism does not, in itself, demonstrate a theoretical or material link. Sometimes authors invoke a notion of resonance, implying some form of structural coupling between events at different levels or linked systems. The spatial contiguity or temporal synchronization of events is taken as evidence for resonance. However, without a detailed account of the way in which influence is transmitted and transduced, the appeal to resonance remains unproductive. Such metaphorical arguments are beguiling and may give the illusion of explanation where there is only vague similarity or impressionistic parallels. We readily conflate disparate domains where the metaphoric connotations cannot apply in the same way or jump across many intervening levels without explicating the processes that link each level.

A useful explanatory model should show us how the processes of one level give rise to structures we perceive at another (through "emergence") or, more dynamically, how processes at two different levels cooperatively influence or constrain each other. We want to be able to trace the causal links up and down this hierarchy in a seamless way, identifying the interactions of specific structures and processes at each level. Otherwise, we cannot know if our analogy speaks of anything more than our limited repertoire of ideas or the power of an arresting image to dominate our thinking about distant, perhaps even unrelated, domains.[1]

A consideration of the nature of metaphor itself suggests a way out of this quandary. Studies of the cognitive processes that underlie metaphor provide models of how events on one level (of representation or experience) can be transformed by representations of another domain and how the body is extended in time and space by metaphoric mappings. Tracing how linguistic tropes and other types of metaphoric constructions both arise from and transform bodily experience provides a bridge between levels of explanation that can allow useful traffic between the disciplines of neuroscience, cognitive science, social science, and comparative studies of art and religion.

Embodied Worlds: Maps, Modules, and Metaphors

Recent work in cognitive science has emphasized the centrality of metaphor and analogy in human thought (Gibbs 1994). On this view, the scope of metaphor extends far beyond literary tropes to include sensory, affective, and conceptual analogies as well as physical enactments. The experientialist approach to cognitive semantics developed by Lakoff and Johnson (1980, 1999; also see Johnson 1987) emphasizes that conceptual structure arises from two main sources: (1) the inherent structure and constraints of bodily action and experience and (2) our capacity to project imaginatively from bodily experience to new conceptual domains.

Metaphors involve processes of thinking with the body, through its sensorimotor systems. Bodily experiences arise from loops of action and perception that also provide core metaphors to structure our thinking. The most elementary forms of knowledge are drawn from basic experiences like pushing, pulling, grasping, standing, walking, and interacting with a physical environment. More abstract concepts are built on a scaffolding of simpler metaphors, which in turn can be traced back to sensorimotor image schemas. As a result, the meaning of abstract words is not arbitrary but grounded in a specific developmental history, which is often reflected in the etymology of the words used.

While Lakoff and Johnson (1999) have emphasized the basis of conceptual structure in bodily experiences of sensing and acting in a physical world, the body also presents us with a world populated by others who matter to us (Gibbs 1999). In his account of the metaphorical language of emotions, Kövecses (2000, 162) suggests that the relationship between the body and conceptual structures involves a series of steps, creating progressively more elaborate models: from actual physiology to conceptualized physiology through metonymy; metaphor; cultural models providing schematic structure; and finally, cultural contexts. In this developmental scheme, physiology enters the conceptual system through metonymy: an aspect of bodily experience reflecting physiological functioning supplies a sign for the whole coordinated pattern of physiological events (e.g., the feeling of heat in the face when one flushes in anger supplies a sign for anger).[2] The metonymic sign is then extended metaphorically to include and explain other features of experience (e.g., anger is viewed as a hot liquid under pressure; hence, we may boil over in anger unless we can let off steam). More complex culture-specific notions derive from cultural narratives and situated practices. (Hence, anger becomes part of complex cultural scripts encompassing notions of honor, shame, and whole moral economy [see Rosaldo 1980].)

This hierarchical view acknowledges the role of basic bodily experiences in developing progressively more elaborate conceptual structures, which reflect metaphorical extensions of basic concepts, templates, or schemas configured by cultural conventions—and at the most complex level, schemas that reflect social contexts of meaning, which include ideologies and practices conveyed through narratives, rituals, and institutional routines. However, this account leaves open the question of how far back into the genesis of bodily experience cultural worlds can reach. Although Lakoff and Johnson tend to present their phenomenology as though it is independent of (or prior to) specific cultural content, one can readily see how culture pervades our earliest development experiences of the body (Kirmayer 1992a; Shore 1996; Gibbs 1999; Benson 2001). Basic image schemas may therefore include salient features of interpersonal interaction, especially attachment and conflict, which are conveyed through the communication of emotion. Over time, interpersonal experiences of affect are also reflected in specific image schemas (Kövecses 2000). These affective schemas are elementary maps of the social world. Such maps then provide analogical spaces, which can be used to layer meaning or transform meanings associated with other representational or action systems.

This view of thinking as based on conceptual metaphor contrasts with a popular contemporary approach to cognition that emphasizes the role of discrete modules in the brain designed to undertake specific types of computation relevant to survival and reproduction (e.g., Baron-Cohen 1995).[3] These modules developed through evolution for their adaptive value (Dennett 1995). As a result, there is a high degree of specificity and specialization in brain function. While they evolved to serve specific cognitive functions, modules can be reconfigured (by stringing them together in new ways or applying them to novel inputs) to yield new cognitive functions or mental faculties. The notion of modules is based on the assumption of relatively isolated or independent cognitive functions working in sequence or in parallel. Experimental paradigms can dissect and reveal these separate functions.[4] In practice, however, bodily control systems and cognition are tightly woven together to create a seamless fabric of experience.

Metaphors provide far more flexible and extensible cognitive structures than those posited by modularity theory. Metaphors may configure processing in such a way as to create the impression of a module but without its isolation from other systems; to the contrary, metaphoric remappings of experience generally reveal bidirectional influences in which the connotations of terms from different domains color cognition and experience. Metaphors cannot be mapped onto specific regions of the brain or functional modules. They do have links to more basic levels of information processing (i.e., maps of affect, action, etc.), which in turn depend on specific brain modules or functions. However, they draw equally from the material circumstances, discourses, and narratives of social worlds. Thus, metaphors bridge the bodily given and the culturally configured social world.

Whatever the relative importance of prewired or emergent modules and more fluid metaphoric constructions in cognition, there is increasing recognition that thought depends on embodiment and is best understood as situated action (Clark 1997; Varela, Thompson, and Rosch 1991). Although much social science has focused on the nature of cultural representations, cognitive science concurs with praxis-based social science theories that experience is more closely related to action systems (including the deployment of attention and bodily dispositions ready to apprehend or take hold of the world) than to any representational system. Within cognitive science there is an emerging view that "the proper units of knowledge are primarily concrete, embodied, incorporated, lived; that knowledge is about situatedness; and that the uniqueness of knowledge, its historicity and context, is not a 'noise' concealing an abstract configuration in its true essence. The concrete is not a step toward something else: it is both where we are and how we get to where we will be" (Varela 1999, 7).

Thus cognition consists not primarily of representations but of embodied action. And the acting body is a social body, because it is always already located in a socially constructed world that provides a sense of space and place. The cultural world is the terrain that the body must navigate, the topography within which it situates itself, and the scaffolding against which it finds purchase to take a stand.

The Body's Compass

> Los howl'd in a dismal stupor,
> Groaning! Gnashing! Groaning!
> Till the wrenching apart was healed. (Blake 1978 [1815])

In its salience, intensity, and urgency, pain serves as a message that something is wrong. Acute pain is a preemptive signal that triggers reflexes, focuses attention, commands cognitive resources, and arrests behavior. Pain that persists demands we pay attention to a part of our body, favor it, guard it, worry at it and about it. When it persists long beyond the initial period of injury and alarm, pain nags and harries us, constricting awareness and shrinking the ambit of our social world.

Pain initiates, organizes, and maintains behaviors of withdrawal and avoidance. Thus, there is at root a link between the bodily language of pain and systems for fear, flight, and defeat. The link of pain to withdrawal and avoidance runs directly counter to exploratory and aggressive behavior that moves us outward to claim new territory. The bipolar organization of approach/avoidance is one of the most basic patterns of adaptive behavior in evolutionary ecology (Schneirla 1959). Even the simplest animals have sensorimotor systems devoted to organizing behaviors to approach what is needed for survival and avoid what is potentially harmful. The approach system is elaborated in terms of various specific appetites (hunger, thirst, sexual desire) as well as novelty seeking, which subserves exploration.[5] The withdrawal/avoidance system is governed by pain and fear, which may be readily associated with specific places. Pain thus allows us to draw and remember a map of hardship and danger.

This map is not only about places but especially about people. There is evidence from animal research that the systems for emotional attachment and for pain share common substrates (Panksepp 1998). Infant animals separated from their mothers express their distress through distinctive cries. These vocalizations and other signs of distress on separation are mediated by endorphin systems similar to those involved in pain and may be blocked by giving the animal opiates. The conservatism of evolution, in which new structures must be built on earlier developmental trajectories, ensures that these basic dimensions found in animals

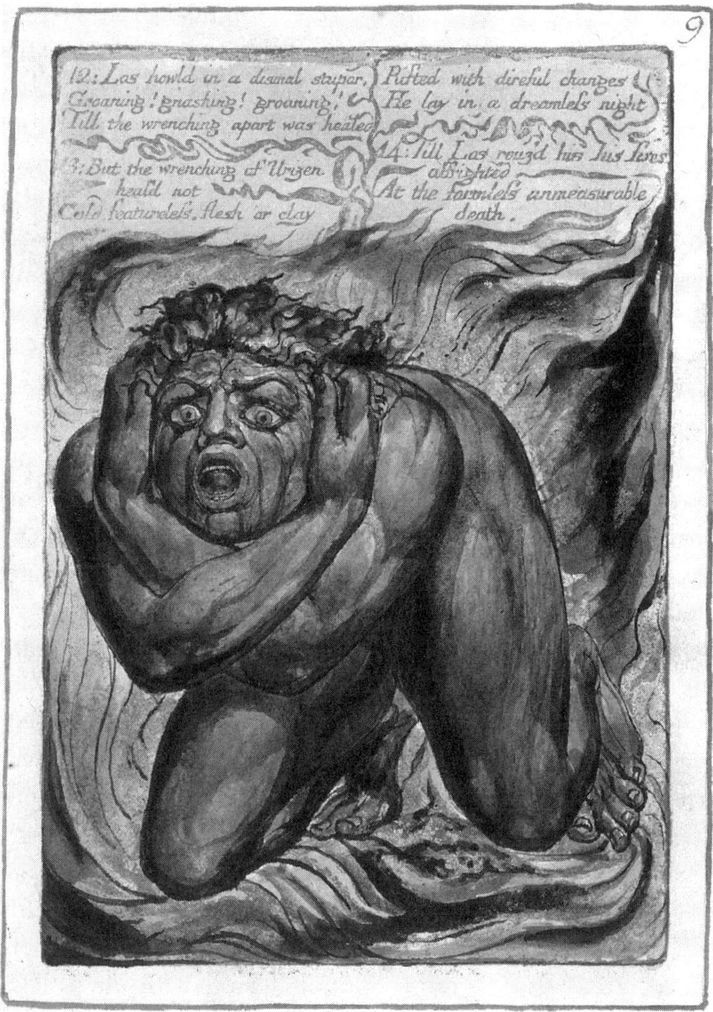
9
12: Los howld in a dismal stupor,
Groaning! gnashing! groaning!
Till the wrenching apart was healed
13: But the wrenching of Urizen
heald not
Cold, featureless, flesh or clay
Rifted with direful changes
He lay in a dreamless night
14: Till Los rouzd his fires
affrighted
At the formless unmeasurable
death.

Figure 13.1. "Los Howl'd here." Figure from William Blake, *The Book of Urizen.*

persist and provide one level of meaning to human experiences. This adaptive organization of experience confers natural metaphoricity on pain, so that we speak of interpersonal loss in terms of pain—although the specific bodily site and sensory quality also reflect ethnophysiological theories and other cultural knowledge about the vicissitudes of love and loss (e.g., our folk theories of "heartache" and "heartbreak").

This speaks to the question of the relationship between physical and emotional pain. Although Clifford Woolf suggests in this volume that the link is *purely* metaphorical, the studies on separation distress indicate that some forms of emotional pain share common substrates with pain-control systems (Panksepp 1998). As well, physical pain has a crucial affective dimension (Casey and Lorenz 2000; Melzack and Casey 1968) that involves different pathways than those that convey the sensory qualities of pain (Rainville et al. 1997). Both anxiety and depression may be caused by physical pain. Negative emotions, in turn, may aggravate acute pain (Meagher, Arnau, and Rhudy 2001) and contribute to its chronicity (Sharp 2001). The crucial observation from cognitive neuroscience is that higher-order processes reach down to modulate incoming sensory information so that larger meanings shape our sensory/perceptual apprehension of the world. This is the essential insight of the gate control theory of pain that has stood the test of time (Melzack and Wall 1965).

The complex relationship between physical and emotional pain is illustrated by the experience of people who deliberately cut or burn themselves in order to experience relief from emotional suffering (Favazza 1989). Such patients often have a history of severe childhood physical abuse (Carroll et al. 1980). They report intense feelings of emotional tension and physical discomfort (usually associated with experiences of loss, rejection, or perceived defeat), which are abruptly relieved when they deliberately cut themselves. In some cases, they describe the experience of self-cutting as causing a pain that is comforting in its definite quality and in the way it displaces other feelings of distress. In other cases, they report feeling little pain—only relief. Self-cutting replaces out-of-control emotional pain with controlled self-inflicted physical pain. The act of self-cutting accentuates individuals' sense of their own boundedness and solidity; it reestablishes body boundaries and a sense of wholeness in individuals who are experiencing fragmentation due to intense feelings of anxiety. Pain cuts through the cloud of anxious feelings that leave the person feeling self-estranged and "disembodied." The effects of self-cutting are not only symbolic—marking the boundary of the self and reasserting self-control over suffering—but also physiological: physical injury activates endogenous pain-control systems that relieve tension and anxiety (Fanselow 1986). By the same mechanisms of activating endorphin systems, pain also suppresses subsequent pain (Willer, Dehen, and Cambier 1981) so that after the first moments of pain on self-cutting the pain of additional acts of self-injury may be diminished. These effects of pain fit with its role in the organization of "fight or flight" behavior.

Pain involves not only the horizontal dimension of approach/avoidance, moving toward or away; for upright bipeds like ourselves, pain also includes the vertical dimension of stance. Our mobility and ability to manipulate the world with our hands depend on being erect, balanced, and unconstrained. The bodily experience of standing gives rise to a series of different image schemas that share in common this bodily origin but that emphasize different elements.[6]

There is a close link between the vertical dimension of bodily stance and emotional experience. Being "up" is generally associated with control, health, consciousness, happiness, and well-being, while being "down" corresponds to the opposite characteristics (Lakoff and Johnson 1980). We soar in ecstasy and sag in abjection and lamentation. Posture thus has fundamental meaning as a social communication. We signal our own emotional state and our stance toward others in the way we carry ourselves before them. This social dimension of posture serves to communicate power, dominance, or submission: standing tall to declare victory over another or cowering in submission.

Pain, suffering, grief, and sorrow are dramatically displayed in posture: the depressed person slumps over; the person in pain pulls back and guards himself or herself and may also shrink down. Blake's image of Los, from *The Book of Urizen*, graphically displays a posture that speaks of fear and agony (see Figure 13.1). We understand this image in all its intensity not just through a universal language of posture and gesture (Barasch 1976) but most basically through our own ability to embody the feeling by imagining or adopting a similar stance.

The value of pain as message, as an imperative to withdraw and immobilize the self and also as a social call for care, is strained and tested in the situation of chronic pain. Chronic pain weighs heavily on us and lays us low. We shrink from it, recoil, and may be cowed and beaten down. But this stance is also constitutive of our pain experience.

I think of a patient injured in a motorcycle accident that left him partially paralyzed and in the grip of chronic leg, back, and arm pain. His pain waxes and wanes with his mood, and he expresses it not only in words but in the way he carries himself. He eases himself gingerly into a chair, anticipating a spasm of pain. Finding no comfortable position in the chair, he asks if he can lie on the floor. There he curls up in a fetal position; his voice becomes thin, his words childlike. Through his posture, he has "regressed," taken the stance of a frightened child, retreating to the meager comfort and safety of the sickbed. In his gestures, we see the movement from an adult stance of upright self-assertion to a childlike stance signaling submission and vulnerability and with it a call for succor.

Though pain forces a stance on us, we retain some freedom in how we respond. In turn, the stance we take toward pain conditions our experience. For example, clinical work with pain patients suggests that fighting pain (tensing and pushing it away, pulling back from or recoiling) may make it worse, whereas accepting it and simply "watching it" may allow it to diffuse and subside (Kabat-Zinn, Lipworth, and Burney 1985). Our stance toward pain is both a specific disposition to act or react in and through the body and an act of positioning in a social world, with communicative value. Standing up to pain tells others we are still in control and intend to vanquish it. Throughout, pain is felt as an adversary external to the self whom we can oppose and defeat, even as it undermines the very solidity and autonomy of that self (Jackson 1999).

The stance we take toward pain reaches down the hierarchy to regulate attention and physiology and up the hierarchy to condition our understanding of and participation in the social world. Hence, the effects of stance on pain influence both our basic bodily experience and our position in the social world.

This vertical dimension of stance that conveys our attitude toward experience is extended to the moral domain: "The 'moral,' rational self is high, while the 'lower' self is associated with the body and bodily functions. This up/down, high/low orientation comes to be correlated with purity versus impurity. The body, with its passions and desires, ties us to that which is dirty, polluted, and impure. The mind, as the seat of reason and will, tries to maintain its purity by rising above and trying to control the body" (Johnson 1993, 51). Much of our vocabulary for moral strength references bodily stance or position: we carry ourselves high with dignity, righteousness, or shrink down in self-abnegation. We speak of core values, close to our position, and peripheral issues where we may readily yield to the views of others. Balance metaphors are used to express the search for harmony and a middle way amid conflicting values. Indeed, the very basis of moral action resides in our ability to take a stance. Moral authority is embodied as the stance one takes toward the world: taking hold of it or shrinking back, being morally upright or skulking and devious.

The basic meanings of stance, which contribute to the experience of pain and the logic of morality, also play a vital role in religious iconography, ritual, and practice. What is godly, spiritual, and transcendent is located upward beyond our gaze, while the fallen world lies at or beneath our feet. When spiritual traditions elaborate a cosmology, they often use the body as a map and divide or subdivide along the vertical axis to indicate levels of transcendence of the mundane or earthly world associated with the lower half of the body. The human body with its limbs extended represents the totality of the world in its order and symmetry. The body bowed or bent down is in a stressed and imperfect state, waiting to be relieved or released. The crucifixion is portrayed in a way that emphasizes the vertical arrangement of Christ. He may sag on the cross, indicating his mortal aspect, while the high placement of the crucifix in churches emphasizes Christ's spiritual ascendancy. The viewer feels both the downward pull of the body in pain and the upward yearning of the spirit for transcendence. Both suffering and its spiritual meaning are graphically displayed.

In many traditions, practitioners bow or prostrate themselves to acknowledge and experience the transcendental power of the divine. While the basic meaning is given in the body's disposition, more complex meanings of prostration come from the religious context of practice, which prescribes specific thoughts and interpretations to the practice. In Tibetan Buddhism, for example, practitioners may commit themselves to perform hundreds of thousands of prostrations as a meditative practice:

> The one hundred thousand prostrations are powerful exercises in humility, security, and—done with a spirit of enlightenment in mind—determination. A creative humility emerges by imprinting the awareness of the dangers of unenlightened living and acknowledging that alone you cannot protect yourself from them. A secure comfort emerges by strengthening the connection to the

> Three Jewels [Buddha, Sangha, and Dharma], considering that they embody freedom from danger, concern for you, and power to protect you from all dangers. (Thurman 1995, 40)

Clearly, the meaning of prostration depends crucially on what the practitioner thinks about it and on how others interpret his actions. These cultural meanings imbue the act with significance and shape the work that it does both in the social world (as a profound statement of devotion) and in the inner realm as a mode of training the self.

All of these correspondences suggest ways in which basic bodily postures or stance build up a vocabulary for moral action and experience as well as spiritual transcendence. These moral and religious languages, in turn, govern our bodily actions and disposition. As a result, our location in space is given added dimensions that reflect our emotional experience, moral position, and social standing. This points toward an understanding of space and place as configured by moral value—a mapping prefigured in the *Sefer Yetzirah* ("Book of Creation," an early Kabbalistic text), which states that there are ten directions to the cosmos: six spatial (up/down, east/west, north/south), two temporal (beginning and end), and the evaluative poles of good and evil. In this cosmology, moral evaluation is a basic dimension that locates experience. There is no compass other than a moral compass.

Facing Pain

> The nakedness of the face is not a figure of speech.
> (Lévinas 1998, 10)

While stance or posture reflects basic dimensions of the response and social meaning of pain, more subtle communication of suffering and experience is conveyed through a wide range of facial expressions, which include blendings (and sequences) of basic emotions. Facial expression can go beyond the basic valences of approach and avoidance expressed through posture to convey nuances of feeling, multiple overlaid feelings, and rapidly changing dynamics.[7]

The face is the most powerful medium for the expression and communication of emotion including pain and fear, as well as pleasure and ecstasy. The expression and communication of emotion are at the center of facial function and experience. As well, the distinctive qualities of the face—and the voice, which emerges from and is synchronized with the movement of the face—are the way we recognize others as themselves (Cole 1999). Face is thus a basic vehicle for organizing interpersonal relationships and, by extension, the social world.

The face is both a transmitter and a receiver of emotion: a transmitter, because it displays our own suffering and broadcasts it to others—not only for them to look at and read but, more palpably, as something that evokes emotions, so that our own expressions are mirrored in their faces. The face is also a receiver of emotion because our own perception of facial expression evokes physiological changes and corresponding emotional states in ourselves (Levenson, Ekman, and Friesen 1990; Zajonc 1985). Our reading and response to the face of others is usually rapid and can occur without conscious awareness. Even brief presentations of another's face showing emotions of happiness or sadness can evoke similar feelings in a viewer. Stronger facial expressions evoke stronger and longer-lasting vicarious emotion (Wild, Erb, and Bartels 2001).

It comes as no surprise, then, to learn that the human brain has specialized systems or modules concerned with recognizing faces and decoding facial expression (Damasio, Tranel, and Damasio 1990). Face perception involves several regions of cortex including an area in the fusiform gyrus that is selectively responsive to faces (Kanwisher, McDermott, and Chun 1997). While the recognition of faces involves modules in the fusiform gyrus, the identification of the familiarity of a person (based on his or her face or voice) involves activity in the posterior cingulate and retrosplenial cortex (Shah et al. 2001). The amygdala, which is involved in fear conditioning, receives inputs from the cortical areas involved in recognition of faces and facial expressions. These connections allow a rapid response to facial expressions; brief presentations of fearful faces may activate the amygdala even in the absence of awareness of the stimulus. Very likely this provides part of the basis for the common phenomenon of emotional contagion in which feelings spread from one person to another simply by exposure to his or her face (Hatfield, Cacioppo, and Rapson 1994).[8]

Infants engage in imitation of the faces of adults looking at them (Meltzoff and Moore 1977). Over the course of early development this imitation and mirroring serve to establish a repertoire of expressions that have social meaning and provide a foundation for knowing the feelings of others and abstracting from that to develop a theory of mind (Gopnik 1993). Following the gaze of others establishes the focus of their attention (as distinct from our own) (Baron-Cohen 1995), and watching (and automatically mirroring) their facial expressions gives us a sense of what they think and feel about what they are watching. A particularly powerful element of this interaction occurs when the gaze of the other is directed toward the self. We then see ourselves mirrored (and evaluated) in the face of the other and come to know ourselves as social beings. This processes of self-definition is reciprocal, occurring in ongoing loops during early development and, indeed, throughout our lives. As a result, "[a] face is not only an expression of a self available for others to read, but to some extent the self is constituted in the face and developed, and experienced, in the interaction between faces" (Cole 1999, 316). Through reading the faces of others, we learn the emotional meaning of social events, including our own actions. The face of the other is the stage on which we watch the play of emotions that gives flesh to abstract notions of personhood implicit in the moral order.

Even our experience of our own body is also mediated by our exchanges with the faces of others. One thinks of the child who injures herself and then looks for the parent to judge how she should respond. If the parent looks anxious or distressed, the child begins to cry. Contrariwise, a parent's indifference may convey an implicit instruction for the child to suppress, deny, or dissociate awareness of her pain. The child comes to know her own bodily and emotional vulnerability (and the desired response) through the parent's face. Though we can learn to use the face to dissimulate, we must first learn the code by accurate mirroring of others; and by their reporting back to us what our face reveals, we learn to be self-consistent or to acknowledge our own inner contradictions and akrasias.

Facial expression is a prime measure of another's pain and suffering. If facial expressions are masked or faked, we have difficulty discriminating real suffering from play-acting. Indeed, when people are asked to pretend they are in pain (or those in pain are asked to pretend they are not), trained clinicians cannot accurately identify those who are in pain and those who are merely play-acting (Poole and Craig 1992).[9]

The face reveals our feelings and responses to others; it is thus the primordial site of our own social presence and identity. And others are most present and compelling for us in their facial expressions, which communicate both their individuality and the immediacy of their unique experiences. This primacy and directness of the face led philosopher Emmanuel Lévinas to give it a privileged moral status: "that bit of absolutely decent skin that is the face" (1998, 32). Lévinas views responsibility for the other as "the essential, primary and fundamental structure of subjectivity" (1985, 95). For this reason, "access to the face is straightaway ethical" (Lévinas 1985, 85). The face is always the face of someone. Hence, it is morally and socially situated. What Lévinas refers to as "the epiphany of the face of the other" provides the origin and ground of ethical concern.[10]

The big ethical question is why we fail to allow ourselves to experience the pain of others—why we turn away and ignore their faces. In large part, this may be due to our inability to tolerate vicarious pain and accept our own powerlessness to alleviate the suffering of others. These are the most obvious explanations for the unsettling finding that health professionals tend to minimize and deny the pain of patients. For example, an ethnographic study on an orthopedic surgery ward for children found that nurses tended to dismiss patients' pain by viewing their complaints as evidence of childish dependency, histrionics, and self-indulgence (Byrne, Morton, and Salmon 2001). Children were enjoined to suppress and deny their pain to be "good patients" and, when they did not respond to such expectations, were sometimes threatened with reprisals. Parents who attempted to convey their child's distress to nurses saw these strategies for discounting, dismissal, and denial directed toward them as well. Throughout, children's unique experiences were subordinated to a generic model of stages of recovery, so that when their experiences did not accord with the nurses' expectations, children could be told: "you can't be feeling that"—their most fundamental experiences effaced by medical routine.

The face is the first site of empathy: the ability to feel something akin to what another feels. Importantly, empathy is strongest for others' negative emotional states or aversive feelings, especially pain, fear, and sadness (Royzman and Kumar 2001). And the failure to empathize with someone in pain is generally recognized as a moral failing. Feeling for others as suffering beings makes possible moral action. But empathy goes beyond sympathetic pain to imaginatively reconstruct the other's world of experience, a process that involves not only apprehending his or her point of view, or way of facing the world, but also his/her position in it.

Empathy can be decomposed into several distinct components: (1) vicarious emotion (e.g., feeling grief because another has facial expressions that evoke that response in oneself either directly or through unintentional mirroring of the other's facial expression); (2) analogical associations to the other's experience (e.g., thinking of one's own losses to evoke a grief that parallels the other's emotion); (3) imaginative reconstruction of the position of another by imagery or story (e.g., imagining in detail what it would be like to lose a parent); and (4) placing oneself in an analogous position to the other (e.g., acting as if one's mother died when one was young). These basic bodily and cognitive-emotional actions are not static responses but must be sustained over time. Thus, empathy further requires (5) regulation of one's own idiosyncratic associations to stay on track with those most pertinent to mirroring the other (e.g., truncating or discarding divergent trains of associations) and especially (6) tolerating negative affect and discomfort and regulating its intensity to continue to track the other person. Excess of "empathy" leads to distancing from feelings that are too intense or appropriating another's experience and, ultimately, occluding it with one's own thoughts and feelings.

We feel empathy only for those we identify as enough like ourselves to evoke such feelings. This recognition of similarity and difference depends on divisions within and between social groups. More fundamentally, it reflects cultural concepts of personhood. The cultural concept of the person conditions who we see as like ourselves—and hence an object of empathy—and who we view as radically other or even inhuman. The naked visage of the other in pain may be unbearable to look on for those unwilling to enter and dwell within the other's world.

The Texture of Time

> Time is a fluid medium for the culture of metaphors.
> (Nabokov 1969)

Pain systems most likely evolved as a mechanism to detect and remember danger (Woolf and Salter 2000). Thus pain organizes both the immediate- and intermediate-term response to injury. The immediate effect is withdrawal followed by immobilization and eventually avoidance. Through the organization of memory and learning, pain forges links between the immediate noxiousness of an event and the longer-term organization of behavioral repertoires—including the complex patterns of self-description and interaction we call personal identity. Pain also contributes to the organization of the social world according to its past history of injury and insults and its potential for future suffering.

Each of these levels of organization is associated with a different temporal span that is reflected in experience. Initially, pain slows us down, insisting that we withdraw from the fray and take time to heal. In the period of recovery, pain maintains immobility needed for tissue repair. Throughout, pain binds time to strong affect, ensuring that we remember what has caused us grief.

At the same time, narrative constructions of temporal experience may modulate these neurophysiological processes. Narration allows us to think of the passage of time differently and so to modify our actual experience of duration. The way we narrate experience may cause certain moments of suffering to endure, whereas others are quickly passed through. This occurs not only through direct reflections on time and temporality but through the way we locate consciousness and deploy our attention through narration (Chafe 1994).

There is a constant circulation between the narrative fashioning of the self, as a social act or interaction, and the experience of interiority. This circulation occurs on many different timescales: on the developmental scale of a lifetime, in the emotional ebb and flow of significant life events, and in the fine-grained structure of a moment of conscious experience. These different timescales each contribute to the texture of experience. The analysis of metaphor can help us to understand how the social enters into and mediates the immediate.

When pain persists, it becomes a problem in its own right as it preempts every aspect of bodily and emotional life, intruding on relationships, narrowing consciousness, and upending our usual hierarchy of values and activities. When pain is planted in memory, it may highlight a whole area or cordon one off. Hence, pain exerts enduring effects even when not present, as something to fear, avoid, and warily anticipate. In relationships, pain may become part of an interactional language that subverts everyday activities and gives central importance to whatever speech or feeling it underscores with its presence.

The suffering of pain is closely related to the apprehension, belief, or conviction that it will persist indefinitely—an experience of duration that is partly given by pain itself (intrinsic to its phenomenology, in the sense that pain makes our experience of time slow down and duration become static or unending) and partly imposed through ongoing interpretations or framing of its meaning. The suffering qualities of pain are directly related to the ability of memory to confer meaning on it.

Our experience of duration is constructed both within the moment and after the fact and so is dependent on memory. Pain and memory are linked in multiple ways: pain cements memory, pain evokes memory, and memory in turn can reevoke pain. The temporal qualities of pain that lead to suffering thus depend on many of the same social processes that govern remembering and forgetting (Kirmayer 1996). We tend to forget pains that had good outcomes and nurse pains that mark some moral violation or unaccepted loss. We may dwell in and prolong pains that allow us to hold on to a valued past. The social processes that underlie memory may work to keep pain alive because it serves collective identity.

This is illustrated by the experience of a man seeking refugee status who suffered from severe low back pain that had begun sometime after his migration to Canada. He spoke of his back pain as a direct result of the torture he had endured. In so doing, he assigned a meaning to the pain that made it a body memory. In truth, he may have had back pain for the same (usually obscure) reasons as many other people without any history of trauma. There was no evidence of lasting injury to his back on physical examination or X-ray. Still, by viewing his back pain this way, he explained it, gave evidence of how severely he had suffered and, in his own mind and to others, justified all of the losses he had endured in coming to Canada, as well as his claim for refugee status. This work of explanation created some closure for him but, perhaps, at the cost of a vicious cycle that aggravated his pain: every twinge of his back would lead his thoughts back to his torture and incarceration, and this would intensify his pain and suffering. He was caught in an endless loop in which the future never arrived.

Memory is not a static repository of knowledge and experience but an active arena of reconstruction, remembering, embodying, and extending experience as it unfolds (Kirmayer 1996). Culture works on and through memory at every step of this process: at the moment of registration by framing experiences as memorable and assigning them specific meanings; in an ongoing way through creating occasions for recollection, retelling, or reenactment; and over the long term, by stabilizing memories through social practices and ritual commemorations or rewriting history to elide or fragment narratives that do not serve dominant interests. To appreciate how ritual can transform painful memory, therefore, we must understand memory not only as representation in an individual but as collective representation, and not only as representation but as individual and collective enactment.

Our sense of duration also is tied to the ways in which we deploy our attention. In states of deep absorption or reverie, we may be unaware of the passage of time (Benson 1993, 2001). Attention in turn may be regulated by social actions and by explicit efforts to train the mind as in meditative practice.

I recall my own brief experience with Vipassana meditation (see Goldstein 1976). As I sat immobile for an hour, my knees began to ache terribly. I had vivid images of jumping up and running from the meditation hall in disgrace. Time seemed to be passing interminably slowly, and I did not think I could stand another second. I had been instructed to keep coming back to simply watching my experience without judging. When my attention was drawn to the pain, I repeated to myself, "Pain, pain, pain . . ." as the meditation teacher had suggested. Suddenly, my experience was radically transformed. The pain in my knees was still there—I could have described its sensory qualities in great detail—but instead of crowding in on me, it fell back to become just a phenomenon I was watching. Sensation was separated from emotional response. A metaphorical space opened up between the observing "I" and the sensory object of pain. And with this space came a sense of distance or detachment from the pain so that it lost its "in your face" urgency, unbearable intensity, and harrying quality. There was no rush to move, no concern that pain would go on building in intensity forever. In its place was a sense of timelessness and spaciousness.

This is not unlike the experience reported by many patients in hypnosis and even the effect of opiate analgesics like morphine. With hypnotic suggestion, it is possible to experience elements of the same experiences achieved through meditation. The clinical use of hypnosis for pain control, for example, allows people to experience themselves as separate from their pain, just watching it. Hypnosis can modify the subjective experience of the passage of time and so prolong a pleasurable state of relaxation or allow us to remember a pain as fleeting and less consequential (Bowers 1979).

The fundamental difference between hypnotic pain control and meditation is the meaning drawn from the experience. Hypnosis exists as a technology devoid of larger moral meaning, and the experiences it offers simply fit within a system of values centered on self-direction and self-control through psychological development. In Buddhist meditation, the lesson on the illusory nature of the self is the important consequence, not the pain control (Collins 1990). These meanings are not simply intrinsic to the experience of meditation but derive from the larger context in which the practice occurs, which shapes both bodily experience and the way that it is interpreted.

Religious experience attempts to help us transcend suffering or give it transcendental meaning. This is achieved through specific practices (prayer, mediation, ritual acts of asceticism, purification, and devotion) oriented toward a transcendental realm of the eternal presented in religious canons, myths, and texts. There is a parallel between the timeless present of myth and the unending time of pain. Hence pain immediately presents itself as a moral-religious problem, not only because its urgency preempts all our other agendas but also because its very quality closely parallels the timeless and eternal presence sought after in "mystical" experience.

The Effectiveness of Ritual

How, then, can we understand the effectiveness of ritual to alleviate (or intensify) suffering and transform its meaning and experience? What are the mediators between the elaborate rituals, trance performances, and other religious practices described in many cultures and alterations in experience that we presume have a neurological substrate?

There are changes in neurophysiological functioning at many levels that may subserve the ritual control of pain. For example, placebo responses (the expectation that one is receiving a potent analgesic) activate endogenous pain-control systems that use endorphins (Levine, Gordon, and Fields 1978; Price and Barrell 2000). Anything that creates expectations for analgesia will have this effect, including both the simple fact of performing the ritual and any of its specific elements or sensory details.[11] But rituals may have effects on pain at many other levels: (1) modifying attention (through distraction or focused attention and absorption); (2) modifying emotion (feeling exaltation or other positive emotions—even, in the case of some famous saints, something approaching erotic transport); (3) modifying expectations (it makes a big difference for pain endurance whether one thinks it is for a good purpose with a desired or positive outcome—compare the expectations associated with pain of childbirth to cancer pain); and (4) modifying the memory of pain, so that whatever qualities it had in the moment of experience are supplanted by later retellings.

Transformations in the experience of pain and suffering may occur at many levels: in social interaction, in cognitive processes, and at many levels or systems within the nervous system (peripheral or central, brain stem, limbic or cortical, and so on). Many transformations take place, sometimes in concert, sometimes in countervailing directions. Any overarching account privileges some few levels and makes them work as metaphors for other levels that may well have quite different dynamics.

Studies of the transformative effects of ritual have focused on the structural organization by which ritual maps the worldly predicament of the sufferer onto a mythic realm (Dow 1986). Metaphoric movements or transformations within the mythic realm are assumed to cause corresponding changes in the sufferer's representation of body and self (Kirmayer 1993). To the extent that these representations, in turn, alter bodily functioning and experience, metaphorical redescriptions can lead to physical and psychological change. At the same time, metaphorical redescriptions shape how others view the sufferer and hence shift the sufferer's social position. The metaphorical actions of ritual thus have the force of performative utterances (Sweetser 2000).

Although, at a basic level, the metaphor of ritual transforms the sensory and affective qualities of experience, in a more extended sense the metaphoric process creates parallel worlds (of imagination or possibility) that can be inhabited as alternatives to the immediacy of pain. These worlds are solipsistic and fragile unless they can move into the social sphere and be stabilized by the active participation of others. This is one purpose of ritual: to externalize and materialize symbolic action so that it engages others and becomes a shared social fact and, ultimately, part of a way of life.

The ritual use of trance and dissociation—of which the contemporary clinical use of hypnosis is but one culture-specific instance—relies on the fact that we have the ability to control our own mechanisms of attention, both directly and indirectly. Trance, hypnosis, and dissociation reflect the coordinated use of the universal human skills or capacities (1) to become deeply absorbed or concentrate attention; (2) to engage in imagery or other internally generated imaginal activity; and (3) to respond to suggestions (ideas, possibilities)[12] from self or other (Kirmayer 1994).[13] These skills can be used to direct attention away from pain, to modify its perception, interpretation, evaluation, and subsequent cognitive and emotional coping responses. This can happen through internal self-directed means or through interaction with external stimuli, the most potent of which are social. In addition to lower-level expectation effects and competition for attention, there are higher-level cognitive faculties that modify our experience of events; these are governed by cultural schemas, narratives, and patterns of social interaction or discourse.

Although hypnosis and trance are often portrayed as involving radical transformations of consciousness with the assumption that there must be some correspondingly profound change in the structure of brain processes, trance and hypnosis are better understood as complex cognitive performances in which expectations, images, and self-direction are used to regulate attention, affect, and the interpretation of experience (Kirmayer 1992b). Culturally prescribed templates for experience combine with ongoing actions of others to reinforce experience. Thus the ritual use of trance and dissociation reveals the social regulation of subjective experience (Kirmayer 1994). Trance serves to change the stance toward the body, both in the moment through the deployment of attention and over longer periods of time (and retrospectively) through attributions of agency in narratives of the self.[14]

This same paradigm can be applied to understand the impact of music on experience. Music and other activities that encourage absorption and that provide a specific rhythm and tempo may also alter temporal experience in ways that transform the urgency and suffering of pain. Music may be arousing or sedating because of its rhythm and intensity, activating central cross-modal mechanisms of orientation and arousal. Engagement in listening to music, like other forms of aesthetic absorption, may not arouse self-awareness with its freight of self-description, discursiveness, self-criticism, and rejection of suggestions for transformation. At the same time, the rhythmic, melodic, and harmonic contours of music convey specific emotions, and the larger temporal organization of music functions as a form of narrative. Musical performances, of course, are embedded in social contexts that confer additional meaning and provide tools for interpreting and responding in culturally prescribed ways (Rouget 1985).

In the actual performance of a ritual, fluctuations in attention and absorption and expectation occur all of the time but are usually not framed as such or consciously recognized, because the microdynamics of experience are replaced by an idealized portrait of experience that conforms to larger cultural templates. In our narratives, then, we recount not the momentary fluctuations of attention but the socially prescribed activities in which we were engaged: watching television on a movie, jogging, reading a book, praying, performing devotions. Closer examination, however, reveals complex shifts in attention and imagination that involve different modes of information processing, with consequent shifts in our experience of self and other.

Hypnosis and other ritual practices frame these fluctuations and make us notice how we are using our own faculties; they also allow people to arrange circumstances to try to maximize performance using explicit suggestions or implicit cues (e.g., control of distraction through use of music, amplifying social support and group solidarity). In many ritual contexts this may not be done self-consciously, but there are overarching narratives and representations of the self that allow for people to be "other" and somewhere else; these provide both permission for dissociation and an implicit model of otherness or "awayness" that is reinforced by specific body practices and modes of interpersonal interaction (Kirmayer and Santhanam 2001).

Western folk psychology does not fully acknowledge these capacities or their power and pervasiveness in everyday life; hence, they appear to us as remarkable, entertaining, magical, or at times, frightening. Certain forms of imaginative involvement and concentrated attention are acceptable to us, for example, aesthetic absorption or heroism in sports or on the battlefield; but religious ecstasy is viewed with ambivalence by those outside such religious systems and contrasted with secular rationality, skepticism, and "tough-mindedness." It is, especially, the image of loss of control or of falling under the influence of others (whether these be gods or mortals) that is disturbing to our own temporary Western notions of autonomy, independence, and self-direction, and these all appear to be contravened in the hypnotic context. We tend to value external vigilance, consensual reality, and a seamless account of our experience and behavior that emphasizes its monological, rational self-direction.

Conclusion

> Alterity's plot is born before knowledge. (Lévinas 1999, 101)

I have tried to show the importance of three sites of metaphoric mediation for our experience of pain and suffering: bodily stance, facial expression, and temporal duration. Each domain of experience is a rich source of metaphors grounded in physiology and specific cultural forms of life. And I have argued that these are not only sites of access to other's experience but the vehicles through which our own experiences of pain and suffering are constructed, articulated, and sustained.

The body's stance expresses our basic approach to the world: moving upward and outward in embrace, or recoiling and withdrawing in pain and fear. This stance constitutes our response to pain. Pain may tear us down and destroy a moral stance or, when less intense, make it possible, as we stand up against oppression.

We recognize others as individuals through their faces (and voices), just as we recognize the moment-to-moment shifts in what they are feeling. The face is thus both the signature of our unique social identity and the sign of our inner disposition and experience. This conflation of personal identity (enduring presence) and moment-to-moment affective response ensures that we understand emotions as always situated in an individual's identity and life history and that we understand personality through the range and rhythm of emotional responsiveness. The face in pain, therefore, is an invitation to engage the suffering of others as a ground for moral life.

The experience of temporal duration makes pain transient and tolerable or never ending and unbearable. Our sense of duration is elastic and shaped by the ways we focus attention and narrate our experience to create a temporal landscape. Meditative practices can clear a space for the experience of the timelessness, even as the global economy encourages us to rush headlong into the future.

Pain willingly endured has a completely different meaning than pain cruelly or arbitrarily inflicted. Indeed, one of its basic meanings is to affirm the very fact of the human capacity to choose to transform our own experience. Thus in the ritual act of self-inflicted pain we have a conjunction between our most basic experience of the body (as a source of inescapable pain) and our most human quality: the self-directed, linguistically shaped fluidity of consciousness and self-awareness.

Culture transforms pain from a signal of injury aimed at promoting withdrawal and avoidance to a prime organizer of memory and identity. Thus, pain and suffering serve powerful symbolic functions themselves, transforming identities, social statuses, and the meaning and value of experience. And as the contributors to this volume make clear, it is not only that culture can transform pain; pain itself serves to transform our cultural worlds.

Our tendency to focus on the elimination or endurance of pain itself may lead us to ignore its broader context and meaning. Although the observer may assume that the transformation of pain and suffering is the goal of practices, often pain and suffering serve as arenas for the working out of larger moral truths. As the chapters in this book show, in many religious contexts it is neither necessary nor desirable to eliminate all pain. Instead, pain may be sought out or ritually inflicted because it serves positive functions: as dramatic testimony to one's devotion, trial, and sacrifice; as training of the self; as evidence of mastery and power; as a marker of transformation of identity; and as a contributor to transformations of consciousness. Beyond its meaning for the individual, pain may work as part of a larger cosmology, moral system, or regulation of the social world—for example, as punishment, penance, or something desired by others and simply endured by the supplicant. From this larger perspective the actual experience of the afflicted individual may even be irrelevant—occluded or eclipsed by its prescribed social meaning.

While we may find it difficult to understand how or why others endure great pain and privation, we can all imagine situations where our own commitments would make such endurance essential and where we would marshal every personal and social resource at our disposal to perform successfully. The problem raised by our sense of the exotic, then, is not one of unique neurological mechanisms or psychological strategies, nor even of spiritual transcendence—but of our own ability to credit, reconstruct, and enter into the cultural world or value systems of another.

Finally, we need to look beyond the immediate moment of dramatic performance to see the dynamics of coping over time and its implications for the person and those around them; in some cases, a dramatic performance is followed by later evidence of suffering, trauma, and other costs for the individual, who may, nevertheless, feel compelled to deny any negative impact because of the larger values and commitments his or her performance represents. Alternatively, the negative outcomes themselves may have positive value as evidence of commitment, devotion, endurance, and the magnitude and seriousness of sacrifice.

We are led to this disturbing conclusion: pain is good to think with. We cannot think and act morally without an intimate understanding of others' pain—and that understanding depends crucially on our own experience with pain. Our inability or unwillingness to enter into the pain of others means that we are free to treat them as objects. Frameworks or forms of life that allow us to encounter and endure the pain of others, without eliding its specificity, open the way to compassionate action.

Notes

1. This use of cross-domain metaphors is basic to all creativity including scientific problem solving (Dunbar 1995) and is common in everyday reasoning as well as in more systematic scholarly argument. As knowledge develops, scientific explanation shifts to using analogies drawn from within the same domain that allow practical problem solving and technical control.
2. The body may enter our conceptual system in other ways than strict metonymy. The body is composed of multiple sensory and action systems that provide modes of transformation of action and perception that are the most basic forms of metaphorical thought. Using these sensorimotor systems to transform our own experience (either through changing the configuration of the environment or through transforming representational structures in the brain) then provides a basis for more elaborate conceptual thought. As well, the body presents multiple experiences (e.g., along different sensory modalities), which have a natural coordination due both to the body's own structure and to the ecological environment. The coordination of bodily experiences may lead to multiple metonyms (each of which can be extended metaphorically), which are mutually coordinated because of the inherent structure of bodily experience. This coordinated structure is reflected in the emergence of more elaborate schemas and modes of thought that link basic bodily actions with larger affective and social meanings (Kirmayer 1992a).
3. Here is how Tooby and Cosmides (1992, xiv) describe modules: "Our cognitive machinery resembles a confederation of hundreds or thousands of informationally dedicated computers (often called modules) designed to solve adaptive problems endemic to our hunter-gatherer ancestors. Each of these devices has its own agenda and imposes its own exotic organization on different fragments of the world. There are specialized systems for grammar induction, for face recognition, for dead reckoning, for construing objects and for recognizing emotions from the face. There are mechanisms to detect animacy, eye direction, and cheating. There is a 'theory of mind' module . . . a variety of social inference-modules . . . and a multitude of other elegant machines."
4. While there is a hope that modules can be mapped neatly onto specific brain structures identified in experimental studies with functional brain-imaging techniques, this is not essential for the viability of the overall theory, since modules could turn out to involve widely distributed circuits in the brain with no simple anatomical localization.

5. Competition between pain/avoidance systems and novelty/approach systems can help account for why many individuals seek out and subject themselves to painful conditions.
6. An experiment by Gibbs and colleagues (1994) provides evidence that awareness of the body conditions our metaphoric language and shows how the wide range of meanings of the word "stand" share common ground in image schemas based on bodily experiences. In Gibbs's experiment, subjects were asked to move (stand up, move around, bend over, crunch, and stretch out on their tiptoes) to become more aware of their bodies and, presumably, of body-related schemas. They were then asked to relate the various different metaphorical uses of "stand" to specific body schemas. The results showed that the most relevant schemas for the diverse metaphorical uses of "stand" were based on notions of *balance,* followed by *verticality, center-periphery, resistance,* and *linkage.* These different metaphorical meanings can work together. For example, *center-periphery,* which reflects an approach/avoidance gradient organized with the location of the body as the center, works together with *verticality* to contribute to the meaning of *stance* as establishing—erecting, situating, and defending—a point of view.
7. Of course, the body can be used in a more differentiated fashion to communicate endless nuance (and metacommentary) through gesture, dance, or sign language. And all that we shall say of the face could apply equally to the voice.
8. When the source of anxiety is misattributed, this process of emotion contagion may give rise to epidemics of bodily distress and disability (Bartholomew and Sirois 2000).
9. The logic of facial expression is revealed in the play of the mask. The mask is an antiface: it cloaks and clothes the face to provide a stylized expression that changes little (except with changing light and shadow or accompanying gestures) across situations, thus freezing the temporal dynamics of feeling. (The fixed mask is also a death mask, a dead face—a primal source of fear for primates; cf. Hebb 1946.) This accentuates the meaning of a single facial expression by rendering it as something divorced from ongoing interaction. The mask hides the true face behind a static caricature, which may be shocking or amusing in its very stasis or exaggeration and distortion. The mask codifies and re-presents feeling at one remove from individual experience; it replaces individuality with collectivity, idiosyncrasy with cultural convention, and so serves to make emotional responses more abstract and formulaic. Thus, the mask allows us aesthetic distance so that we can modulate the intensity of our emotions in response to the other (Scheff 1979). So it is that the surgeon's mask or the blank face of the clinician maintaining therapeutic "neutrality" protects them from the intensity of their own emotional response to the other. But the mask adds its own freight of strangeness and alienation.

10. This underwrites the widespread moral language of honor and duty to others that is couched in metaphors of the maintenance or loss of face. To save face is to maintain social standing, moral presence, and social capital; to lose face is to endure the pain of shame, dishonor, and social marginalization.
11. Of course, this applies equally well to taking an active analgesic agent. In clinical and experimental settings the response to analgesics is highly variable. Much of the variability of individual response to analgesics can be accounted for by differences in the activation of the endorphin system (Amanzio et al. 2001). Maximizing positive expectations is an important element of effective analgesic treatment (Pollo et al. 2001).
12. Studies of potential neurophysiological correlates of hypnosis suggest relatively high-level effects involving more specific activation of regions associated with focused attention (De Pascalis 1999). The pattern of activation depends on the particular task the subject is performing. Individuals who are highly hypnotizable may show differences in patterns of activation outside the hypnotic context, reflecting their greater ability to focus attention and become deeply absorbed. Participants in healing rituals that involve trance may tend to be more highly hypnotizable, and this could contribute to their success in achieving subjectively compelling experiences and enjoying therapeutic benefit (Biswas et al. 2000).
13. Although Judith Becker (in this volume, Chapter 8) associates trance with strong emotion, in fact there is no need for any specific emotion or level of intensity to elicit trance. Strong emotion may add something to trance behavior and experience, perhaps increasing the likelihood of dissociation and amnesia as a result of affective-state-dependent learning. However, complete amnesia is the exception rather than the rule in hypnotic trance and, like all other aspects of trance, depends on the subject's expectations.
14. Ritual activities may reinforce this shift in agency by arranging coordinating or synchronizing events inside and outside the body, blurring boundaries and creating a sense of extension or continuity between the self and the external world. An example is provided by Becker's account of the synchrony between the Balinese barong dancer and the gamelan musicians. We readily extend our sense of the body, even to incorporate inanimate prostheses, when temporal coordination suggests we have control (Ramachandran and Blakeslee 1998).

References

Amanzio, M., A. Pollo, G. Maggi, and F. Benedetti. 2001. "Response Variability to Analgesics: A Role for Non-Specific Activation of Endogenous Opioids." *Pain* 90: 205–215.

Barasch, M. 1976. *Gestures of Despair in Medieval and Early Renaissance Art.* New York: New York University Press.

Baron-Cohen, S. 1995. *Mindblindness: An Essay on Autism and Theory of Mind.* Cambridge, Mass.: MIT Press.

Bartholomew, R. E., and F. Sirois. 2000. "Occupational Mass Psychogenic Illness." *Transcultural Psychiatry* 37(1): 495–524.

Basbaum, A. I., and H. L. Fields. 1978. "Endogenous Pain Control Mechanisms: Review and Hypothesis." *Annals of Neurology* 4: 451–462.

Bateson, G. 1979. *Mind and Nature: A Necessary Unity.* New York: E. P. Dutton.

Ben-Dov, G., and A. Carmon. 1976. "On Time, Space and the Cerebral Hemispheres: A Theoretical View." *International Journal of Neuroscience* 7(1): 29–33.

Benson, C. 1993. *The Absorbed Self: Pragmatism, Psychology and Aaesthetic Experience.* New York: Harvester Wheatsheaf.

———. 2001. *The Cultural Psychology of Self: Place, Morality and Art in Human Worlds.* London: Routledge.

Biswas, A., D. See, M. M. Kogon, and D. Spiegel. 2000. "Hypnotizability and the Use of Traditional Dhami-Jhankri Healing in Nepal." *International Journal of Clinical and Experimental Hypnosis* 48(1): 6–21.

Blake, W. 1978 [1815]. *The Book of Urizen.* Boston: Shambhala.

Blood, A. J., and R. J. Zatorre. 2001. "Intensely Pleasurable Responses to Music Correlated with Activity in Brain Regions Implicated in Reward and Emotion." *Proceedings of the National Academy of Sciences USA* 98: 11818–11823.

Bowers, K. S. 1979. "Time Distortion and Hypnotic Ability: Underestimating the Duration of Hypnosis." *Journal of Abnormal Psychology* 88(4): 435–439.

Byrne, A., J. Morton, and P. Salmon. 2001. "Defending against Patients' Pain: A Qualitative Analysis of Nurses' Responses to Children's Postoperative Pain." *Journal of Psychosomatic Research* 50: 69–76.

Carroll, J., C. Schaffer, J. Spensley, and S. I. Abramowitz. 1980. "Family Experiences of Self-Mutilating Patients." *American Journal of Psychiatry* 137(7): 852–853.

Casey, K. L., and J. Lorenz. 2000. "The Determinants of Pain Revisited: Coordinates in Sensory Space." *Pain Research and Management* 5(3): 197–204.

Chafe, W. 1994. *Discourse, Consciousness and Time.* Chicago: University of Chicago Press.

Clark, A. 1997. *Being There: Putting Brain, Body, and World Together Again.* Cambridge, Mass.: MIT Press.

Cole, J. 1999. "On Being Faceless: Selfhood and Facial Embodiment." In S. Gallagher and J. Shear, eds., *Models of the Self.* Thorveton, U.K.: Imprint Academic, 301–318.

Collins, S. 1990. *Selfless Persons: Imagery and Thought in Theravada Buddhism*. Cambridge: Cambridge University Press.

Damasio, A. R., D. Tranel, and H. Damasio. 1990. "Face Agnosia and the Neural Substrates of Memory." *Annual Review of Neuroscience* 13: 89–110.

Delvecchio Good, M.-J., P. E. Brodwin, B. J. Good, and A. Kleinman, eds. 1992. *Pain as a Human Experience: An Anthropological Perspective*. Berkeley: University of California Press.

Dennett, D. 1995. *Darwin's Dangerous Idea: Evolution and the Meanings of Life*. New York: Simon and Schuster.

De Pascalis, V. 1999. "Psychophysiological Correlates of Hypnosis and Hypnotic Susceptibility." *International Journal of Clinical and Experimental Hypnosis* 47(2): 117–143.

Dow, J. 1986. *The Shaman's Touch: Otomí Indian Symbolic Healing*. Salt Lake City: University of Utah Press.

Dunbar, K. 1995. "How Scientists Really Reason: Scientific Reasoning in Real-World Laboratories." In R. J. Sternberg and J. Davidson, eds., *The Nature of Insight*. Cambridge, Mass.: MIT Press, 365–396.

Ekman, P., W. V. Friesen, and R. J. Davidson. 1990. "The Duchenne Smile—Emotional Expression and Brain Physiology." *Journal of Personality and Social Psychology* 58(2): 342–353.

Ervin, F. R., R. M. Palmour, B. P. Murphy, R. H. Prince, and R. C. Simons. 1988. "The Psychobiology of Trance: II. Physiological and Endocrine Correlates." *Transcultural Psychiatric Research Review* 25(4): 267–284.

Fanselow, M. S. 1986. "Conditioned Fear-Induced Opiate Analgesia: A Competing Motivational State Theory of Stress Analgesia." *Annals of the New York Academy of Sciences* 467: 40–54.

Favazza, A. R. 1989. "Normal and Deviant Self-Mutilation: An Essay-Review." *Transcultural Psychiatric Research Review* 26(2): 113–127.

Gibbs, R. W., Jr. 1994. *The Poetics of Mind: Figurative Thought, Language and Understanding*. Cambridge: Cambridge University Press.

———. 1999. "Taking Metaphor Out of Our Heads and Putting It into the Cultural World." In R. W. Gibbs, Jr., and G. J. Steen, eds., *Metaphor in Cognitive Linguistics*. Amsterdam: John Benjamins, 145–166.

Gibbs, R. W., Jr., D. Beitel, M. Harrington, and D. Sanders. 1994. "Taking a Stand on the Meanings of Stand: Bodily Experience as Motivation for Polysemy." *Journal of Semantics* 11: 231–251.

Goldstein, J. 1976. *The Experience of Insight: A Natural Unfolding*. Santa Cruz, CA: Unity Press.

Gopnik, A. 1993. "How We Know Our Minds: The Illusion of First-Person Knowledge." *Behavioral and Brain Sciences* 16(1): 1–14.

Hatfield, E., J. T. Cacioppo, and R. L. Rapson. 1994. *Emotional Contagion*. Cambridge: Cambridge University Press.

Hebb, D. O. 1946. "On the Nature of Fear." *Psychological Review* 53: 259–276.

Henningsen, P., and L. J. Kirmayer. 2000. "Mind beyond the Net: Implications of Cognitive Neuroscience for Cultural Psychiatry." *Transcultural Psychiatry* 37(4): 467–494.

Hilgard, E., and J. Hilgard. 1975. *Hypnosis in the Relief of Pain.* Hillsdale, N.J.: Erlbaum.

Hoffman, M. L. 1978. "Toward a Theory of Empathic Arousal and Development." In M. Lewis and L. Rosenblum, eds., *The Development of Affect.* New York: Plenum Press, 227–256.

Holroyd, J. 1996. "Hypnosis Treatment of Clinical Pain: Understanding Why Hypnosis Is Useful." *International Journal of Clinical and Experimental Hypnosis* 44(1): 33–51.

Jackson, J. 1999. *Camp Pain: Talking with Chronic Pain Patients.* Philadelphia: University of Pennsylvania Press.

Johnson, M. 1987. *The Body in the Mind: The Bodily Basis of Meaning, Imagination, and Reason.* Chicago: University of Chicago Press.

———. 1993. *Moral Imagination: Implications of Cognitive Science for Ethics.* Chicago: University of Chicago Press.

Kabat-Zinn, J., L. Lipworth, and R. Burney. 1985. "The Clinical Use of Mindfulness Meditation for the Self-Regulation of Chronic Pain." *Journal of Behavioral Medicine* 8(2): 163–190.

Kanwisher, N., J. McDermott, and M. M. Chun. 1997. "The Fusiform Face Area: A Module in Human Extrastriate Cortex Specialized for Face Perception." *Journal of Neuroscience* 17: 4302–4311.

Kirmayer, L. J. 1992a. "The Body's Insistence on Meaning: Metaphor as Presentation and Representation in Illness Experience." *Medical Anthropology Quarterly* 6(4): 323–346.

———. 1992b. "Social Constructions of Hypnosis." *International Journal of Clinical and Experimental Hypnosis* 40(4): 276–300.

———. 1993. "Healing and the Invention of Metaphor: The Effectiveness of Symbols Revisited." *Culture, Medicine and Psychiatry* 17(2): 161–195.

———. 1994. "Facing the Void: Social and Cultural Dimensions of Dissociation." In D. Spiegel, ed., *Dissociation: Culture, Mind and Body.* Washington, D.C.: American Psychiatry Press, 91–122.

———. 1996. "Landscapes of Memory: Trauma, Narrative and Dissociation." In P. Antze and M. Lambek, eds., *Tense Past: Cultural Essays on Memory and Trauma.* London: Routledge, 173–198.

———. 2000. "Broken Narratives: Clinical Encounters and the Poetics of Illness Experience." In C. Mattingly and L. Garro, eds., *Narrative and the Cultural Construction of Illness and Healing.* Berkeley: University of California Press, 153–180.

Kirmayer, L. J., and R. Santhanam. 2001. "The Anthropology of Hysteria." In P. W. Halligan, C. Bass, and J. C. Marshall, eds., *Contemporary Approaches to the Study of Hysteria: Clinical and Theoretical Perspectives.* Oxford: Oxford University Press, 251–270.

Kövecses, Z. 2000. *Metaphor and Emotion: Language, Culture, and Body in Human Feeling.* Cambridge: Cambridge University Press.

Lakoff, G., and M. Johnson. 1980. *Metaphors We Live By.* Chicago: University of Chicago Press.

———. 1999. *Philosophy in the Flesh: The Embodied Mind and Its Challenge to Western Thought.* New York: Basic Books.

Levenson, R. W., P. Ekman, and W. V. Friesen. 1990. "Voluntary Facial Action Generates Emotion-Specific Autonomic Nervous System Activity." *Psychophysiology* 27(4): 363–384.

Lévinas, E. 1985. *Ethics and Infinity.* Pittsburgh: Duquesne University Press.

———. 1998. *Entre Nous: Thinking of the Other.* New York: Columbia University Press.

———. 1999. *Alterity and Transcendence.* New York: Columbia University Press.

Levine, J. D., N. C. Gordon, and H. L. Fields. 1978. "The Mechanism of Placebo Analgesia." *Lancet* 23: 654–657.

Meagher, M. W., R. C. Arnau, and J. L. Rhudy. 2001. "Pain and Emotion: Effects of Affective Picture Modulation." *Psychosomatic Medicine* 63: 79–90.

Meltzoff, A. N., and M. K. Moore. 1977. "Imitation of Facial and Manual Gestures by Human Neonates." *Science* 198: 75–78.

Melzack, R., and K. L. Casey. 1968. "Sensory, Motivational and Central Control Determinants of Pain." In D. R. Kenshalo, ed., *The Skin Senses.* Springfield, Va.: C. C. Thomas, 423–443.

Melzack, R., and P. D. Wall. 1965. "Pain Mechanisms: A New Theory." *Science* 150: 971–979.

Montgomery, G. H., K. N. DuHamel, and W. H. Redd. 2000. "A Meta-Analysis of Hypnotically Induced Analgesia: How Effective Is Hypnosis?" *International Journal of Clinical and Experimental Hypnosis* 48(2): 138–153.

Nabokov, V. 1969. *Ada.* New York: McGraw-Hill.

Needleman, J. 1985. *The Way of the Physician.* New York: W. W. Norton.

Panksepp, J. 1998. *Affective Neuroscience: The Foundations of Human and Animal Emotions.* New York: Oxford University Press.

Panksepp, J., E. Nelson, and M. Bekkedal. 1999. "Brain Systems for the Mediation of Social Separation-Distress and Social-Reward: Evolutionary Antecedents and Neuropeptide Intermediaries." In C. S. Carter, I. I. Lederhendler, and B. Kirkpatrick, eds., *The Integrative Neurobiology of Affiliation.* Cambridge, Mass.: MIT Press, 221–243.

Pollo, A., M. Amanzio, A. Arslanian, C. Casadio, G. Maggi, and F. Benedetti. 2001. "Response Expectancies in Placebo Analgesia and Their Clinical Relevance." *Pain* 93: 77–84.

Poole, G. D., and K. D. Craig. 1992. "Judgments of Genuine, Suppressed, and Faked Facial Expressions of Pain." *Journal of Personality and Social Psychology* 63(5): 797–805.

Price, D. D., and J. J. Barrell. 2000. "Mechanisms of Analgesia Produced by Hypnosis and Placebo Suggestions." *Progress in Brain Research* 122: 255–271.

Price, D. D., L. S. Milling, I. Kirsch, A. Duff, G. H. Montgomery, and S. S. Nicholls. 1999. "An Analysis of Factors that Contribute to the Magnitude of Placebo Analgesia in an Experimental Paradigm." *Pain* 83: 147–156.

Prince, R. 1982. "Shamans and Endorphins." *Ethos* 10: 409–423.

Rainville, P., G. H. Duncan, D. D. Price, B. Carrier, and M. C. Bushnell. 1997. "Pain Affect Encoded in Human Anterior Cingulate But Not Somatosensory Cortex." *Science* 277(5328): 968–971.

Ramachandran, V. S., and S. Blakeslee. 1998. *Phantoms in the Brain.* New York: William Morrow.

Rosaldo, M. Z. 1980. *Knowledge and Passion: Ilongot Notions of Self and Social Life.* Cambridge: Cambridge University Press.

Rouget, G. 1985. *Music and Trance: A Theory of the Relations between Music and Possession.* Chicago: University of Chicago Press.

Royzman, E. B., and R. Kumar. 2001. "On the Relative Preponderance of Empathic Sorrow and Its Relation to Commonsense Morality." *New Ideas in Psychology* 19: 131–144.

Scheff, T. J. 1979. *Catharsis in Healing, Ritual, and Drama.* Berkeley: University of California Press.

Schneirla, T. C. 1959. "An Evolutionary and Developmental Theory of Biphasic Processes Underlying Approach and Withdrawal." In M. R. Jones, ed., *Nebraska Symposium on Motivation.* Lincoln: University of Nebraska Press, 1–42.

Shah, N. J., J. C. Marshall, O. Zafiris, A. Schwab, K. Zilles, H. J. Markowitsch, and G. R. Fink. 2001. "The Neural Correlates of Person Familiarity: A Functional Magnetic Resonance Imaging Study with Clinical Implications." *Brain* 124: 804–815.

Sharp, T. J. 2001. "Chronic Pain: A Reformulation of the Cognitive-Behavioural Model." *Behaviour Research and Therapy* 39: 787–800.

Shore, B. 1996. *Culture in Mind: Cognition, Culture, and the Problem of Meaning.* Oxford: Oxford University Press.

Simons, R. C., F. R. Ervin, and R. H. Prince. 1988. "The Psychobiology of Trance: I. Training for Thaipusam." *Transcultural Psychiatric Research Review* 25(4): 249–266.

Sweetser, E. 2000. "Blended Spaces and Performativity." *Cognitive Linguistics* 11(3–4): 305–333.

Thurman, R. A. F. 1995. *Inside Tibetan Buddhism: Rituals and Symbols Revealed.* San Francisco: Collins.

Tooby, J., and L. Cosmides. 1992. "The Psychological Foundations of Culture." In J. Barkow, L. Cosmides, and J. Tooby, eds., *The Adapted Mind.* Oxford: Oxford University Press.

Varela, F. J. 1999. *Ethical Know-How: Action, Wisdom, and Cognition.* Stanford: Stanford University Press.

Varela, F. J., E. Thompson, and E. Rosch. 1991. *The Embodied Mind: Cognitive Science and Human Experience.* Cambridge, Mass.: MIT Press.

Villemure, C., and M. C. Bushnell. 2002. "Cognitive Modulation of Pain: How Do Attention and Emotion Influence Pain Processing?" *Pain* 95: 195–199.

Wild, B., M. Erb, and M. Bartels. 2001. "Are Emotions Contagious? Evoked Emotions While Viewing Emotionally Expressive Faces: Quality, Quantity, Time Course and Gender Differences." *Psychiatry Research* 102: 109–124.

Willer, J. C., H. Dehen, and J. Cambier. 1981. "Stress-Induced Analgesia in Humans: Endogenous Opioids and Naloxone-Reversible Depression of Pain Reflexes." *Science* 212: 689–691.

Woolf, C. J., and M. W. Salter. 2000. "Neuronal Plasticity: Increasing the Gain in Pain." *Science* 288: 1765–1768.

Zajonc, R. B. 1985. "Emotion and Facial Efference: A Theory Reclaimed." *Science* 228: 15–21.

Discussion:
The Notion of Face

ARTHUR KLEINMAN: I thought Laurence Kirmayer's use of the idea of face was very interesting. In the Chinese setting, face signifies your social and moral status in the society, but losing face is also an experience of shame, and regaining face and being given face are moralizing experiences. It is very important for us to take into account that, through relationships, moral meanings enter into the bodily experience of affect related to pain. That is a part of the suffering component of pain, and it is impossible to leave that out of the equation.

HOWARD FIELDS: This might be an appropriate point to bring in some very interesting new neurobiology of the amygdala, the area that's critical in human beings to the conditioned fear phenomenon and to the recognition of emotion in faces. People who have bilateral lesions of the amygdala have no trouble identifying a person's face, but they lose the ability to recognize the emotional communication of facial expression.

Professor David Amaral at the University of California at Davis has access to one of the largest communities of primates, who live in groups and roam free (see Prather et al. 2001). He has made bilateral amygdala lesions in some of these primates. When tested, they seem to have much less fear than normal. But when interacting with other primates, Amaral sees much bigger differences in the behavior of primates without amygdala lesions when they are in the presence of a primate that does have the lesion. For example, the normal primates are much more likely to approach a dominant male who has bilateral amygdala lesions. So there must be something in their facial expressions or gestures or posture that other members of the group are picking up.

Another set of experiments done by Linda Watkins relates to emotional memories and the concept of a safety signal (Watkins et al. 1998). If you put rats in a box and shock them, when you later return them to the box, they show fear behaviors. But if you change the experiment by turning a light on that signals the end of the shock, and then bring the animals into the room when the light is on, they no longer are afraid of the room. A transformation has taken place. We are now coming to a neurobiology of transformation. If you want to label it reductionism, okay, but we can't argue with the observations.

LUIS GÓMEZ: I was also taken by the reference to face, which interests me a lot. In the context of psychotherapy (which is usually conceived, I think erroneously, as individual rather than interpersonal work), the face of the psychotherapist, as well as the tone of voice, is critical to the process. Yet there are some theories of psychotherapy, such as the more traditional Freudian psychotherapies, that assume that not seeing the face is critical to the process. As a historical note, apparently the only reason that Freud used the couch was because he himself could not tolerate the emotions generated by the face of the patient.

SARAH COAKLEY: I wonder whether medical practitioners dealing with intense pain give any thought to how they can effectively present themselves facially to their patients? Psychiatrists think about this to some extent; they're not avoiding direct eye-contact, like Freud, but doctors in the wards don't generally think about it as far as I know. And yet if the evidence that we've seen is to be believed, it is a vital factor in the capacity for recovery or response to painful states. Can anyone tell us more about this?

SHAHRAM KHOSHBIN: I take issue with the assertion that the medical profession is not sensitive to the issue of pain. Nursing schools and even medical schools have made strides in recent years to correct those past mistakes. Pain is now its own specialty in medicine, beyond the realm of psychiatry and neurology. Information such as what hopefully will come out of our deliberations here is gobbled up by people who teach our students to be better caretakers or managers of pain.

The fact that there have been mistakes in the past doesn't mean that the same mistakes are currently taking place. The understanding of biology is now in a very advanced form. Twenty-five hundred years of studying pain has led to a better conclusion than we are making it sound.

COAKLEY: I didn't mean that there wasn't interest in pain. Even if there is great interest in pain in a specialized ward, that doesn't always mean that the person who comes with the syringe has a sympathetic face.

TU WEIMING: The term for pain in Chinese is linked to the idea of blockage, which is very much related to the question of sympathy. In other words, pain means that the natural flow is being blocked somewhere, so that intervention is needed. If we broaden that to include not only your own physiology but also the interpersonal relationships between the patient and other persons or even society, it becomes very interesting. I don't know whether or not it is part of an enabling language, but it is interesting to see how pain is perceived by one culture or tradition.

There are two terms for the face in Chinese. One means presence. When you have a big face it means you have a big, humorous presence. The other meaning is really facial expressions, which can be perceived by others as an indicator of your inner emotions. These two meaning are interconnected in strange ways.

One of the intriguing issues is whether our study of the brain can bring new insights into the very difficult concept of mind. Yet there is something that flows beyond what we can study in terms of the actual. If we take learning or unlearning relationality seriously, as part of the process of growing up or being human, then the question becomes very intriguing whether there is indeed a social dimension of the mind that cannot be understood in simply subjectivist terms. That is an intriguing question for the philosophy of mind that our conversations are revealing.

References

Prather, M. D., P. Lavenex, M. L. Mauldin-Jourdain, W. A. Mason, J. P. Capitanio, S. P. Mendoza, and D. G. Amaral. 2001. "Increased Social Fear and Decreased Fear of Objects in Monkeys with Neonatal Amygdala Lesions." *Neuroscience* 106: 653–658.

Watkins L. R., E. P. Wiertelak, M. McGorry, J. Martinez, B. Schwartz, D. Sisk, and S. F. Maier. 1998. "Neurocircuitry of Conditioned Inhibition of Analgesia: Effects of Amygdala, Dorsal Raphe, Ventral Medullary, and Spinal Cord Lesions on Antianalgesia in the Rat." *Behav. Neurosci.* 112: 360–378.

The Place of Pain in the Space of Good and Evil

14

Nicholas Wolterstorff

Among the most important aspects of cultural perspectives on pain are the assessments we make of pain as good, evil, or indifferent. Is pain always an evil, or is it sometimes indifferent? Might it sometimes be a good? Might it sometimes even be inherently, and not just instrumentally, good? And what do we mean in calling it "evil" or "good"? In short, what is the place of pain in the space of good and evil? That is the issue I propose introducing, mainly by presenting a few contrasting perspectives on the matter.

Among the most prominent topics in one of the fields in which I do a good deal of my own work, namely, philosophy of religion, is the so-called problem of evil. The "problem" consists, strictly, in several distinct problems, united in that all of them have to do, in one way or another, with the relation between God and evil. In discussions of these various problems, pain is regularly taken as a paradigmatic example of an evil. Seldom is there any recognition of the possibility that perhaps some pain is not an evil but indifferent or even good; just as seldom is there any discussion of what is meant in calling pain an "evil." Of course it might just be in some cases that the philosopher has nonetheless reflected seriously on the matter and that the results of his reflections are manifested not in explicit theory but in the examples he gives; possibly such reflection lies behind what is often cited in recent literature as an obvious example of an evil, namely, the excruciating pain of a young deer burned to death in a forest fire. But as we shall see, there have been major evaluative perspectives that would deny that even such pain is an evil.

1. It will be important for my subsequent purposes to begin with a bit of phenomenology in which I distinguish two dimensions of the self. One fundamental and ineradicable dimension of us human beings is that we invest ourselves in one thing and another: actualities or presumed actualities, possibilities or presumed possibilities. We love our children, attach ourselves to some baseball team, care about the fate of some political party, concern ourselves over the progress of our career, and so forth. It is standard practice to identify this aspect of the self with desire; but that seems to me a mistake. Desire is a manifestation and species of the phenomenon in question, not the phenomenon itself. For one thing, though one's love of one's children will no doubt manifest itself in desire for one thing and another with respect to them, one's love for them is broader than any particular desire. Relevant desires come and go, depending on circumstances, while the love remains and gets manifested in the desires. Second, that particular mode of investment in something that constitutes admiration for the thing sometimes has nothing to do with desire. And third, when one's desire, say, to hear once again some piece of music to which one is attached is satisfied, by virtue of one's actually hearing the piece, one's desire to hear it ceases, whereas one's love for hearing it remains. One desires what one loves but does not presently enjoy; when one then actually enjoys it, the desire ceases on account of being satisfied, but the love remains.

To point us toward the aspect of the self that I have in mind, I have used a variety of words: "investment," "attachment," "care," "concern," "love." The word Plato preferred was "eros," standardly translated as "love." Unfortunately, somewhere between Plato and us the word "eros" got captured for speaking of the sexual. When one sees the sign "Erotica Shop" on an establishment in Amsterdam, one does not expect upon entering to find oneself among philosophers talking about love for the Good as such. Nonetheless, "eros," as Plato used it, does capture the phenomenon in question precisely; accordingly, I propose every now and then using it with the Platonic meaning, hoping that its present-day sexual connotations can be, for the time being, suppressed.

Much of the joy of human life is located in the satisfaction, or perceived satisfaction, or perceived imminent satisfaction, of eros. Since childhood the St. Louis Cardinals have been my favorite baseball team; it is because I am attached to them that their winning gives me satisfaction, and their slugging home runs by the multiples gives me joy. Others, who are not attached to the Cardinals, view their winning, and their slugging prowess, with indifference, or even dismay. Too bad for them, I say!

The other dimension of the self of which we must take note is this: each of us finds certain experiences pleasant, certain others unpleasant, and some just neutral, neither here nor there. Almost all of Brahms's chamber music I very much like listening to; almost all of Wagner's music I quite strongly dislike listening to. I recognize certain excellences in it; but listening to it makes me feel uneasy. It is not to my taste.

Among the experiences we like is that of our desires being satisfied; among the experiences we dislike is that of our desires being frustrated. That is but one of the many ways in which these two dimensions of the self are intertwined. The intertwinement presupposes, however, the distinctness. Among the many different sorts of things we desire is the having of certain experiences; and prominent among the reasons for desiring an experience of a certain sort is that one expects to enjoy the experience. Anticipated enjoyment could not constitute a reason for desiring some experience if the enjoyable character of the experience were not distinct from the desire and the enjoyment of its satisfaction.

When one's desire for an enjoyable experience is gratified, then one's joy is double: one enjoys having the experience one desired, and one also enjoys having the experience of desire satisfied. I very much enjoy listening to Brahms's Three Intermezzos, Opus 117. When I first heard them, my enjoyment had nothing to do with the experience of desire satisfaction; I just happened to hear them being played one day. Right now, when listening to them, I both enjoy hearing them and am happy that my desire to hear them once again is presently being satisfied.

For the sake of convenience, let me call these two dimensions of the self that I have distinguished the *erotic* and the *hedonic* dimensions, respectively—"hedonic" borrowed from the Greek word for pleasure, *hedonê*, as "erotic" is from the Greek word for love, *eros*.

Where is pain to be located in this phenomenology? Well, pain is an experience; and for most people most of the time, it is an unpleasant experience. It is like the experience of tasting bitter medicine, like the experience of hearing fingernails scratching across a blackboard, like the experience of feeling depressed, like the experience of disappointed desire: most of us most of the time do not like it. It is my impression, however, that some people enjoy certain pains. I do not mean that they are glad they are having the pain—that for one reason and another they desire the pain and are experiencing the joy of satisfied desire. I mean that they find the pain itself enjoyable. Or actually—generalizing from my own case—I would guess that this is true not just for a few of us but for most of us. Sometimes, when there is something mildly wrong with one of my fingers, I rather enjoy pressing on the sore spot to feel the pain. It is rather like enjoying the taste of some mildly bitter food—a salad of young dandelion greens, perhaps.

2. All this so far is purely descriptive, purely phenomenological; it is time to move on to the evaluative perspectives. I shall have to confine myself entirely to Western perspectives—partly because there is no time on this occasion to branch out beyond those, partly because my expertise does not extend any farther.

For us in the modern West the most alien evaluative perspective on pain represented in the Western tradition is that of the Neoplatonists and Stoics of late antiquity. So alien is their perspective that it jolts us; that is a good reason for beginning there. The perspective of the Neoplatonists was significantly different from that of the Stoics; shortly I will explain the difference. But for our purposes here, the similarities are more important than the differences. Both hold that the person who sees things in their true light—the sage—will regard pain as a matter of indifference.

A large part of the thought of all the ancient philosophers, including then the Neoplatonists and the Stoics, revolved around the question of what constitutes *eudaimonia* and how we human beings can attain it. The word is customarily translated "happiness"; a better translation in contemporary English is probably "well-being." What constitutes human well-being, and how is it to be attained?

The answer of both the Neoplatonists and the Stoics is, for us, striking: human well-being is located entirely in the erotic dimension of the self. It is constituted entirely by the proper orientation of one's desires, and more generally, of one's eros, and of the enjoyment experienced in the satisfaction of one's love. What is striking for us about this claim is the implied negation: well-being has nothing to do with the hedonic dimension of the self, except, of course, for the delight of experiencing the satisfaction of properly oriented desires. With that exception, well-being has nothing to do with enjoyable and distasteful experience: nothing to do with enjoying listening to music and reading poetry, nothing to do with the pain of cancer or the suffering of depression.

What led the Stoics to this view was their conviction that the only life worthy of a human being is a life in which one's well-being is not hostage to fortune: a life in which one's well-being is, on the contrary, in one's own hands. A life in which one's well-being is entirely in one's own hands would have to be, in the first place, a life in which pleasant and unpleasant experiences are a matter of indifference—since whether I will suffer physical pain, and whether I will experience the enjoyments of sex, fine food, and so forth, lies in good measure outside my control. Positively, a life in which one's well-being is entirely in one's own hands will be a life in which one's desires are focused entirely on ends whose attainment one can be assured of. Desires to manipulate the world or society in certain ways do not qualify, since we can seldom be assured of being able to satisfy such desires. In fact the only end whose attainment lies entirely in one's own hands is one's own virtue. Whether I shall do what I ought to do, so that my will is a good will and my character virtuous—this is entirely up to me. It follows that human well-being consists in striving to do what one ought to do and finding enjoyment therein. The virtuous man has achieved well-being, *eudaimonia,* whether or not he is on the torture rack.

The Stoics often put the point by saying that the only thing that is a *good* for oneself is one's own virtue—by which they meant that the only thing that is desire worthy for oneself is one's own virtue. Of course the sage, the virtuous man, would *prefer* not being on the torture rack; but the preferable is not to be identified with the good. The good, to say it again, is the desire-worthy. And the absence of pain is not desire-worthy, since by and large it is not within one's control whether one will or will not experience pain. To desire the absence of pain is to allow oneself to be taken hostage by fortune.

The Neoplatonists agreed with the Stoics that well-being consists in the satisfaction of properly oriented desires and that the person who has oriented her desires aright—the virtuous person, the sage—will be happy even on the torture rack. The goal that the Neoplatonists proposed was different, however: not one's own virtue but "mystical union" with the divine. What recommended this goal was not that its achievement lies entirely within one's own hands, since it does not. One can prepare oneself for the mystical union; but then, preparations finished, one can only await its happening. No guarantees. What recommended this goal was rather that the divine is the supreme good and that the most excellent relationship to the supreme good available to a human being is mystical union therewith. Pain is an evil for one only if it hinders one from achieving that ultimate form of well-being; it hinders one from that only if one lets it do so.

3. I dare say that all of us would readily second Kant's response to the Stoics and Neoplatonists—namely, that it is inhumane to hold that well-being is compatible with being on the torture rack. Yet it is not as if the Stoics and Neoplatonists had never thought about what it is to be human. Quite to the contrary: they saw themselves as drawing out the implications of what it is to be fully human. So something deep has changed between them and us. What might that be?

What is changed is that whereas the Stoics and Neoplatonists saw the therapy of desire—to use Martha Nussbaum's nice phrase (Nussbaum 1994)—as the path toward well-being, we in the modern world place much more confidence in the satisfaction of desire as the path toward well-being. The evidence is all about us, for example, in the view that democratic politics ought to be the politics of preference satisfaction.

Why, in turn, has this alteration in attitude taken place? No doubt in part because the expansion of our technological capacity for altering nature, society, and self to the measure of our desire has enabled us to satisfy, a great many more of our desires than was possible in antiquity. But that cannot be the whole story. Many of our desires we still cannot satisfy; and often when one desire is satisfied, a new one emerges to take its place. The therapy of desire remains a live candidate as the road to happiness.

No doubt the alteration has also taken place, in part, because it is characteristic of theorists and laypeople alike in the contemporary world to invert what most of the ancients saw as the relation between excellence and desire. Most of the ancients believed that there is an objective structure of excellence and that well-being is to be found in conforming one's eros to that objective structure, admiring what is admiration worthy, desiring what is desire worthy, and so on. Our theorists, by contrast, have struggled to develop the view that what is good is determined somehow by what people desire or by what they would desire in one or another idealized situation. But this too cannot be the whole story, since the conviction that even for the righteous person pain may be an evil precedes the emergence of such value subjectivism.

Somewhere along the line what took place was a revaluation of values, with the consequence, among others, that whereas pain was seen by the Stoics and the Neoplatonists as a matter of indifference for the virtuous person, it is no longer so seen.

Not all the ancient philosophers agreed with the Stoics in their insistence that the well-being worthy of a human being must be immune to the vicissitudes of fortune, nor with the Stoics and Neoplatonists in their insistence that the road to well-being consists entirely in the therapy of desire. But it is my own judgment that it was Christianity, especially in its Augustinian form, that is principally responsible for altering our valuation of pain and making the perspective of the Stoics and Neoplatonists profoundly alien.

Dominant in the writings of Augustine's early middle career—I have in mind particularly *Of True Religion* (Augustine 1991 [1959]), the *Confessions* (1961), and the first book of *On Christian Doctrine* (1987 [1958])—was a fascinating appropriation of both Stoic and Neoplatonist emphases to Christian purposes. Assuming without question that happiness is for each of us our sole end in itself, Augustine argued that the only assured path to unalloyed and uninterrupted happiness is fixing one's love on that which is not only worthy of love but cannot change or disappear. God is the only candidate. Augustine urges his readers to take delight in the enjoyable experiences that come one's way and to give God thanks both for those experiences and for the absence of unpleasant experiences when they are absent. But do not, he said, make the presence of the enjoyable and the absence of the unenjoyable the object of one's love; for that way lies disappointment. Love God alone and one's fellow human beings *in* God.

This, I say, was the dominant note in the writings of Augustine's early middle career. Now and then, however, in addition to this dominant note, one encounters a different note, more softly sounded; this different note is a radical departure from anything the Stoics or Neoplatonists said. Augustine enjoins his readers to grieve over the sins of their fellow human beings—and over their own. The fact that "everyone wants to be happy" should not be taken to imply, he remarks, that "we must arm ourselves against compassion. There are times when we must welcome sorrow on behalf of others" (1961, 56).

In his final book, *The City of God*, this theme of empathic grieving is sounded much more emphatically than it was in his earlier writings, and the scope of what it is appropriate for us to grieve over is expanded. Now Augustine allows, and sometimes even enjoins, his readers to grieve not just over the sins of themselves and their fellow human beings but over their misery as well: the misery of poverty, the misery ensuing on the death of friends, the misery of intractable pain. Let me quote at length what he says in one remarkable passage:

> The more friends we have, and the more places we have them in, the further and more widely do we fear that some evil may befall them out of all the mass of the evils of this world. . . . And when such things do happen (and the more numerous our friends, the more often they happen) and the fact is brought to our knowledge, who, save one who has experienced the same thing, can understand the burning sorrow which then afflicts our hearts? Indeed, we would rather hear that our friends were dead; although this also we could not hear without pain: for if their life delighted us with the solace of friendship, how could it be that their death should not bring us grief? Anyone who forbids such grief must forbid, if he can, all friendly conversation; he must prohibit or

> extinguish affection; he must with ruthless disregard sever the ties of all human companionship, or else stipulate that such companionship must merely be made use of, without giving rise to any delight of soul. But if this can in no way be done, how can the death of one whose life has been sweet to us not bring us bitterness? (1998, 929–930)

Thus Augustine angrily rejects the imperturbability of the Stoic sage:

> They believe that their wise man . . . even if he becomes blind, deaf and dumb; even if he is enfeebled in limb and tormented with pain; even if he falls victim to every other ill that can be described or imagined; even if he is compelled to put himself to death: that such a man would not shrink from calling such a life, beset with such ills, a happy one. (1998, 922)

"Oh happy life," Augustine replies with sarcastic irony, "that seeks the aid of death to put an end to it!"

It was mainly Augustine's reading of the Christian Bible that accounts for this radical rejection of the Stoicism and Neoplatonism that dominated his intellectual environment. What he found in the Bible was a picture of two ages: this present age and the age to come. In the age to come, to which we look forward, there will be no suffering, no wrongdoing, no death; suffering, wrongdoing, and death are evils conquered by God at the inauguration of the new age. But if suffering, wrongdoing, and death are evils conquered by God at the inauguration of the new age, what else could they be now than evils not yet overcome? Augustine is manifestly reluctant to enjoin us to work to diminish the evil of suffering. When it comes to the evil of wrongdoing we are not just to grieve empathically but to struggle to eliminate such evil; not so for the evil of suffering. Probably he saw small prospect of success in such a struggle; hence he stops with urging empathic grieving. But there can be no doubt that his manifest reluctance to urge the alleviation of suffering has lost all theoretical basis and is now a matter of purely practical considerations. The power of Augustinian Christianity in subsequently shaping the West has meant that henceforth the indifference of Stoics and Neoplatonists to pain and suffering has forever seemed alien.

The only way to articulate what Augustine has done in this overturning of Stoicism and Neoplatonism is to understand him as tacitly distinguishing between the *moral excellence* of a person, on the one hand, and the *well-being* or *happiness* of a person, on the other, and as arguing that here in this present age these regularly come into conflict with each other. The person who grieves and the person whose endeavors are frustrated are, so far forth, not happy, given Augustine's understanding of happiness. Yet we are morally required to grieve empathically over the suffering and wrongdoing of ourselves and our fellow human beings and morally required to invest ourselves in the alleviation of suffering and wrongdoing, morally allowed if not required to grieve over their suffering and ours, and morally required to invest ourselves in the alleviation of wrongdoing, knowing full well that our efforts in this regard will in good measure prove in vain. Whereas the Stoics and the Neoplatonists allowed no gap between excellence and well-being—well-being for them just *was* moral excellence—suffering now becomes a moral requirement. Certain modes of suffering are a condition of moral excellence. Present-day philosophers are best acquainted with this use of the distinction between excellence and well-being from Kant's argument for the existence of a *summum bonum.* But Kant was doing no more than embracing this part of the Augustinian tradition. Of course Augustine, in turn, was enjoining a variant on the biblical lament: why do the ungodly prosper and the righteous suffer?

4. What would Augustine have meant in calling suffering an *evil?* Augustine embraced the Platonic account of excellence according to which the excellence of something is determined by its degree of resemblance to the paradigmatically good being, this in Augustine's case being God, rather than Plato's impersonal *eidos,* The Good Itself. Augustine was emphatic in his insistence, however, that this account of excellence is not at the same time an account of evil; in particular, a thing is not evil on account of being located near the low end of the scale of excellence. The account of evil espoused by Augustine was the account that was standard in antiquity and on through the high Middle Ages. Evils are never evils per se; an evil is always an evil *for something.* More precisely, things are evils for the beings of a certain nature.

Not being able to see is an evil for a human being but not for a tree; not being able to fly is an evil for a robin but not for a human being. Something is an evil for things of a certain nature if it is an impairment of the proper formation or the proper functioning of things of that nature. Evils are malformations and malfunctionings.

On this account, a good deal of pain is not an evil but is, on the contrary, a case of the body's proper functioning. We are meant to feel pain when we develop an inflamed appendix, break a leg, or touch a hot object; should we not feel pain in such circumstances, *that* would be a case of malfunctioning. Rather than the pain being a malfunction, it is the *indicator* of a malfunction in some part of the body: an indicator of something wrong with one's appendix, of something wrong with one's leg, of something wrong with the flesh of one's finger. Pain serves thus as a warning: a warning to see a doctor immediately, a warning to beware of jumping from heights and of touching hot objects.

That we feel pain under such circumstances is thus an excellence in our design plan, not a defect; life would be vastly more precarious if we did not feel pain in such circumstances. Of course the pain is an unpleasant experience; if it were not, it would not serve as effectively as it does as a warning. But on this way of seeing things it is not, to say it once again, the pain that is the evil but the malformation of which the pain is an indicator.

Not all pain is of this sort, however; sometimes pain acquires, as it were, a life of its own, so that it is no longer an indicator of bodily malformation but is itself the malformation. In such cases, pain itself is the evil.

Earlier I argued that on the Augustinian perspective, in contrast to that of the Stoics and Neoplatonists, pain in particular and suffering in general is incompatible with full well-being. Well-being is not confined to the proper orientation of the erotic dimension of the self; it includes delight in the hedonic dimension as well. Just now we have seen that a good deal of pain, probably most, is not itself an evil on the classical understanding of evil that Augustine embraced. But are not these two perspectives in conflict with each other? How can something be incompatible with well-being if it is not an evil?

Part of the answer is that, as we have seen, bodily malfunction, and pain as the indicator thereof, typically, though not invariably, come as a package; it is that package that is incompatible with full well-being even though the pain itself is not an evil but that of which the pain is an indicator. The rest of the answer is that well-being includes, but goes beyond, proper formation and proper functioning.

5. Experience and literature, both secular and religious, teach us that the relation of pain to the good is by no means confined to the fact that one of the excellences of our makeup is that we have a design plan in which pain is an indicator of bodily malformations and malfunctions. From experience and literature we learn of cases—many cases—in which pain, along with other forms of suffering, contributes significantly and even indispensably to the sufferer's becoming a more excellent person. That diminution of well-being that pain is, on Augustine's account and accounts similar, becomes a means to the formation of a better person. Pain contributes to soul making. Of course it does not inevitably do this; there are other cases, perhaps more, in which pain embitters.

Obviously this point could be developed in great and moving detail. But I want instead to close with a question suggested by the point. It is the ultimate question in a discussion of the place of pain in the space of good and evil, both repellant and irresistible. Pain, I said, sometimes becomes a means to the sufferer's becoming a more excellent, more admirable, person than she was before the pain and than she would in all likelihood have been without it. Could it sometimes be that pain serves not as a means to excellence, or not *just* as a means, but that it is itself an excellence in a human being? It will always, on an Augustinian perspective, be an impairment in well-being—though even that assumption would be worth exploring. Might it nonetheless, in this world of ours, sometimes be an excellence, that is, an *inherent,* and not merely instrumental, excellence in the person?[1] Grief, as we have seen, is sometimes such an excellence, both original and empathic. But is *pain* ever that? As we have already seen several times, well-being and excellence do, all too often, part ways in this present world of ours.

Presumably pain *as such, sheer* pain, will never be an excellence in a person; if pain is ever an excellence in a person, it will be so on account of *how* the person experiences the pain—her mode of pain. The mode of experiencing pain that is inherently excellent—if any such there can be—will not be that in which the pain becomes a *means* to excellence; for in that case it is not the pain that is inherently excellent but that which pain yields. Neither will the mode be the virtuous way in which the person *bears* the pain—with patience, with fortitude, whatever. For then it is the mode of bearing pain that is inherently excellent, not the pain itself.

Does anything remain? Can pain be an inherent good in a person, something inherently admirable? Can pain itself be transformed into something good, and not merely be an agent for transforming a person into something good? I do not know; perhaps such a place in the space of the excellent can never be occupied by pain. But let me make a suggestion. One finds cases in the Christian tradition in which a person describes herself as in her pain participating—in a way I do not profess to understand—in Christ's pain. One finds hints of this way of experiencing pain already in the New Testament writings of St. Paul; it is also how the martyrs sometimes spoke. If we are to find cases of pain as an inherent excellence, I think it is to such cases that we will have to look—and perhaps to similar cases in other religious traditions. For what is excellent in such cases is neither the virtuous way in which the sufferer endures the pain nor the excellence of character that the pain yields. Of course Christ's pain would itself have to be an excellence if one's participation in it by one's own pain were to be an inherent excellence in the sufferer. Whether Christ's pain would also have to be inherently excellent is not clear to me.

6. I have offered very little by way of conclusions; my aim on this occasion has rather been to loosen the straps on imagination, so that what once seemed obviously to be the place of pain in the space of the good and the evil now seems problematic rather than obvious.

Note

1. This problem is addressed in the final discussion of Chapter 6, "The Instrumentality of Pain in Christianity and Buddhism."

References

Augustine. 1961. *Confessions.* Trans. R. S. Pine-Coffin. New York: Penguin Books.

———. 1987 [1958]. *On Christian Doctrine.* Trans. D. W. Robertson. New York: Macmillan

———. 1991 [1959]. *Of True Religion.* Trans. J. H. S. Burleigh. Chicago: Regnery Press.

———. 1998. *The City of God.* Trans. R. W. Dyson. Cambridge: Cambridge University Press.

Nussbaum, M. 1994. *The Therapy of Desire.* Princeton: Princeton University Press.

Response:
The Problem of Action

Charles Hallisey

I wanted to make some general concluding comments locating Nicholas Wolterstorff's paper within the context of the last few days' discussion. I was struck by how much of what Clifford Woolf and Howard Fields had said seemed to be echoed in his own comments, even though his angle of vision is the most abstract and philosophical of the three, and the most concerned with the context of meaning, whereas the papers of the other two are more concerned with the small bits that are the conditions for the experience of pain.

In his title, Nick indicates that he is concerned about where is pain to be located, then he adds "in the space of good and evil." I want to focus my attention on the question: Where is pain to be located? This seems to be a question that we've been worrying over. Is it located in molecules or in the brain, and in which part of the brain? Is it located in contexts of meaning, whether scientific or religious, musical or cultural? Is it located in one's own experience or in the reduplication of experience communally in ritual and literature? Part of our problem with communicating pain has to do with defining which layer of the phenomenon of pain we're addressing.

Within the Buddhist tradition, as Luis Gómez explained, there is a consistent assumption that the description of the four Noble Truths implies a course of action. This also struck me in thinking about Howard Fields's and Clifford Woolf's presentations, on the one hand, and Nicholas Wolterstorff's, on the other: their descriptions imply courses of action.

In Nick's view, there is an implied course of action whether you think of pain within a therapy of desire or pain within the satisfaction of desire. Those two descriptions imply very radically different courses of action.

Clifford Woolf's work on the receptors of pain is clearly about alleviating pain. The description is dedicated to a course of action to remove it. But Howard Fields's comment that pain is one of the ways that we interact with the environment clearly makes the case that we don't want to alleviate *all* pain, because then the world would become a very dangerous place, as it is for people with congenital analgesia.

So we make a kind of evaluative judgment, which Nick referred to as distinguishing what counts as good or bad pain. One of the things that makes our discussion difficult is that it is difficult for us not only to communicate the experience of pain but also to communicate what the assumptions are that allow us to distinguish good pain from bad pain.

The other thing that struck me in listening to Nick was how often our discussion seems to hinge on a distinction between pain in oneself and pain in others. That distinction occurs in every layer, whether we see pain located in receptors to the world, at the molecular level, or in the amygdala. Clifford talked about how we want to alleviate pain by somehow interrupting the receptors, blocking the transmission of pain. But in apes in which the amygdala is severed, this interruption is a disastrous thing. This is connected, I think, to the experience of pain in oneself and in others.

Nick's discussion of Augustine led me to think that the implied courses of action are based on midlevel, cultivated forms of ethical behavior. Elaine Scarry referred to the necessity of doctors and nurses working with severely injured people to cultivate the ability to not turn away or flinch. I think there is a whole range of midlevel behaviors that needs to be cultivated according to different broad-level contexts of meaning about pain. In thinking about pain in another person, we recognize that the problems of communication have an integrity of their own and that we shouldn't try to find a detour around them. We should respect that pain silences and in some ways *cannot* be communicated.

But at the same time, we have an ambiguity in that pain both generates sympathy and also repulses. How do those two things fit together? From what Howard Fields has said, I'm sure it must have something to do with the amygdala at the physiological level; but seemingly we cannot yet explicate this fully.

Nick made the point that you don't try to alleviate patient or empathetic grieving for the suffering of others. There are certain kinds of pain that are not to be alleviated but, rather, are to be dwelled in, and this contributes to an excellence.

On the other side, in the world of CAT scans, problems of communication are somehow to be removed so that we have a more accurate description of the pain that someone can't talk about. Reduction here is a value, and we describe things not to dwell in them but, in the end, to remove the pain.

So we have almost the same question we began this conference with: How do we build a bridge between molecules and contexts of meaning? There are rival or parallel contexts of meaning operating at every level. The bridge is a problem when those of us in the same room are talking about the same thing but within very different paradigms of disciplinary behavior.

My last point is something that just came to mind about the conference title: the transformation of pain. In an unreflective way I had been thinking about it only as how pain is transformed into something else, something that can be valued. (Obviously, there are ways that pain can't be transformed into something good; at the level of medicine, pain is not good, and it is good that we can remove it.) But Nick added that "the transformation of pain" can be interpreted in terms of how we are transformed *by* pain. In this case, pain is not the object to be transformed; pain is the agent of transformation. It's not a question of what we do to pain but what pain does to us, in that it can make us into something better than we otherwise have a right to be. In short, it seems that the problem of pain cannot avoid becoming a moral and religious question.

Afterword 15

Sarah Coakley

Even since the original conference that spawned this book, remarkable new discoveries about pain at the molecular level have been made.[1] These discoveries suggest that we can now foresee being able to create effective *individualized* pain remedies for human patients, closely correlated to their individual genetic, neurobiological, and circumstantial states. But how, exactly, will the full range of such states be investigated, quantified, and assessed? How in particular will the multifaceted question of "meanings"—cultural, moral, metaphysical, and religious—that we have probed in this volume be factored into such assessments? How can such meanings be related, in research terms, to the exacting biological details of current pain investigation from the "bottom up"?

At the heart of this book's interdisciplinary exchange has been a focal question: how is pain "transformed"? We close with an enumeration of some of the ways in which we believe the book has suggested new ways forward for research on pain: pain research can itself be "transformed." Inevitably, these new ways themselves cut across the disciplines.

As our Introduction indicated at the outset, we cannot go far in the discussion of the meaning of pain without hitting seemingly intractable problems in the philosophy of mind. Ultimately these philosophical riddles cannot be averted, for they are intrinsic to the questions we have surveyed and therefore to the theorization of future research protocols. Is there a "mind," or even a "soul," dualistically distinct from brain and body states and operative in the experience and interpretation of pain? Or are mental states in some more subtle sense "supervenient" on brain states, allowing us to speak of the reality of pain within the context of a "nonreductive" physicalism? Or is it perhaps that neither option is true (as is sometimes now claimed by philosophers), and pain as "subjective experience" is therefore a "myth" that can simply be dispelled by a more ardent and reductive physicalism?

This book has not attempted to *solve* this highly technical debate—nor could it within its particular bounds. But by setting molecular, neuroscientific, "hermeneutical," and cultural evidences on pain closely alongside each other, it has at least *suggested* a fresh philosophical investigation of the topic of mental "emergence."[2] Where pain is concerned, we confront an extremely subtle layering and interaction of different possible levels of investigation, explanation, and causal interaction; and neither a simple "bottom-up" account nor a simple "top-down" one is sufficient in itself to do justice to the total phenomenon of pain. Certainly a disjunctive choice between them is a false one. It is where biology and culture meet (and interact, in the enigmatic realm of "consciousness") that the mystery of pain resides, and especially—as this book has been concerned to illuminate—in the crucial area of the relation of neural substrates to meaning ascription.

Here is the really interesting realm for continuing neuroscientific and philosophical research. Any nuanced and convincing philosophy of mind must, therefore, strive to give a convincing account of the *complexity* of the phenomenon of pain, as here explicated by molecular biologists, neuroscientists, anthropologists, and religionists, among others. Moreover, the philosophy of mind, alone and as such, cannot exhaust even the philosophical implications of pain and its transformations. Inexorably, this book has argued, the problem of pain becomes, on closer investigation, a transindividual and intersubjective one, replete with ethical, social, religious, and political ramifications that themselves demand philosophical analysis. The potential absence of physical pain from human life (a prospect not completely unforeseeable), as well as its searing presence, raises existential questions of great moral moment. This book has attempted to draw attention to such unavoidable features of philosophical debate that remain pressingly au courant and to give new interdisciplinary "texture" to their discussion.

As will also have emerged in the course of this book, there is in addition a great deal of potential new medical research that is suggested by our findings, some of which is already in process under a variety of guises. An implicit lesson of this volume is that the phenomenon termed "placebo" in medical circles is clearly too blunt and broad a category to do justice to the many dimensions of pain and its transformations that now demand further close, clinical investigation. As was noted in an important earlier volume in this series devoted to the "placebo effect" (Harrington 1997), the "placebo response" can often still be viewed in medical circles as a "dirty contaminant in the research process" (234). Yet if this present book has shown anything, it is surely that hermeneutical, contextual, and interpersonal variables in a pain event are of *crucial* significance, both for diagnosis and treatment, and as worthy therefore of funded research as that undertaken right "down" at the molecular level. The challenge here resides, first, in deconstructing the notion of placebo as a monolithic, immovable, and intrinsically suspect category. Rather than allowing "placebo" to remain as the undiscriminating "dumping" ground for the remaining mysteries of pain, future research must distinguish carefully between discrete areas of significant investigation for its interpretative modulation: trust (or lack thereof) in medical personnel; belief (or lack thereof) in the power of "pills" or medical interventions; the significance of interpersonal relations in hospital and at home (including gender, class, and race relations, as variables); the vital importance of varied cultural and religious meaning systems for pain (including some of those involving non-Western theories about the "subtle body," but currently categorized under another catchall term, complementary and alternative medicine [CAM]); and the impact of meditative, musical, and other ritual practices as relievers or transformers of pain. Such investigations must, as we have attempted to show, enroll perforce the interdisciplinary insights of social scientists, religionists, and musicologists, among others, if precise physiological and neuroscientific investigations are to be conducted in an intrinsically open-minded—but also nongullible—mode.

Such imaginative suggestions as these are not, of course, without difficulty. Some of this type of research, as this book has indicated en passant, is already beginning in small or exploratory ways. But many of the early forays, as we have also noted, have suffered from poor methodology, underfunding, lack of imagination, lack of interdisciplinary assistance, or sheerly crass *theological* presumptions.[3] An additional difficulty is that many of the pain-relieving public events described in this volume are, one must admit, seemingly nonsusceptible to investigation by precise biomedical methods. They remain for now in the realm of anthropological, historical, aesthetic, or sociological research. Yet as fMRI and other forms of imaging become more accurate and illuminating, some researchers have begun to imagine, for instance, how particular religious practices and attendant beliefs, in their *precise* relation to pain events, could be brought within the orbit of detailed laboratory investigation. Indeed, we already know, as discussed earlier,[4] that different forms of relief from pain can be achieved by *different* sorts of "meditative" practice, a research arena in which the question of the meditator's spiritual maturity is also a variable of some significance; and this relates closely to the whole matter of the sense of "control" in pain management (actual control or control by voluntarily losing control). The issue of control is one of the most interesting and important in current pain research and vitally related, as we now see, to questions of cultural, moral, and religious meaning.[5]

Such investigations as we have briefly suggested here, however, must ultimately relate their findings to the exacting research at the molecular level with which we started our discussion. This is a task that will demand all the methodological sophistication and ingenuity that this book has itself attempted to foster. Just as top-down pain researchers met bottom-up ones in our original conference, and went away mutually changed by the discussion, so—we dare to claim—pain research will itself only be transformed by a similar, and continuing, creative interaction between scholars across the disciplinary spectrum.

Notes

1. A recent article in *Harvard Magazine* (Koman 2005) describes the advancements of pain research made at Harvard since our original conference, particularly by Clifford Woolf and his colleagues in the area of explaining, and treating, genetic and "central sensitivization" variables in pain events. Forthcoming work suggests, for instance, that a person's pain threshold and

the risk of developing chronic pain together have an important inherited genetic component. For a recent general statement of Woolf's novel approach to pain, see Woolf 2004.

2. The possibility of an "emergence" solution to the mind-body problem was already suggested in Chapter 1 of this volume. It is hoped that, considered together, the scientific and hermeneutical materials presented in this volume might act as significant new "intuition pumps" for philosophy of mind and perhaps as a spur to bringing (mostly continental) hermeneutical philosophy and phenomenology into closer interaction with analytic philosophy's exacting investigations in this area. For one recent volume that does attempt to bring phenomenology and philosophy of mind into close relation, see Woodruff Smith and Thomasson 2005.
3. Some of these problems are adumbrated in Chapter 1.
4. See again the introductory Chapter 1 and Chapter 5.
5. The work of David Borsook and his research associates in Boston has been particularly important in this regard: see again Koman 2005 for a brief account of Borsook's pathbreaking work with fMRI and pain.

References

Harrington, A., ed. 1997. *The Placebo Effect: An Interdisciplinary Exploration.* Cambridge, Mass.: Harvard University Press.

Koman, K. 2005. "The Science of Hurt: Medical Researchers and Doctors Work to Close the 'Gates' on Pain." *Harvard Magazine* 108(2): 46–54.

Woodruff Smith, D., and A. L. Thomasson, eds. 2005. *Phenomenology and Philosophy of Mind.* Oxford: Clarendon Press.

Woolf, C. J. 2004. "Pain: Moving from Symptom Control toward Mechanism-Specific Pharmacologic Management." *Annals of Internal Medicine* 140: 441–451.

Contributors

Judith Becker is the Glenn McGeoch Collegiate Professor of Music at the University of Michigan.

Herbert Benson, M.D., is the founding President of the Mind/Body Medical Institute and the Mind/Body Medical Institute Associate Professor of Medicine at Harvard Medical School.

John C. M. Brust, M.D., is the Director of the Department of Neurology, Harlem Hospital Center, and Professor of Clinical Neurology, Columbia University Medical Center, College of Physicians and Surgeons.

Sarah Coakley is the Edward Mallinckrodt, Jr., Professor of Divinity at Harvard Divinity School. In 2007 she becomes the Norris-Hulse Professor of Divinity at the University of Cambridge.

Jennifer Cole is Associate Professor in the Department of Comparative Human Development, as well as a cultural anthropologist and member of the Committee on Human Development, at the University of Michigan.

Howard L. Fields is Professor of Neurology, Physiology, and Psychiatry at the University of California, San Francisco, and is Vice Chair of the Department of Neurology and Director of the Wheeler Center for the Neurobiology of Addiction.

Luis O. Gómez is Charles O. Hucker Professor of Buddhist Studies in the Department of Asian Languages and Cultures and Adjunct Professor of Psychology in the Department of Psychology at the University of Michigan.

Charles Hallisey is a Senior Lecturer in Buddhist studies at Harvard Divinity School.

Anne Harrington is Loeb Harvard College Professor and Professor for the History of Science at Harvard University.

Jean Jackson is Professor of Anthropology and Head of the Anthropology Program at the Massachusetts Institute of Technology.

Shahram Khoshbin, M.D., is Director of the Teaching and Education Division at Brigham and Women's Hospital and an Associate Professor of Neurology at Harvard Medical School.

Laurence J. Kirmayer, M.D., is James McGill Professor and Director of the Division of Social and Transcultural Psychiatry, Department of Psychiatry, at McGill University.

Arthur Kleinman is the Esther and Sidney Rabb Professor of Anthropology at Harvard University and Professor of Medical Anthropology and Psychiatry at Harvard Medical School.

Jon D. Levenson is the Albert A. List Professor of Jewish Studies at Harvard Divinity School.

Elaine Scarry is the Walter M. Cabot Professor of Aesthetics and the General Theory of Value and Senior Fellow of the Society of Fellows at Harvard University.

Martha Ann Selby is Associate Professor of Asian Studies at the University of Texas, Austin.

Kay Kaufman Shelemay is the G. Gordon Watts Professor of Music and Professor of African and African American Studies at Harvard University.

Stanley Tambiah is Esther and Sidney Rabb Research Professor Emeritus of Anthropology at Harvard University.

Elizabeth Tolbert is Professor of Ethnomusicology at the Peabody Conservatory of the Johns Hopkins University, with a joint appointment in the Department of Anthropology.

Tu Weiming is the Director of the Harvard-Yenching Institute and Harvard-Yenching Professor of Chinese History and Philosophy and of Confucian Studies at Harvard University.

Richard K. Wolf is the Harris K. Weston Associate Professor of the Humanities at Harvard University.

Nicholas Wolterstorff is the Noah Porter Professor Emeritus of Philosophical Theology at Yale University.

Clifford J. Woolf, M.D., Ph.D., MRCP, is the Richard J. Kitz Professor of Anaesthesia Research at Harvard Medical School.

Figure Credits

4.1. Reprinted with permission from Howard L. Fields and Donald D. Price, "Toward a Neurobiology of Placebo Analgesia," in Anne Harrington, ed., *The Placebo Effect: An Interdisciplinary Exploration* (Cambridge, Mass.: Harvard University Press, 1997), 93–116, figure 5.2.

4.2. Reprinted with permission from Howard L. Fields, "Is There a Facilitating Component to Central Pain Modulation?" *American Pain Society Journal* 1 (1992): 139–141, figure 1.

7.1. Musical excerpt adapted from Elizabeth Tolbert, "The Voice of Lament," in Leslie Dunn and Nancy Jones, eds., *Embodied Voices: Representing Female Vocality in Western Culture* (Cambridge: Cambridge University Press, 1994, 189). Reprinted with permission from Cambridge University Press.

8.1–8.3. Photographs by Judith Becker.

8.4–8.5, 8.7, 8.9. Reprinted with permission from Antonio Damasio, *The Feeling of What Happens: Body and Emotion in the Making of Consciousness* (San Diego, New York, and London: A Harvest Book, Harcourt Inc., 1999), 61 (figure 8.4), 199 (table 8.5), 155 (figure 8.7), 181 (figure 8.9).

8.6, 8.8, 8.10–8.12. Drawings by Angela Youells. Used with permission.

8.13. Transcription by Judith Becker.

8.14. Graphic by Judith Becker.

R8.1. Collection of Kay Kaufman Shelemay.

11.1. Pieter Paul Rubens (with Franz Snyders), *Prometheus Bound.* Philadelphia Museum of Art: Purchased with the W. P. Wilstach Collection Fund, 1950. W1950-3-1. Photograph by Graydon Wood.

11.2. Pacecco de Rosa, *Massacre of the Innocents.* Philadelphia Museum of Art: Purchased with the John D. McIlhenny Fund, 1973. 1973-253-1.

11.3. Francis Bacon, *Three Studies for Figures at the Base of a Crucifixion* (1944), central panel. Copyright © Tate, London 2004.

11.4 Edvard Munch, *The Sick Girl.* Lithograph. Courtesy of the Fogg Art Museum, Harvard University Art Museums. Purchased through the generosity of Lynn and Philip A. Straus, Class of 1937. Photo: Photographic Services. Copyright © President and Fellows of Harvard College.

11.5. Käthe Kollwitz, O *Nation, You Bleed from Many Wounds.* © 2004, Artists Rights Society (ARS), New York / VG Bild-Kunst, Bonn.

11.6. Käthe Kollwitz, *The Downtrodden.* © 2004, Artists Rights Society (ARS), New York / VG Bild-Kunst, Bonn.

11.7. Käthe Kollwitz, *The Downtrodden,* detail. © 2004, Artists Rights Society (ARS), New York / VG Bild-Kunst, Bonn.

11.8. Andrea Mantegna, *The Lamentation over the Dead Christ.* Milan, Brera Gallery. Permission granted by Ministero per i Beni e le Attività Culturali.

11.9. Aubrey Beardsley, "Girl, Wounded Tree, and a Book Shop" (title is Elaine Scarry's). Poster for T. Fisher Unwin Books, Pseudonym and Autonym Library.

11.10. Aubrey Beardsley, cover and spine, *Morte D'Arthur.* Reproduced from David Colvin, *Aubrey Beardley: A Slave to Beauty* (New York: Welcome Raine, 1998), 54.

11.11. Aubrey Beardsley, letter with cover design for Balzac's *Père Goriot.* "Letter to Leonard Smithers, 13 March l897," reproduced from *The Letters of Aubrey Beardsley,* ed. Henry Maas, J. L. Duncan, and W. G. Good (Rutherford, N.J.: Fairleigh Dickinson University Press, 1970), 275. Reprinted, Henry Maas, J. L. Duncan, and W. G. Good, eds., *The Letters of Aubrey Beardsley* (Oxford: Plantin Publishers, 1990).

R12.1–R12.4. Photographs by Richard K. Wolf.

13.1. "Los Howl'd here." Figure from William Blake, *The Book of Urizen.* Library of Congress. Copyright © 2003, The William Blake Archive.

Index

Note: Page numbers followed by *f* indicate figures.